Mycoplasma Infection of Cell Cultures

CELLULAR SENESCENCE AND SOMATIC CELL GENETICS

Series editors: **Warren W. Nichols**   **Donald G. Murphy**
Institute for Medical Research *National Institute on Aging*
Camden, New Jersey   *Bethesda, Maryland*

Mycoplasma Infection of Cell Cultures

Edited by
Gerard J. McGarrity
Institute for Medical Research
Camden, New Jersey

Donald G. Murphy
National Institute on Aging
Bethesda, Maryland

and
Warren W. Nichols
Institute for Medical Research
Camden, New Jersey

PLENUM PRESS · NEW YORK AND LONDON

Library of Congress Cataloging in Publication Data

Main entry under title:

Mycoplasma infection of cell culture.

(Cellular senescence and somatic cell genetics; v. 3)
Bibliography: p.
Includes index.
1. Mycoplasmatales. 2. Culture contamination (Biology) 3. Cell culture. I. McGar-
ity, Gerard J. II. Murphy, Donald G. III. Nichols, Warren W. IV. Series. [DNLM: 1.
Cells, Cultures. 2. Mycoplasma infections. 3. Mycoplasma—Pathogenicity. 4. Bacterio-
logical technics. W1 CE1295 v. 3/QW143 M997]
QR352.M88   574.8'028   77-25003
ISBN 0-306-32603-5

Proceedings of the Institute for Medical Research
Workshop on Mycoplasma Infection of Cell Cultures
held in Camden, New Jersey, March 22-23, 1977

© 1978 Plenum Press, New York
A Division of Plenum Publishing Corporation
227 West 17th Street, New York, N.Y. 10011

Organizing Committee

Michael F. Barile
   Bureau of Biologics
   Food and Drug Administration

Jack Gruber
   National Cancer Institute

Gerard J. McGarrity
   Institute for Medical Research

Donald G. Murphy
   National Institute on Aging

Warren W. Nichols
   Institute for Medical Research

Joseph G. Tully
   National Institute of Allergy and
   Infectious Diseases

Preface

If one were to design the ideal nuisance for cell cultures,
the resultant might well be similar to mycoplasmas. These microorganisms are very prevalent in nature, being found in the oral
cavity, blood, the mucous membranes of the respiratory and urogenital tract and other tissues of both man and animals. They are
relatively difficult to detect microbiologically and chemically.
Lacking cell walls, they do not routinely produce turbidity in
cell cultures and are resistant to antibiotics that act on cell
walls.

Mycoplasmas grow to high titers in cell cultures. Concentrations of 10^7-10^8 colony forming units per ml of supernatant
medium are representative. Additionally, more numbers are attached
to cell membranes. Further, mycoplasmas have been shown to mimic
in vitro effects of viruses and toxic chemicals. In various cell
culture systems, mycoplasmas have been known to cause cell death,
decrease or increase cell growth, affect virus titers, induce
interferon, cause chromosome damage, induce transformation, cytopathic effects, alter phenotypic expression, and significantly
alter metabolic pathways and products of cells. The presence of
such high concentrations of mycoplasmas in cell cultures constitutes
a true in vitro infection. Such infected cell cultures, with a
total of 10^8-10^9 or more actively metabolizing mycoplasmas, have
no place in controlled, standardized cell culture procedures.

Numerous reports have been published on mycoplasma assay procedures, effects of infection, and preventive and elimination
measures. The purpose of this workshop is to present a current
state of the art evaluation of mycoplasmal infection of cell cultures. Special emphasis is placed on detection methods, effects on
infection, and preventive measures. It is believed that the pre-
sentations in this text summarize the latest available information
gathered by recognized workers in the field. Also included is a
bibliography listing references on cell culture mycoplasmas.

The institutions which sponsored this workshop--the Bureau of Biologics, the National Institute on Aging, and the National Cancer Institute--are among those with substantial commitment to research and biologics production utilizing cell cultures. The workshop was encouraged by these organizations in an appreciation of the probable existing compromise of published data attributable to unrecognized mycoplasma contamination of cell cultures and the reduction in laboratory productivity incurred with the belated diagnosis of infection. The rapid expansion of the cell culture field and technologies indicates that the potential for substantial time and effort loss to laboratories due to mycoplasma contamination is high. Further, it is appreciated that the field of mycoplasmology is underdeveloped relative to the sister disciplines of virology and bacteriolgy. This situation, combined with a current knowledge of the field, suggests that a major expansion of knowledge of these organisms is overdue, and that the problems these organisms cause to cells in culture and to man and his laboratory animals are likely more complex than currently understood.

The editors hope this text will serve as both a thorough reference and a practical guide to cell culturists. The ultimate goal is that, through strict adherence to detection, prevention and control practices described herein, accidental mycoplasmal infection of cell cultures can be eliminated.

Contents

BIOLOGY OF THE MYCOPLASMAS

Joseph G. Tully

Mycoplasma Section, Laboratory of Infectious
Diseases, National Institute of Allergy &
Infectious Diseases, National Institutes of
Health, Bethesda, Maryland

INTRODUCTION

There are, in my opinion, three major milestones in
the current history of the mycoplasmas. The first concerns the recovery and description of the first organism
in this group in 1898 (1), later to be designated
Mycoplasma mycoides and shown to be the etiologic agent
of contagious bovine pleuro-pneumonia. The second involves the recognition (2) and subsequent cultivation
(3) of the etiologic agent of primary atypical pneumonia
(4). This organism, designated Mycoplasma pneumoniae,
became the first mycoplasma shown to be pathogenic for
man. Finally, the third event concerns recent observations that a group of helical, motile mycoplasmas,
termed spiroplasmas (5), exist in nature as plant and
insect pathogens (6-8), and possess capabilities of
provoking disease in vertebrate hosts (9).

It is not possible to present a comprehensive cover-
age of the very extensive biology of mycoplasmas in this
space, especially when one observes in a recent three
volume mycoplasma bibliography (10) that more references
were listed for a recent five-year period (1970-75) than
the number of references tabulated for the previous 118
years (1852-1970). Therefore, an attempt will be made
here to select some of the important points on the basic
biology of mycoplasmas that relate to the central theme
of this conference. At this meeting we shall undoubtedly
hear of many things mycoplasmas can do to tissue cells,

1

TABLE 1

CHARACTERISTICS OF MYCOPLASMAS

1. Can replicate in a cell-free environment.
   (exception noted of certain cell-adapted
   strains of <u>Mycoplasma</u> <u>hyorhinis</u>).

2. Minimal reproductive unit in size range
   near 300 nm.

3. Lack a rigid cell wall or chemical
   precursors of cell wall peptidoglycan.
   Possess only a limiting, triple-layered,
   plasma membrane.

4. Exhibit a more or less characteristic
   colonial form on solid growth medium
   (the so-called "fried egg" colony).

5. Most species require cholesterol or
   native serum proteins as a supplement for
   growth (exceptions noted for the acholeplasmas).

6. Resistant to most forms of penicillin
   and other antibiotics directed to
   inhibition of cell wall synthesis.

and a few things tissue cells might be doing to mycoplasmas. Much has been learned in the past twenty years
since mycoplasma infection of cell cultures was first
demonstrated and we know now how mycoplasmas can produce
direct cytopathic effects on cells, how they can deplete
arginine and alter the pH of cell culture fluids, and
affect virus-cell interactions in a variety of ways.
There are still other very important, and unanswered
questions such as whether mycoplasmas adsorbed to
tissue cells might alter cell culture membrane organization or chemical structure. These are fundamental
questions of very practical significance to those looking
at the chemical nature and orgainization of membranes
from virus-transformed cells, or other malignant cells,
under <u>in</u> <u>vitro</u> conditions.

MYCOPLASMAS - GROUP CHARACTERISTICS AND TAXONOMY

In the broadest context, what are the characteristic
properties of mycoplasmas that make them a distinct

group of organisms and how can they be distinguished
from other prokaryotic microbial forms with which they
share some basic attributes? Table 1 lists some of the
most fundamental properties of mycoplasmas, and subsequently comments will amplify the rather unique features
of these organisms. A comparison of several basic
features of mycoplasmas to those of other prokaryotes
is presented in Table 2.

The current basis for the classification and nomen-
clature of mycoplasmas was proposed in 1956 (11), and
this scheme has been modified and extended with
international cooperation as new information became
available. In 1967, a recommended extension of the
system placed the mycoplasmas in a new and separate
class (Mollicutes)(12), the ultimate effect of which
was to elevate them to a toxonomic level equivalent
to the true bacteria, viruses, etc. As can be seen in
Table 3, the current classification provides for three
families, with the Mycoplasmataceae being the largest
group. Species of the genus Mycoplasma number 50 now,
and these represent isolations from almost all types of
animal hosts. We have little indication now that we
have reached the point where the mycoplasma flora of
any one animal host is completely known, since new
isolates now appear from newly-explored tissue sites
(recently, for example, in the intestinal tract), or
following the use of new media formulations which might
satisfy more fastidious growth requirements of previously
uncultivated species. This progression is to be encouraged for it might provide significant clues to the
nutritional requirements of new and potentially pathogenic mycoplasmas for man. The genus Ureaplasma was
created to provide more adequate status for those mycoplasmas previously referred to as T-strain or T-mycoplasmas. They represent unique mycoplasmas which are
able to hydrolyze urea but under the usual culture
conditions do not attain colony sizes on agar much larger
than 10 um (± 5) in diameter. It is unclear at present
how the classification scheme of this group should
proceed and, although ureaplasmas have been isolated from
man and a variety of other animals, their interrelationships are not well understood at this point. The most
logical plan seemed to provide the group with a single
species designation (Ureaplasma urealyticum) and a set
of serotype designations for the first eight serologically distinct ureaplasmas found in man (13).

TABLE 2

CHARACTERISTICS OF MYCOPLASMAS AND SOME OTHER PROKARYOTIC ORGANISMS

Property	Mycoplasmas	Schizomycetes	Chlamydiae	Rickettsiae	Viruses
Growth on cell-free medium	+	+a	-	-a	-
Absence of cell wall or cell wall peptidoglycan	+	-	-	-	+
Generation of metabolic energy	+	+	-	+	-
Dependent on host cell nucleic acid for multiplication	-	-	-	-	+
Can synthesize proteins by own enzymes	+	+	+	+	-
Sterol requirement	+b	-	-	-	-
Visible in optical microscope (1500 X)	+	+	+	+	-
Filterability through 450 nm pore size filters	+	-a	+	+	+
Contain both RNA and DNA	+	+	+	+	-
Growth inhibited by antibody alone	+	-	+	+	+
Growth inhibited by antibiotics acting on protein synthesis	+	+	+	+	-

a) with few exceptions

b) except Acholeplasma species

From Tully, J.G. and Razin, S.: The Mollicutes "Mycoplasmas". In: Handbook of Microbiology, Vol. 1, 2nd edition CRC Press, Cleveland, Ohio, 1977.

TABLE 3

TAXONOMY OF THE CLASS MOLLICUTES

Class: Mollicutes

  Order: Mycoplasmatales

    Family I: Mycoplasmataceae

        1. Sterol required for growth

        2. Genome size about 5.0×10^8 daltons

        3. NADH oxidase localized in cytoplasm

      Genus I: Mycoplasma (about 50 species current)

        1. Do not hydrolyze urea

      Genus II: Ureaplasma (single species with serotypes)

        1. Hydrolyzes urea

    Family II: Acholeplasmataceae

        1. Sterol not required for growth

        2. Genome size about 1.0×10^9 daltons

        3. NADH oxidase localized in membrane

      Genus I: Acholeplasma (6 species current)

    Family III: Spiroplasmataceae

        1. Helical organisms during some phase of growth

        2. Sterol required for growth

        3. Genome size about 1.0×10^9 daltons

        4. NADH oxidase localized in cytoplasm

      Genus I: Spiroplasma (1 species current)

Genera of Uncertain Taxonomic Position

    Thermoplasma (single species)

    Anaeroplasma (two species)

Mycoplasmas now classified as <u>Acholeplasma</u> <u>laidlawii</u> were a taxonomic dilemma for a number of years since these organisms were known to have no sterol require- ments for growth and could grow at temperatures as low as 22-25 C. The concept of a much larger group of non- sterol requiring mycoplasmas became evident when another <u>Mycoplasma</u> species (<u>M</u>. <u>granularum</u>) was found to grow independent of serum or cholesterol (14). Sub- sequently (15), it became clear that other mycoplasmas from a variety of animals belonged to this group and that these organisms also possessed other, and more fundamental, distinctions from mycoplasmas - namely a genome size of 1×10^9 daltons (16), the ability to synthesize fatty acids from acetate (17), the presence of reduced nicotinamide adenine dinucleotide (NADH) oxidase in membranes instead of in the cell cytoplasm (18), and lactate dehydrogenases (LDHs) specifically activated by fructose-1,6-diphosphate (19). There are now about eight distinct species of <u>Acholeplasma</u>, separated primarily by serological differences. The most unique feature of the acholeplasmas is their ecology (20). The acholeplasmas were initially re- covered from sewage and soil over forty years ago and were considered at that time to be free-living sapro- phytes. We have no evidence at this point that acholeplasmas are saprophytic or that they could long survive under conditions necessary to establish this relationship. The rather wide distribution of achole- plasmas in animals, and their recent recovery from animal feces and intestinal contents (21,22), provides a more logical explanation for their occurrence in soil and sewage.

The designation "spiroplasma" was first given to helical, wall-free prokaryotes observed in corn plants infected with the insect-borne corn stunt disease (5). Subsequently, a mycoplasma-like agent was visualized, and eventually cultivated, from citrus plants infected with "stubborn disease" (6,23). The organism was found to be a motile, helical form similar to the corn stunt agent and the complete characterization of the "citrus stubborn" agent as <u>Spiroplasma</u> <u>citri</u> was the first plant mycoplasma to be described and classified (24). Culti- vation of the corn stunt spiroplasma was accomplished shortly thereafter by two independent groups (7,8). The third spiroplasma to be cultivated was from tick- derived, egg-passaged material containing an infectious entity termed the "suckling mouse cataract agent" (9). This organism, and a second related isolate (GT-48), are of fundamental importance since they represent the first

spiroplasmas exhibiting pathogenicity for vertebrates
and having the capability of replicating at 37°C.
Spiroplasmas also have been observed in other insect
and plant hosts. These include certain Drosophila
species where spiroplasmas (termed the sex ration
organism) are associated with a maternally-inherited
syndrome leading to an absence of males in the progeny
of infected females (25). More recently, other spiroplasmas have been recovered in culture from cactus
plants (26) and in a lethal infection in honey bees (27).
Serological comparisons of a number of the cultivated
spiroplasmas revealed considerable sharing of antigens
with S. citri and so more extensive characterization
procedures, possibly involving new techniques, may be
required before species designations can be assigned
to spiroplasmas other than S. citri. Preliminary characterization of S. citri indicated that the organism
had a requirement for sterol and possessed a genome
size of 1 x 10⁹ daltons (24).

Finally, two additional groups of organisms are
included in the Mollicutes. In each instance, the
amount of information necessary to provide a proper
classification is somewhat limited and so they have been
given genus and species designations without further
taxonomic assignments. Thermoplasma acidophilum is an
obligate thermophilic and acidophilic wall-free prokaryote
recovered from burning coal refuse piles (28). Sterols
are not required for growth and the organism grows well
over a temperature range of 45 to 62 C (optimum at 59 C),
and at an optimum pH of 1.0 to 2.0 (29). Lastly, the
anaeroplasmas are a group of obligately anaerobic,
wall-free prokaryotes recovered from the bovine and ovine
rumen (30,31). Two species have been proposed with some
differences noted in their biological and serological
properties (31).

MORPHOLOGY

The cellular morphology of mycoplasmas has frequently
been described as pleomorphic and one might expect this
of wall-free and plastic organisms. However, there are
suggestions that preparative techniques used to examine
the morphology of these agents, specifically the osmol-
arity of fixatives and some buffers, frequently alters
the size and shape of mycoplasmas (32,33). Selection
of materials used in these techniques should be based
upon correlation with how much they alter the morphology
of cells observed under darkfield or phase-contrast

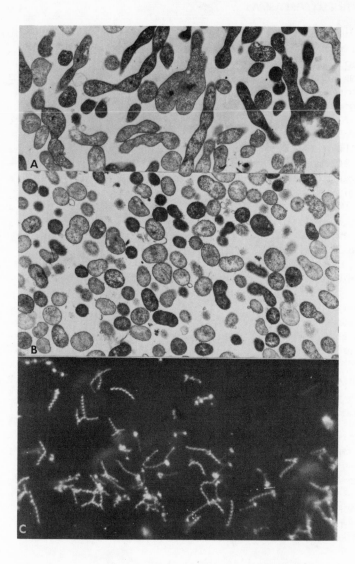

FIGURE 1 - Morphology and ultrastructure of various mycoplasmas.
(A) - Electron micrograph of thin section of M. neurolyticum PG-28
strain. Cells were grown 16 hrs. in broth culture, sedimented by
centrifugation, and pellets fixed in 2.5% glutaraldehyde. Cells
then washed in 0.2 M sucrose and 0.1 M phosphate buffer, secondarily
fixed in 1% osmium tetroxide, block-stained in uranyl acetate, and
embedded in Spurr's medium. X16,000. (B) - M. neurolyticum Type A
strain. Cells cultured and fixed as above. X16,000. (C) - Log
phase culture (unfixed) of Spiroplasma citri cells as seen in
darkfield microscopy. Note helical filaments. X3,750.
Reduced 45% for reproduction.

microscopy.   Mycoplasmas will usually exhibit either
spherical or coccoid structures of 300 to 800 nm in
diameter or slender, and sometimes branched, filaments
of uniform diameter (100 to 800 nm) which may vary in
length from 3-10 um to almost 150 um.   Figure 1 (A and B)
demonstrates variations in cellular morphology of two
strains of M. neurolyticum, cultivated, fixed, and examined under identical conditions.   The cellular morphology
of spiroplasmas also varies from pleomorphic, sperical
cells of 200 to 300 nm in diameter, to helical and
branched, non-helical filaments.   Helical forms, usually
3-12 um in length and 100 to 200 nm in diameter, predom-
inate in logarithmic phase cultures (Figure 1C).   Cultures
in the late logarithmic or in the stationary phases tend
to show few helical forms and will consist primarily of
non-helical filaments, some greatly elongated and with
irregular round bodies at various points on the filament.
Much of the earlier data which suggested viable mycoplasma
cells in the range of 100 to 150 nm in diameter were based
upon sizing data obtained from filtration techniques or
observations by electron or phase-contrast microscopy.
The limitations with these procedures in regard to wall-
free organisms has been recorded (34,35).   There seems to
be general consensus now that the minimal reproductive
unit of mycoplasma cells is around 300 nm (36).

     Thin section of mycoplasma cells reveals a rather
simple ultrastructure consisting essentially of the cell
membrane and cytoplasm, the latter containing ribosomes
and the characteristic prokaryotic genome.   However, in
several species specialized terminal structures of considerable importance have been observed.   A highly struc-
tured polar body, termed the "bleb" has been noted to
protrude from one or both ends of M. gallisepticum cells
(Figure 2A) (37).   While the blebs and near-associated
regions (infrableb) seem to be devoid of nucleic acids,
portions of these areas contain basic proteins and appear
to be sites of enzymatic activity (38).   The bleb also
appears to function as an attachment site of M. gallisepticum to animal cells (39).   A terminal organelle
has been observed in M. pneumoniae when cells are grown
in human fetal or hamster tracheal organ cultures
(Figure 2B) (40,41).   More recently, these terminal
cultures have been observed in M. pneumoniae parasitized
respiratory epithelium cells from sputum of patients
with primary atypical pneumonia (42).   The terminal
point is characterized by an electron dense central
rod in the long axis of the tip, which ends on a

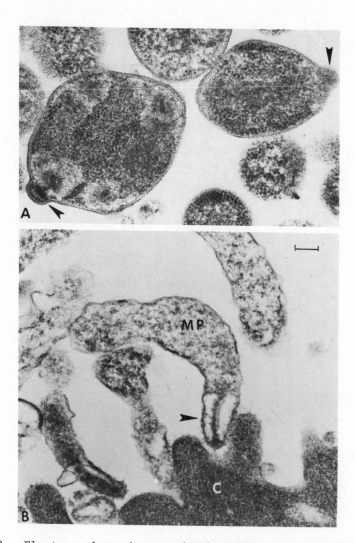

FIGURE 2 - Electron photomicrographs demonstrating the specialized
terminal structure on some mycoplasmas. (A) - Thin section of M.
gallisepticum A5969 cells showing terminal "blebs" (arrows) as
densely stained protrusions from cell membrane. X70,000 (from
Maniloff and Quinlan, Annals of the N.Y. Acad. of Sci. 225:181-189,
1973 - with permission of the publisher). (B) - Section of M.
pneumoniae (MP) cells from infected hamster tracheal ring showing
classical filamentous structure of organism. Note orientation of
specialized tip (arrow) of organism to nonciliated tissue cell and
the central rod and lucent area of terminal structure. Bar marker
represents 0.1 μm. (From Wilson & Collier, J. Bacteriology 125:332-
339, 1976 - with permission of publisher). 10mm = 0.1 μm.
Reduced 30% for reproduction.

plate-like structure at the tip. There is a lucent
space around the central rod which ends at the organism's
unit membrane. The tapered terminal tip is always
oriented to that end of the organism which is attached
to host cell membrane (42). Special terminal structures
have also been observed in at least one other mycoplasma
(M. pulmonis) (43), but detailed information on structure
and function is lacking. Intracytoplasmic structures,
designated rho fibers, have been observed in two sub-
species of M. mycoides and in several other caprine and
bovine mycoplasmas (44). These structures consist of
apparently rigid, rod-like striated fibers extending
axially through the cell and terminate in a knob-like
structure. The function and significance of these
organelles are unknown but they have been observed in
cells after artificial cultivation and in vivo (45).

        The cell membrane of mycoplasmas is undoubtedly
the most useful model available in biological membrane
studies. Membranes are relatively easy to isolate, are
free from other types of intracytoplasmic membrane or
cell wall components, and can be fairly easily altered
in chemical composition by growing mycoplasma cells in
various culture media. Extensive reviews are available
on isolation and characterization of mycoplasma membranes
(46-48) and their reconstitution (49). Extracellular
material on the membrane of mycoplasmas has been of
interest as a possible component in virulence or of
unique antigenic significance. A slime layer of
galactan has been identified on the surface of M. mycoides
cells (50) and a capsule-like material was observed in
electron microscopic examination of cells from M. mel-
eagridis (51) and M. dispar (52) cultures. A hexosamine
polymer isolated from A. laidlawii cells has been
described (53) and indirect studies with plant lectins
have suggested that small quantities of other carbohydrate-
containing materials are probably present on the membranes
of many mycoplasmas (54). The role of these substances
might play in pathogenic or immunological reactions is
not clear.

        The colonial morphology of mycoplasmas varies con-
siderably, depending upon species and strain variability,
culture medium components, hydration of agar, atmospheric conditions (aerobic or anaerobic incubation), and
a number of other known and unknown factors. The appearance of the basic "fried egg" colony is demonstrated in
Figure 3A, and the variation noted in another strain of
the same species is shown in Figure 3B. The most

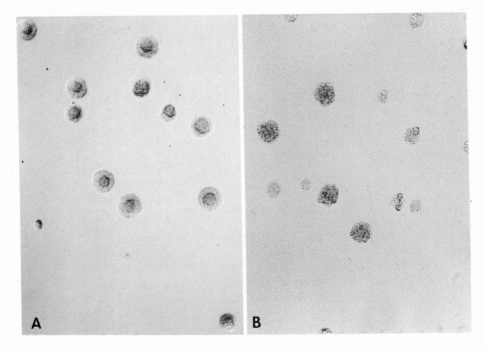

FIGURE 3 - Colony morphology of two strains of M. edwardii.
(A) - PG-24 strain. (B) - Dog G strain. Both strains grown under
similar conditions, including the same agar medium. Note the typical
"fried egg" colony for the PG-24 strain.

distinctive feature of the mycoplasma colony is that
growth occurs down into the agar in the central
portion of the colony, while the periphery of the colony
is associated more with growth on the surface of the
agar. These conditions permit the colony to be transferred to other solid media only when an explant of
colony and agar is removed, inverted onto fresh agar,
and pushed over the surface of the new medium. Colonial
morphology of spiroplasmas and most other mycoplasmas
demonstrate similar variability. For some organisms
in the group special circumstances are required to
demonstrate growth on solid medium, or manipulations
in medium components are necessary to produce the usual
colony types. For instance, with ureaplasmas the
addition of certain buffers (HEPES) to the agar medium
or incubation of inoculated plates in an atmosphere of
100 percent CO_2 not only results in colony sizes typical
of other mycoplasmas (100 to 300 um), but in the
formation of classical "fried egg" colonies (55,56).
Higher concentrations of purified agar (up to 3 percent)
are sometimes necessary to demonstrate colony growth
of some spiroplasmas and thermoplasmas.

MOTILITY AND MODE OF REPRODUCTION

Flagella, axial filaments, or other organelles
associated with motility have not been detected in
mycoplasmas. However, at least three mycoplasmas
(M. gallisepticum, M. pneumoniae, and M. pulmonis) have
been described as exhibiting motility and there appears
to be a direct correlation between this so-called gliding movement of mycoplasmas and the specialized terminal
structures observed in these three organisms (57). The
leading direction of movement is always oriented tip
first and, at least with M. pneumoniae, the movement is
frequently in a circular pattern. Although the mechanism
of motility is not well understood, the movement of
these cells is of considerable interest - especially in
light of the small size of the cells and their lack of
apparent structures or materials to mediate energy
transfer. The motility observed in spiroplasmas is much
different from the gliding movement of some mycoplasmas.
Helical spiroplasma filaments may exhibit both rapid,
rotary "screw" motion and flexional movements, the latter
evident when the filaments or a portion of the filament
bends and twists at the midpoint of the filament while
a portion remains stationary (33). Each type of motility
has been observed with spiroplasmas in culture or with

organisms observed directly in plant fluids or insect hemolymph. There is still some question whether trans- lational movement occurs in spiroplasmas, as opposed to the clear directional movement observed with M. pneumoniae. Again no evidence of any organelles assoc- iated with motility has been seen on spiroplasmas. There is some preliminary evidence that an actin-like protein is present in both M. pneumoniae and S. citri and may play some part in motility (58).

The mode of reproduction of mycoplasmas has been of some dispute. There seems to be clear evidence now that replication of the prokaryotic genome, which must precede cell division, follows a pattern much like other prokaryotes dividing by binary fission (59). Cytoplasmic division must, therefore, be synchronized with genome replication for binary fission to occur - and this synchrony is not always present in mycoplasmas. Consequently, when cytoplasmic division lags behind genome replication, multinucleated filaments occur and subsequent division of the cytoplasm results in char- acteristic chains of coccoid cells which later fragment into individual cells. Budding cells are also observed in mycoplasmas and this may also be considered a form of binary fission in which the cytoplasm is not equally divided between daughter cells (60). Less information is available about the mode of reproduction for spiro- plasmas, although cells apparently in final stages of binary fission have been observed (D.L. Williamson, personal communication).

THE MYCOPLASMA GENOME

All mycoplasmas examined to date have circular genomes built of double stranded DNA (59). DNA repli- cation is semi-conservative, proceeding unidirectionally, probably from a single growing point, as is seen in bac- teria. Estimates of the genome size of Mycoplasma species, based upon measurement of circular DNA strands in electron micrographs (59) or in renaturation studies (16), gave values clustered around 5.0×10^8 daltons. Acholeplasma species, examined primarily by renaturation kinetics (16) represented a distinct group with genome sizes approximately 1×10^9 daltons. Spiroplasmas also tend to have genome sizes around 1×10^9 daltons (24), as do Thermoplasma acidophilum (61,62).

In addition to its relatively small size the mycoplasma genome is also characterized by a low guanosine
and cytosine (G+C) content (63). Thus, in Mycoplasma
species values range from a high of about 40 moles
percent G+C in M. pneumoniae to a low of about 23 moles
percent G+C for M. neurolyticum. Most acholeplasmas
possess G+C ratios in the range of 30-34 moles percent,
while those of S. citri are recorded at 26 moles percent,
the anaeroplasmas from 29-40 moles percent, and T.
acidophilum at 45 moles percent (see reference 20) for
more extensive tabulation and associated bibliography).

DNA hybridization studies have been very useful
with mycoplasmas, especially in early studies when there
was some question about the relationship of these organisms to L-phase bacterial variants. In no instance was
any evidence obtained of a relationship, whereas the
L-phase variants showed complete homology with their
expected parental forms (64,65). More recently DNA
hybridization tests have been useful in providing some
additional information of the taxonomic position of
specific mycoplasmas or confirming questioned serological
relationships among certain strains or species (15).

Discussions on the mycoplasma genome also lead into
the intriging observations that viruses exist that are
capable of infecting prokaryotes the size of mycoplasmas.
Although a few reports appeared in the 1960's suggesting,
on morphological grounds, that viruses occurred in mycoplasmas, the presence of satellite DNA (20-30 x 10^6
daltons) in several mycoplasmas offered more firm evidence. The first direct confirmation of plaque-forming
viruses in A. laidlawii was reported in 1970 (66) and
this was eventually followed by an extensive series of
reports on at least three morphologically and serologically distinct viruses in A. laidlawii (67). Studies
carried out after the isolation and cultivation of S.
citri revealed that this organism also contained three
morphologically distinct virus-like agents, and all
spiroplasmas described to date appear to be infected
with viruses (68). Insufficient evidence exists at this
time to state whether there is any serological relationship between the mycoplasmaviruses and virus-like agents
found in spiroplasmas (see references 68 and 69 for
recent reviews.

MYCOPLASMA METABOLISM AND NUTRITION

Most mycoplasmas can generally be separated into
fermentative or nonfermentative classes in regard to
energy needs. The fermentative group derives its carbon

and energy from the dissimilation of hexoses, especially
glucose, whereas nonfermentative species appear to carry
out amino acid degradation, fatty acid oxidation, or
metabolism of short-chain carbon compounds. The carbo-
hydrate-fermenting strains generally catabolize glucose
by homolactic or heterolactic glycolytic pathways and
production of acid can be measured by appropriate pH
indicators incorporated into carbohydrate-containing
media. A few non-glycolytic nonfermentative mycoplasmas
have been observed to produce a slight fall in medium
pH, even in control cultures in the absence of glucose.
More sensitive tests for glucose metabolism are available,
especially a procedure for detection of glucose phospho-
transferase and hexokinase systems (70).

    Most of the nonfermentative mycoplasmas possess
enzymes for the arginine dihydrolase pathway and arginine
supplementation of undefined growth media generally results in marked increase in growth yields in these
strains (71). This pathway yields ATP, ammonia, and
carbon dioxide, and the liberated ammonia released into
the medium produces a rise in medium pH which is used as
an indicator of arginine hydrolysis.

    A few mycoplasmas appear not to have either glyco-
lytic or arginine dihydrolase pathways (i.e. M. bovis,
M. agalactiae, M. bovigenitalium, and M. verecundum).
Conversely, a few Mycoplasma species (M. fermentans,
M. alvi, M. bovoculi, M. capricolum, and M. moatsii) are
able to carry out both fermentation of glucose and hydrolysis of arginine. The ureaplasmas are notable among
mycoplasmas for their ability to hydrolyze urea, but the
physiological role of urea hydrolysis in these organisms
is uncertain at the moment. All species assigned to the
Acholeplasma, Spiroplasma, Thermoplasma and Anaeroplasma
genera catabolize glucose and none appears to hydrolyze
arginine (72).

    Nutritional requirements of most mycoplasmas are
not well defined, partly because of difficulties involved
in developing a defined media for growth of these organisms. Defined media sufficient to meet the needs of
M. mycoides (73) and A. laidlawii (74) have been developed
but for most mycoplasmas nutritional needs have been
derived from studies in undefined media with the use of
labeled precursors. Cholesterol is the most distinctive
nutritional requirement of mycoplasmas and standardized
procedures to establish this requirement are available
(75,76). More extensive discussion of the requirements

of mycoplasmas for lipids, amino acids, nucleic acid
precursors, vitamins, urea, etc. can be found in several
recent reviews or monographs (46,72,77,78).

ACTION OF PHYSICAL AND CHEMICAL FACTORS ON MYCOPLASMAS

The lack of a rigid outer wall on mycoplasmas would
suggest extreme sensitivity to a variety of chemical and
physical agents. However, these organisms adapt surprisingly well to some fairly severe alterations in
their environment, and the significant amounts of
sterol present in the membrane of most species is thought
to play a role in protection. Despite these notations,
most mycoplasmas, except the thermoplasmas, are fairly
sensitive to heat. A half-life of generally less than
2 minutes is noted at temperatures above 50°C. The use
of temperatures in the range of $39-45^{\circ}$C to selectively
inactivate mycoplasmas in infected cell cultures (79) is
not uniformly successful, although recommendations for
the inactivation of mycoplasmas in animal sera used for
propagation of cell cultures by heating to 56°C for 1
hour (in volumes no larger than 100 ml) can be an effective control procedure (80).

Mycoplasmas stored at temperatures of 4 to 25°C show
much variation in half-life. Acholeplasmas might survive
under these conditions for 2 weeks to several months,
while ureaplasmas and other sterol-requiring mycoplasmas
will show viability loss in 1 to 7 days. Mycoplasmas
maintained at temperatures around -20°C show extended
viability, usually averaging 6 months to several years,
while optimum long-term storage temperatures are nearer
-65 to -70°C. Optimal conditions also depend upon pH
and the constituents of the suspending medium, with the
usual mycoplasma culture medium containing 20 percent
horse serum providing satisfactory storage conditions
(81). Alternate freezing and thawing of mycoplasmas in
broth culture suspensions are not generally detrimental
to viability, although a slight decrease in number of
viable cells might occur. However, mycoplasma suspensions
in deionized water subjected to freezing will undergo
almost complete lysis (78).

Most mycoplasmas readily survive lyophilization in
the usual culture medium but may show a one to four log
drop in colony-forming units/ml after drying. Freeze-
drying directly from incubated broth cultures is generally preferred to most concentration procedures.
Pertinent references and a review of various lyophilizat-

ion techniques have been given in several recent reports
(80, and FAO/WHO Program on Comparative Mycoplasmology,
Document VPH/MIC/74.1, WHO, Geneva, Switzerland).

A few studies have been directed to airborne transmission of pathogenic mycoplasmas and the conditions
necessary for survival upon aerosolization. However,
the number of parameters, including suspending medium,
relative humidity, particle size, temperature, etc.
make meaningful comparisons difficult. Even sudden
changes in relative humidity were found to increase
biological decay of aerosolized M. pneumoniae (82).
Aerosolization of mycoplasmas from a variety of techniques, including pipetting, centrifugation, filtration,
etc. have been shown to increase the chance of cell
culture contamination with mycoplasmas (83-86), as well
as contaminate cell lines with other types of tissue
cells. Under these conditions, the consequences of
seeding the environment with mycoplasmas, particularly
in commercial organizations where raw animal sera, re-
fined animal sera, and dehydrated culture media components are being handled, can have some very undesirable
and long-range effects (87).

Mycoplasmas are generally resistant to changes in
osmotic environment, in spite of the absence of a cell
wall. The sterol-requiring mycoplasmas have greater
osmotic stability than the acholeplasmas, apparently
from the higher sterol content of their cell membrane.
However, osmotic shock, carried out under specific conditions whereby cells sedimented from culture media are
transferred directly to deionized water, is a useful
method for preparation of mycoplasma membranes (46).
The spiroplasmas appear to have some specific need for
a much higher osmotic pressure in culture media used for
primary isolation from plant and insect materials (24,33).

Mycoplasmas are especially sensitive to a variety
of compounds which lower surface tension. Again, this
activity appears related to the sterol content of the
mycoplasma membrane. Anionic detergents give more
ready lysis of mycoplasmas over a wider range of concentrations than cationic detergents. Nonionic detergents
have been used frequently to inactivate mycoplasmas in
cell cultures or virus suspensions since they possess
lower toxicity for animal cells, but the action of these
substances on mycoplasmas varies considerably (88). Some
nonionic detergents (Tween 80) have been reported to be
effective in inactivating mycoplasmas in cell cultures

but the in vitro activity of many of the nonionic
detergents does not correlate well with their action in
cell cultures (89). Selective inactivation of mycoplasmas in virus suspensions or in cell culture materials
has been observed with other compounds, including phen-
ethyl alcohol (90), sodium polyanethol sulfate (91), and
Tricine (92). Mycoplasmas are more susceptible to the
effects of lysolecithin (in concentrations of 125 to
250 ugm/ml) than acholeplasmas, which appear to show
little inhibition when grown in concentrations of
$\geq$500 ugm/ml (93).

The differential activity of certain heavy metal
salts, particularly those of gold and thallium, on
mycoplasmas and bacteria has been of some value.
Mycoplasmas, except the ureaplasmas and some acholeplasmas, are more resistant to thallium acetate than bacteria
and are able to grow in the presence of concentrations
up to 2 mg/ml. This observation has been used to advantage in the preparation of culture media for the selective recovery of mycoplasmas in the presence of heavy
bacterial loads (94-97). Gold salts, in the form of
sodium aurothiomalate, have been shown to have an
inhibitory effect on some experimental mycoplasma infections, but there are variable effects on the elimination
of mycoplasmas from infected cell cultures (98). A
recent report also advocated the use of peracetic acid
(in concentrations of 0.05 to 0.1 percent) for the
sterilization of animal sera and other cell culture in-
gredients that might contain mycoplasmas (99).

Recent summaries on the sensitivity or resistance of
mycoplasmas to various antibiotics are available (100-102).
In general most mycoplasmas are resistant to those
antibiotics with activity directed to cell wall synthesis,
such as penicillin, cycloserine, polymyxin, bacitracin,
etc. A few mycoplasmas have been reported to be sensitive
to penicillin (M. neurolyticum, M. flocculare, and M.
suipneumoniae) and the presence of this antibiotic has
definitely been shown to reduce the primary isolation of
M. dispar from animal tissues (103). Since ampicillin
is not inhibitory under these same conditions, it is
thought that molecular forms of penicillin or other unknown components involved in the preparation of the drug
are involved in the inhibitory activity. Polyene antibiotics have variable effects on mycoplasmas depending
again on the content of sterol in the mycoplasma membrane
or the molecular size of the polyene. Thus, amphotericin
B at concentrations of 20 ugm/ml is inhibitory to

TABLE 4

MYCOPLASMA SENSITIVITY TO TETRACYCLINE

Mycoplasma species	No. Strains	\(\leq\)0.1	0.25	0.4	0.5	0.8	1.0	1.5	5.0	6.25	10	25	50	100	>100
M. gallisepticum [a]	12	7			5										
M. hominis [b]	44		15		29										
M. canis [c]	55	1			3		6		34		10		1		
M. spumans [c]	11				1		2		4		3		1		
M. pneumoniae [d]	152	4	(0.2) 60	48		29		(1.6) 11							
M. orale [e]	10									7		3			
M. salivarium [e]	84			3				28		27		5		6	15

Number of strains with minimum inhibitory concentrations (in ugm/ml) of:

a) Newnham and Chu (1965) Ref. 106
b) Blyth (1962) Ref. 105
c) Kato et al.(1972) Ref.108
d) Niitu et al.(1974) Ref. 109
e) Steward et al. (1969) Ref. 107

sterol-requiring mycoplasmas but does not affect the growth of the acholeplasmas (104). Two additional observations on the response of mycoplasmas to antibiotics requires emphasis. The first involves the concept that various Mycoplasma species have different sensitivities to certain antibiotics and many strains within a given species may exhibit a very broad range of responses to given drug levels, as is depicted in Table 4. The second point of note involves recent and confirmed observations that tetracycline-resistant ureaplasmas exist in nature (109-111). These findings, while probably of little significance to cell culturists or virologists, have important implications to clinical studies on the role of ureaplasmas in certain genito-urinary tract (non-gonococcal urethritis) diseases.

MYCOPLASMA-HOST RELATIONSHIPS

A recent tabulation of all recognized species in the class Mollicutes has been presented, along with information on their habitat and pathogenicity (20). Comments on host-parasite relationships will be limited to some broad generalizations and possible mechanisms of mycoplasma pathogenicity. Mycoplasmas were initially recognized as important animal-pathogens. They were found to involve a variety of organs and tissues, and to be associated with acute and chronic respiratory disease, mastitis, polyarthritis, and genitourinary tract infections (113). The concept of a vast normal flora of mycoplasmas in animals (and including man) was not well appreciated until major advances occurred in the cultivation of the more fastidious mycoplasmas, such as M. pneumoniae (3). From that time in the early 1960s, we have seen a continual extension of the number of mycoplasmas in each animal host selectively surveyed. The great majority of these mycoplasmas appear to be strictly part of the normal microbial flora. However, it is important to stress that limited information is available on the interrelationships of normal mycoplasma flora and other microbial agents, including virulent as well as avirulent bacteria, viruses, etc. Thus, normal flora might still play some role in human or animal diseases when acting in concert with other microbial agents or when the host is compromised in some way.

To gain some flavor of the current status of the distribution of mycoplasmas in specific hosts, I have tabulated those species identified as part of the mycoplasma flora of man, along with sites of their

TABLE 5

MYCOPLASMA FLORA OF MAN AND NON-HUMAN PRIMATES

Mycoplasmas	Recovery Sites
Mycoplasma buccale (orale 2)	Oropharynx (rare)
M. faucium (orale 3)	Oropharynx (rare)
M. fermentans	Genitourinary tract
M. hominis	Oropharynx, genitourinary tract, blood
M. lipophilum	Oral cavity (rare)
M. orale	Oropharynx (common)
M. pneumoniae	Oropharynx, upper and lower respiratory tracts, middle ear, and spinal fluid (usually only in disease)
M. primatum	Urogenital tract (rare in man)
M. salivarium	Oral cavity (common)
Acholeplasma laidlawii	Oral cavity (rare)
Ureaplasma urealyticum	Urogenital tract, oral cavity, blood, and intestinal tract

recovery (Table 5). The mycoplasma flora of the bovine (Table 6) is of special interest here because of the frequent occurrence of bovine mycoplasmas in cell culture infections. Thirdly, the acholeplasmas are also very high on any list of mycoplasmas involved as cell culture contaminants and a summary of the host distribution and recovery sites of these organisms is included (Table 7).

The mechanisms involved in the pathogenicity of mycoplasmas are not well defined at present, although there are a few factors present in mycoplasmas (toxins,

TABLE 6

MYCOPLASMA FLORA OF THE BOVINE

Mycoplasmas	Recovery Sites
M. alvi	Intestinal tract and feces
M. alkalescens	Nasal cavity, serum
M. arginini	Nasal cavity, respiratory tract, lung, eye, udder, joint, serum, and semen
M. bovigenitalium	Urogenital tract
M. bovirhinis	Respiratory tract, lung, synovial fluid and milk
M. bovis	Respiratory tract, joints and udder
M. bovoculi	Eye
M. canadense	Urogenital tract, joint, milk and semen
M. dispar	Pneumonic lung
M. mycoides subsp. mycoides	Respiratory tract and lung (in contagious bovine pleuropneumonia)
M. verecundum	Eye
A. axanthum	Nasal cavity, lymph nodes, kidney
A. laidlawii	Oral cavity, lymph nodes, respiratory and urogenital tracts
A. modicum	Lung and lymph nodes
An. bactoclasticum	Rumen
An. abactoclasticum	Rumen
Ureaplasma species or serotypes	Urogenital tract, lung, conjunctivae

hemolysins, etc.) which undoubtedly contribute to pathogenicity (113). For the most part mycoplasmas do not
contain or secrete many of the extracellular factors
or the aggressive enzyme systems that virulent bacteria
possess to promote their invasion and dissemination
within the host. The absence of a cell wall also puts
the mycoplasma cell at a disadvantage since cell wall
constituents frequently prevent or inhibit phagocytosis
by normal cellular defenses of the host, or they may
provoke additional host stress through release of
endotoxins.

TABLE 7

HOST DISTRIBUTION AND HABITAT- ACHOLEPLASMAS

Acholeplasma species	Host	Recovery Sites
A. axanthum	Bovine	Nasal cavity, lymph nodes, kidney
	Equine	Oral cavity
	Porcine	Peribronchial lymph nodes
A. equifoetale	Equine	Nasopharynx and trachea
A. granularum	Porcine	Nasal cavity
	Equine	Conjunctivae
A. laidlawii	Avian Bovine Canine Caprine Equine Feline Murine Ovine Porcine Primates	Oral cavity, lymph nodes respiratory and uro- genital tracts
A. modicum	Bovine	Lung and lymph nodes
A. oculi	Caprine	Eye
	Equine	Nasopharynx

Although it might appear from these comments that all mycoplasmas should be easily handled by the normal health host, the evidence for pathogenic mycoplasmas certainly indicates that while these organisms might be deficient in some virulence factors other components are present in sufficient amounts to produce disease. The very subtle invasion of the host by mycoplasmas, the absence of most microbial factors which actively and rapidly stimulate the host's humoral and cellular defenses, and the ability of pathogenic mycoplasmas to adsorb to cells and to rapidly colonize the mucosal surfaces of the host, all appear to be important factors in their ability to incite disease.

Also, recent observations that certain M. hyorhinis strains in cell culture infections have reached a stage in cell adaptation that prevents their growth on artificial (or cell-free) media (114) raises important questions about mycoplasma-host relationships. Although this cell-associated state has not been completely confirmed in other Mycoplasma species, it is very important to understand the mechanisms involved in a situation whereby mycoplasmas can reach a state of parasitism apparently sufficient to lead to a shut down in their own "metabolic machinery." Thus, the important question is whether this state of parasitism can occur with other known mycoplasmas, or possibly with new and previously uncultivated mycoplasmas, and does it play some role in human diseases of unknown etiology (115)? Recent observations (9) that a number of newly isolated spiroplasmas would not replicate on conventional mycoplasma media, nor on previously developed spiroplasma media, should provide a strong stimulus to continue not only experimental studies on the nutritional requirements of mycoplasmas but to pursue the development of new cultural and non-cultural methods for the detection and identification of these organisms.

ACKNOWLEDGMENT

I wish to thank A.M. Collier and J. Maniloff for their generosity in supplying electron photomicrographs of M. pneumoniae and M. gallisepticum, respectively. I also thank T.J. Popkin for his efforts in the ultrastructural examination of the M. neurolyticum cells and in the preparation of photographs.

REFERENCES

1. Nocard, E., E.R. Roux, M.M. Borrel, Salimbeniet, and E. Dujardin-Beaumetz. 1898. Ann. Inst. Pasteur 12:240-262.

2. Marmion, B.P. and G.M. Goodburn. 1961. Nature 189: 247-248.

3. Chanock, R.M., L. Hayflick and M.F. Barile. 1962. Proc. Nat. Acad. Sci. (USA), 48:41-48.

4. Couch, R.B., T.R. Cate, and R.M. Chanock. 1964. J. Am. Med. Assoc. 187:442-447.

5. Davis, R.E. and J.F. Worley. 1973. Phytopathol. 63:403-408.

6. Saglio, P., LaFleche, D., C. Bonissol, and J.M. Bove. 1971. Physiol. Veg. 9:569-582.

7. Chen, T.A. and C.H. Liao. 1975. Science 188:1015-1017.

8. Whitcomb, R.F. and D.L. Williamson. 1975. Ann. N.Y. Acad. Sci. 266:260-275.

9. Tully, J.G., R.F. Whitcomb, H.F. Clark, and D.L. Williamson. 1977. Science 195:892-894.

10. Domermuth, C.H. and J.G. Rittenhouse. 1976. Mycoplasma Bibliography, Research Div. Bulletin No. 114, Virginia Polytechnic Institute, Blacksburg, Va.

11. Edward, D.G.ff and E.A. Freundt. 1956. J. Gen. Microbiol. 14:197-207.

12. Edward, D.G.ff and E.A. Freundt. 1967. Int. J. Syst. Bacteriol. 17:267-268.

13. Shepard, M.C., C.D. Lunceford, D.K. Ford, R.H. Purcell, D. Taylor-Robinson, S. Razin, and F.T. Black. 1974. Int. J. Syst. Bacteriol. 24:160-171.

14. Tully, J.G. and S. Razin. 1968. J. Bacteriol. 95: 1504-1512.

15. Tully, J.G. 1973. Ann. N.Y. Acad. Sci. 225:74-93.

16. Bak, A.L., F.T. Black, C. Christiansen, and E.A. Freundt. 1969. Nature 224:1209-1210.

17. Herring, P.K. and J.D. Pollack. 1974. Int. J. Syst. Bacteriol. 24:73-78.

18. Pollack, J.D. 1975. Int. J. Syst. Bacteriol. 25: 108-113.

19. Neimark, H.C. 1973. Ann. N.Y. Acad. Sci. 225:14-21.

20. Tully, J.C. and S. Razin. 1977. The Mollicutes in Handbook of Microbiology vol. 1, 2nd edition (in press), A.I. Laskin and H. Lechevalier (Eds.) Chemical Rubber Co., Cleveland, Ohio.

21. Gourlay, R.N. and S.G. Wyld. 1975. Vet. Record 97: 370-371.

22. Roberts, D.H. and T.W.A. Little. 1976. Vet. Record 99:13.

23. Fudl-Allah, A.A., E.C. Calavan and E.C.K. Igwegbe. 1972. Phytopathol. 62:729-731.

24. Saglio, P., M. L'Hospital, D. Lefleche, G. Dupont, J.M. Bove, J.G. Tully, and E.A. Freundt. 1973. Int. J. Syst. Bacteriol. 23:191-204.

25. Williamson, D.L. and R.F. Whitcomb.1974. In: Les Mycoplasmes, 33:283-290, J.M. Bove and J.F. Duplan (Eds.) Colloques Inst. Nat. Sante Recher Med.(Paris).

26. Kondo, F., A.H. McIntosh, S.B. Padhi and K. Maramorosch. 1976. Proc. Electron Microscopic Soc. Amer., p. 56.

27. Clark, T.B. 1977. J. Invert. Pathol. 29:112-113.

28. Darland, G., T.D. Brock, W. Sansonoff, and S.F. Conti. 1970. Science 170:1416-4117.

29. Belly, R.T., B.B. Bohlool, and T.D. Brock. 1973.

30. Robinson, J.P. and R.E. Hungate. 1973. Int. J. Syst. Bacteriol. 23:171-181.

31. Robinson, I.M. and M.J. Allison. 1975. Int. J. Syst. Bacteriol. 25:182-186.

32.   Lemcke, R.M. 1972. J. Bacteriol. 110:1154-1162.

33.   Cole, R.M., J.G. Tully, T.J. Popkin, and J.M. Bove.
      1973. J. Bacteriol. 115:367-386.

34.   Razin, S. 1969. Ann. Reve. Microbiol. 23:317-356.

35.   Lemcke, R.M. 1971. Nature 229:492-493.

36.   Maniloff, J. 1969. J. Bacteriol. 100:1402-1408.

37.   Maniloff, J. and H.J. Morowitz. 1967. Ann. N.Y.
      Acad. Sci. 143:59-65.

38.   Maniloff, J. and H.J. Morowitz. 1972. Bacteriol.
      Rev.36:263-290.

39.   Zucker-Franklin, D., M. Davidson, and L. Thomas.
      1966. J. Exp. Med. 124:521-532.

40.   Biberfeld, G. and P. Biberfeld. 1970. J. Bacteriol.
      102:855-861.

41.   Collier, A.M. and W.A. Clyde, Jr. 1971. Infect.
      Immun. 3:694-701.

42.   Collier, A.M. and W.A. Clyde, Jr. 1974. Am. Rev.
      Resp. Dis. 110:765-773.

43.   Richter, C.B. 1970. In: U.S. Atomic Energy Commis-
      sion Symp. Series vol. 21, p. 365-382, Oak Ridge
      Tenn.

44.   Rodwell, A.W., J. E. Peterson, and E.S. Rodwell.
      1973. Ann. N.Y. Acad. Sci. 225:190-200.

45.   Rodwell, A.W., J.E. Peterson, and E.S. Rodwell.
      1974. In: Les Mycoplasmes 33:43-46, J.M. Bove
      and J.F. Duplan (Eds.), Colloques Inst. Nat. Sante
      Recher. Med. (Paris).

46.   Razin, S. 1973. In: Advances in Microbial Physiology,
      vol. 10, p. 1-80, A.H. Rose and D.W. Tempest (Eds.)
      Academic Press, N.Y.

47.   Razin, S. 1975. In: Progress in Surface and Membrane
      Science, vol. 9, p. 257-312, D.A. Cadenhead, J.F.
      Danielli, and M.D. Rosenberg (Eds.), Academic
      Press, N.Y.

48. Razin, S. and S. Rottem. 1976. In: Biochemical
    Analysis of Membranes. p. 3-26, A.H. Maddy (Ed.),
    Chapman Hall Ltd., London.

49. Razin, S. 1974. J. Supramolecular Struct. 2:670-681.

50. Gourlay, R.N. and K.J. Thrower. 1968. J. Gen.
    Microbiol. 54:155-159.

51. Green, F. and R.P. Hanson. 1973. J. Bacteriol.
    116:1011-1018.

52. Howard, C.J. and R.N. Gourlay. 1974. J. Gen.
    Microbiol. 83:393-398.

53. Gilliam, J.M. and H.J. Morowitz. 1972. Biochem.
    Biophy. Acta 274:353-363.

54. Kahane, I. and J.G. Tully. 1976. J. Bacteriol. 128:
    1-7.

55. Manchee, R.J. and D. Taylor-Robinson. 1969. J.
    Bacteriol. 100:78-85.

56. Razin, S., G.K. Masover, M. Palant, and L. Hayflick.
    1977. Appl. Environ. Microbiol. (in press).

57. Bredt, W. 1974. In: Les Mycoplasmes, 33:47-52.
    J.M. Bove and J.F. Duplan (Eds.), Colloques Inst.
    Nat. Sante Recher Med. (Paris).

58. Neimark, H.C. 1976. Abstracts of the Annual Meeting
    of American Soc. Microbiology, p. 61.

59. Morowitz, H.J. and D.C. Wallace. 1973. Ann. N.Y.
    Acad. Sci. 225:62-73.

60. Bredt, W., H.H. Heunert, K.H. Hofling, and B.
    Milthaler. 1973. J. Bacteriol. 113:1223-1227.

61. Cristiansen, C., E.A. Freundt, and F.T. Black. 1975.
    Int. J. Syst. Bacteriol. 25:99-101.

62. Searcy, D.G. and E.K. Doyle. 1975. Int. Syst. Bac-
    teriol. 25:286-289.

63. Neimark, H.C. 1970. J. Gen. Microbiol. 63:249-263.

64. McGee, Z.A., M. Rogul, and R.G. Wittler. 1967. Ann.
     N.Y. Acad. Sci. 143:21-30.

65. Somerson, N.L., P.R. Reich, R.M. Chanock, and S.M.
     Weissman. 1967. Ann. N.Y. Acad. Sci. 143:9-20.

66. Gourlay, R.N. 1970. Nature 225:1165.

67. Gourlay, R.N. 1974. Critical Reviews in Microbiol-
     ogy 3:315-331.

68. Cole, R.M. 1977. In: Handbook of Microbiology, vol.
     2, 2nd edition (in press), A.I. Laskin and H.
     Lechevalier (Eds.), Chemical Rubber Co., Cleveland.

69. Maniloff, J. 1977. In: Advances in Virus Research,
     vol. 21, p. 343-380, K.M. Smith and M.A. Lauffer
     (Eds.), Academic Press, N.Y.

70. Cirillo, V.P. and S. Razin. 1973. J. Bacteriol.
     113:212-217.

71. Barile, M.F., R.T. Schimke and D.B. Riggs. 1966.
     J. Bacteriol. 91:189-192.

72. Rodwell, A.W. 1977. In: Handbook of Nutrition and
     Food, Part IV, vol. 1 (in press), M. Rechcigl
     (Ed.), Chemical Rubber Co., Cleveland.

73. Rodwell, A.W. 1969. J. Gen. Microbiol. 58:39-47.

74. Tourtellotte, M.E., H.J. Morowitz, and P. Kasimir.
     1964. J. Bacteriol. 88:11-15.

75. Razin, S. and J.G. Tully. 1970. J. Bacteriol. 102:
     306-310.

76. Edward D.G.ff. 1971. J. Gen. Microbiol. 69:205-210.

77. Rodwell, A.W. 1974. In: Les Mycoplasmes 33:79-85,
     J.M. Bove and J.F. Duplan (Eds.), Colloques Inst.
     Nat. Sante Recher. Med. (Paris).

78. Smith, P.F. 1971. In: The Biology of Mycoplasmas,
     Academic Press, N.Y.

79. Hayflick, L. 1960. Nature 185:783-784.

80.   Barile, M.F. and J. Kern. 1971. Proc. Soc. Exp.
      Biol. Med. 138:432-437.

81.   Raccach, M., S. Rottem, and S. Razin. 1975. Appl.
      Microbiol. 30:167-171.

82.   Hatch, M.T., D.N. Wright, and G.D. Bailey. 1970.
      Appl. Microbiol. 19:232-238.

83.   Stanbridge, E. 1971. Bacteriol. Rev. 35:206-227.

84.   Barile, M.F. 1973. In: Contamination in Tissue
      Cultures, p. 131-172, J. Fogh (Ed.), Academic
      Press, N.Y.

85.   McGarrity, G.J. 1976. In Vitro 12:634-648.

86.   Low, I.E. 1976. Health Lab. Sci. 13:129-136.

87.   Low, I.E. 1974. Appl. Microbiol. 27:1046-1052.

88.   Wolford, R.G. and F.M. Hetrick. 1972. Appl. Micro-
      biol. 24:18-21.

89.   Reynolds, R.K. and F.M. Hetrick. 1969. Appl.
      Microbiol. 17:405-411.

90.   Staal, S.P. and W.P. Rowe. 1974. J. Virol. 14:1620-
      1622.

91.   Mardh, P-A. 1975. Nature 254:515-516.

92.   Spendlove, R.S., R.B. Crosbie, S.F. Hayes and
      R.F. Keeler. 1971. Proc. Soc. Exp. Biol. Med.
      137-258-263.

93.   Mardh, P-A and D. Taylor-Robinson. 1973. Med. Micro-
      biol. Immun. 158:219-226.

94.   Edward, D.G.ff. 1947. J. Gen. Microbiol. 1:238-243.

95.   Morton, H.E. and J.G. Leece. 1953. J. Bacteriol.
      66:646-649.

96.   Taylor-Robinson, D., M.H. Williams and D.A. Haig.
      1968. J. Gen. Microbiol. 54:33-46.

97.   Kunze, M. 1972. Zbl. Bakt. Hyg. I. Abt. Orig. 222-
      535-539.

98.   Shedden, W.I.H. and B.C. Cole. 1966. J. Pathol.
        Bacteriol. 92:574-576.

99.   Wutzler, P., M. Sprossig, and H. Peterseim. 1975.
        J. Clin. Microbiol. 1:246-249.

100. Braun, P., J.O. Klein, and E.H. Kass. 1970. Appl.
        Microbiol. 19:62-70.

101. Niitu, Y., S. Hasegawa and H. Kubota. 1974.
        Antimicrob. Ag. Chemother. 5:513-519.

102. Mardh, P-A. 1975. Chemotherapy 21:47-57 (Supplement
        1).

103. Andrews, B.E., R.H. Leach, R.N. Gourlay, and C.J.
        Howard. 1973. Vet. Record 93:603.

104. Rottem, S. 1972. Appl. Microbiol. 23:659-660.

105. Blyth, W.A. from Klieneberger-Nobel, E. 1962.
        Pleuropneumonia-like Organisms (PPLO) Mycoplas-
        mataceae, Academic Press, London.

106. Newnham, A.G. and H.P. Chu. 1965. J. Hyg. 63:1-23.

107. Steward, S.M., M.E. Burnet and J.E. Young. 1969. J.
        Med. Microbiol. 2:287-292.

108. Kato, H., T. Murakami, S. Takase, K. Ono. 1972.
        Japan J. Vet. Sci. 34:197-206.

109. Niitu, Y., H. Kubota, S. Hasegawa, S. Komatsu, M.
        Horikawa, and T. Seutake. 1974. Japan J. Micro-
        biol. 18:149-155.

110. Ford, D.K. and J. R. Smith. 1974. Brit. J. Vener.
        Dis. 50:373-374.

111. Spaepen, M.S., R.B. Kundsin and H.W. Horne. 1976.
        Antimicrob. Ag. Chemother. 9:1012-1018.

112. Prentice, M.J., D. Taylor-Robinson, and G.W. Csonka.
        1976. Brit. J. Ven. Dis. 52:269-275.

113. Whittlestone, P. 1972. In: Microbial Pathogenicity
        in Man and Animals, Soc. Gen. Microbiol. Symp.
        No. 22, p. 217-250, H.Smith and J.H. Pearce
        (Eds.) Cambridge Univ. Press, London.

114.   Hopps, H.E., B.C. Meyer, M.F. Barile and R.A.
        Del Guidice. 1973. Ann. N.Y. Acad. Sci. 225:
        265-276.

115.   Stanbridge, E.J. 1976. Ann. Rev. Microbiol. 30:
        169-187.

INCIDENCE AND SOURCES OF MYCOPLASMA CONTAMINATION: A BRIEF REVIEW

Michael F. Barile, Hope E. Hopps and Marion W. Grabowski

Bureau of Biologics, FDA
Bethesda, Maryland 20014

In 1956, Robinson and colleagues (1) reported the first isolation
of a mycoplasma from a contaminated cell culture. Subsequently,
mycoplasmas have been shown to be common and bothersome contaminants capable of altering the activity of cells and affecting the
results of study. Because many of the vaccines prepared for human
use are produced in cell cultures and are subject to mycoplasma
contamination, the Bureau of Biologics has maintained a continuing
study for the past 18 years to examine various aspects of mycoplasma
contamination. This report will review some of our findings and
present a brief, updated status report on the incidence, prevalence
and sources of mycoplasma contamination. The subject has been
reviewed in detail elsewhere (2-5).

Contamination of primary and continuous cell culture substrates.
It has been known for many years that primary cell cultures are
rarely contaminated (0 to 4 percent), whereas continuous, stable
cell lines are frequently contaminated, from 57 to 92 percent (3,6).
These findings indicate that the original organs and tissues used
to prepare a primary cell culture are not major sources of contamination, and that most contamination occurs during cell propagation
and comes from exogenous sources. Because primary cell cultures
are rarely contaminated, and continuous cell lines are frequently
contaminated, primary cell cultures should be used whenever
possible.

The larger the volume the greater the risk. The risk and/or
frequency of contamination from exogenous sources is directly pro-
portional to the volume of cells and to the number of containers
used. Because laboratories that use cells for virus propagation

and the commercial suppliers either use or produce large volumes of cells, these laboratories are subject to the highest risk, and should have the highest incidence of contamination and, in fact, this is precisely what our studies showed many years ago (7). The cell culture producers had 91% contamination, and the investigators using large numbers of containers and large volumes of cells had 76% contamination, whereas the investigators who carried just a few cell lines and carefully examined their cells microscopically every few days for overt changes had minimal (<5%) contamination. When cytopathic changes or differences in cell activity were noted, the cell cultures became suspect and were examined for mycoplasma contamination. Contaminated cells were discarded immediately and an earlier passage of the cell culture was revived from the freezer. Because large-scale usage and production present greater risks of contamination, the producers and the large-scale users must establish vigorous quality control procedures in order to reduce the risk and eliminate the sources of contamination. Prevention and elimination of contamination have been discussed in detail in this monograph and elsewhere (3, 5).

Sources and prevalence of contamination. In 1958 we initiated a continuing program to isolate, detect, identify, speciate, and classify the mycoplasma contaminants of cell cultures. An updated status report of our findings is summarized in Table 1. In brief, over 17,000 continuous cell culture specimens were examined during

TABLE 1

MYCOPLASMAS ISOLATED FROM
CONTAMINATED CELL CULTURES:
SOURCE AND PREVALENCE[*]

Source	Number of Isolations	Percent
Bovine	1262	44.7
Human	927	32.9
Swine	590	20.9
Avian	17	0.6
Murine	16	0.6
Canine	5	0.1
Total	2817	100

[*]From over 17,000 continuous cell
cultures examined 1960-1976.
Extension of studies reported
earlier (2-7).

the period 1960-1976, and over 2800 mycoplasma contaminants were
isolated and identified by the epi-immunofluorescence procedure (9).
Approximately 10 percent of these cell culture specimens examined
had mixed contamination with two or more mycoplasma species (2).
The majority, 99 percent, of the contaminants were mycoplasma
species of either human, bovine or swine origin, and, therefore,
the major sources of contamination were either from human, bovine,
or swine origin.

   Bovine mycoplasma contaminants of cell cultures.   The bovine
species of mycoplasmas are presently the largest group of contaminants (Table 2).   At least 7 distinct bovine species of *Mycoplasma* and *Acholeplasma* have been isolated and identified during
these studies.   The two most frequent contaminants were *Mycoplasma
arginini* (26%) and *Acholeplasma laidlawii* (8.5%).

   Contaminated commercial bovine sera.   In 1971 we reported that
commercial bovine serum was frequently contaminated and that it was
the major source of bovine mycoplasma contamination (8).   To date,
285 of 888 lots of sera tested (32 percent) were found contaminated
(Table 3).   These include 22 lots of raw calf sera; 159 lots of raw
fetal bovine sera obtained from either the abattoir directly or
from a supplier; and 104 final lots of sera produced for market by
five different manufacturers.   Successful isolations were made only
when our large volume broth culture procedure was used.   In brief,
a large volume, 25 ml or more of serum specimen, is tested in a 100-
1000 ml volume of broth medium (3-5).   The incidence of bovine serum

TABLE 2

MYCOPLASMA CONTAMINATION OF CELL CULTURES: BOVINE STRAINS[*]

Species	Natural Habitat	Number of Isolation	Percent
M. arginini	oral, genital	739	26
A. laidlawii	oral, genital	240	8.5
Mycoplasma, strain 70-159	?	197	7.0
Acholeplasma sp. (unspeciated)	?	60	2.1
M. agalactiae var. bovis	respiratory	23	0.8
A. axanthum	nasal	2	0.07
M. bovoculi	conjunctivae	1	0.03
Totals		1262	44.7

[*]Extension of studies reported earlier (2-7)

TABLE 3

ISOLATION OF MYCOPLASMAS FROM
CONTAMINATED COMMERCIAL BOVINE SERA[†]

Sera[*] Source	Origin	Isolations[†]
Supplier	Calf	22/55
Supplier	Fetal bovine	159/438
Manufacturer	Fetal bovine	104/395
TOTALS		285/888

[*] Supplier denotes unprocessed sublots of raw sera and
manufacturer denotes final lots of sera produced for
market.
[†] Number positive/number tested. Lots were not selected
at random and data do not reflect incidence of contamination.
[†]From: Barile et al.(1973).

contamination was dependent on whether or not aseptic procedures
were used for collection of blood and for the processing of serum.
Serum from blood obtained by using sterile cardiac puncture was
rarely contaminated. Because most abattoirs in this country collect
blood by using rapid, non-sterile assembly-line procedures, about
50 percent of the raw, unprocessed lots of sera tested were found
contaminated (8). Normal and infected mucosal tissue of cattle are
frequently colonized by mycoplasmas and, therefore, the probable
source of contamination is from the oral, genital, and intestinal
secretions of these animals which contaminate the blood and or
serum during collection and harvest under poor quality controlled
and septic conditions.

Processing bovine serum. Most manufacturers in this country
process raw sera by filtering twice through 220 nanometer membrane
filters, using high pressures. Although filtration markedly reduces
contamination, it does not necessarily eliminate every single mycoplasma cell. Since cell cultures are an exquisitely sensitive
substrate for growth of mycoplasmas, very small numbers of the
mycoplasma contaminant can reach high population titers within a
few days. High pressures can also force the pliable mycoplasma
cells through very small bacteria-retaining filters. Thus, commercial sterilization of serum presents difficult technical problems
to the industry, and rigid quality control procedures must be used.

It is far easier to remove small numbers of contaminants using small volumes of serum for laboratory use. In our institute, we have effectively eliminated bovine mycoplasma contamination of cell cultures by pretesting and pretreating each lot of bovine serum. In brief, a large lot of serum pretested by the manufacturer and by us (using our large volume broth culture procedure and found free of mycoplasmas) is purchased and stored frozen at -20°C in 100 ml volumes. Cell cultures are then monitored weekly for myco- plasma contamination. If cells become contaminated with a bovine mycoplasma, the serum lot becomes suspect, and if found contaminated, it is replaced. In addition, every bottle of serum is routinely pretreated by either heat-inactivation at 56°C for 45 min and/or by filtration twice through a 220 nanometer filter. If heat- inactivation is unsuitable for growth of a given cell culture, we then filter the complete medium containing the serum through a 220 nanometer filter twice (Nalgene Filter Unit, Nalge Sybron Corp., Rochester, NY). This can be accomplished using small, 100 ml, volumes of media without the use of high pressure filtra- tion.

   Mycoplasma contaminants of commercial bovine sera. The bovine mycoplasma species isolated from contaminated commercial bovine sera were similar to or identical to the bovine mycoplasmas isolated from contaminated cell cultures (Table 4). At least 8 distinct species were isolated and identified. The most frequent contami- nants were *Acholeplasma laidlawii*, 45 percent, and *Mycoplasma*

TABLE 4

MYCOPLASMA CONTAMINATION OF COMMERCIAL
BOVINE SERA: IDENTIFICATION & SPECIATION†

Species	Natural Habitat	Numbers of Isolations	Percent
M. arginini	bovine; oral & genital	65	33.7
M. alkalescans	bovine; oral & genital	6	3.1
M. bovis	bovine, genital	5	2.6
M. bovoculi	bovine, conjunctivae	3	1.6
Mycoplasma sp 70-159*	cell cultures	3	1.6
M. hyorhinis	swine, nasal	1	0.5
A. laidlawii	bovine, genital	87	45.1
A. axanthum	bovine, genital	1	0.5
Acholeplasma sp	unknown	22	11.4
TOTALS		193	100.1

* Distinct unspeciated serotypes unrelated to established
  species.
† From: Barile et al. (1973).

arginini, 34 percent. In addition, a swine strain of *Mycoplasma hyorhinis* was also isolated, a finding which suggested to us that bovine sera may also be a source of swine mycoplasma contamination of cell cultures.

Human mycoplasma contaminants of cell cultures. The human oral and genital mycoplasma species are the second major group of contaminants and, therefore, the laboratory personnel and their environment are a major source of contamination. The use of poor or inadequate quality control procedures by the laboratory investigators is also a very important factor in the spread of contamination. The most frequent contaminant isolated during these studies was *Mycoplasma orale*, causing 29 percent of all contamination observed (Table 5). Mouth pipetting is still a major vehicle of oral mycoplasma contamination. Saliva containing both bacteria and mycoplasmas is introduced into the cell culture. The antibiotics present, generally penicillin and streptomycin, destroy the bacteria but may not destroy the mycoplasmas. In cells grown without antibiotics, the bacteria destroy the cells, and the contaminated culture along with the traveling mycoplasma contaminants is discarded. Thus, antibiotics may tend to mask mycoplasma contamination and should be avoided. Mouth pipetting should also be avoided. Contamination by human genital mycoplasmas may also occur occasionally, and is probably due to inadequate sterile procedures.

Swine mycoplasma contaminants of cell cultures. The third major group of contaminants are the swine mycoplasmas (Table 6). Although the source of swine mycoplasma contamination has not been established, trypsin and contaminated bovine sera have been incriminated as probable sources. However, all attempts to grow mycoplasmas from commercial trypsin have failed, and only one strain of *M. hyorhinis* has been isolated from one lot of contaminated bovine serum (2-5). Because swine and cattle are frequently processed

TABLE 5

MYCOPLASMA CONTAMINATIONS OF CELL
CULTURES: HUMAN STRAINS

Species	Natural Habitat	Number of Isolations	Percent
M. orale	oral	832	29.5
M. hominis	genital	63	2.2
M. fermentans	genital	28	1.0
M. salivarium	oral	4	0.14
M. buccale	oral	2	0.07
TOTALS		929	32.9

TABLE 6

MYCOPLASMA CONTAMINATION OF CELL
CULTURES: SWINE STRAINS

Species	Natural Habitat	Number of Isolations	Percent
M. hyorhinis	nasal	590	21
TOTAL		590	21

through the same abattoir, it is possible that bovine sera may also
become contaminated with swine mycoplasmas during collection and
manufacture.

*Murine, avian and canine mycoplasma contaminants of cell
cultures.* Occasionally, cell cultures are contaminated with mycoplasmas derived from murine, avian and canine origin (Table 7).
Because these mycoplasma contaminants have been isolated only from
primary cell cultures derived from homologous murine, avian and
canine tissues, and because these same contaminants are rarely
found in continuous and/or heterologous cell culture lines, the
probable sources of these contaminants were the original organs or
tissues used to produce the primary cell cultures.

TABLE 7

MYCOPLASMA CONTAMINATION OF CELL CULTURES:
MURINE, AVIAN AND CANINE STRAINS*

Species	Natural Habitat	Number of Isolations	Percent
MURINE			
M. arthritidis	respiratory	5	0.36
M. pulmonis	respiratory	4	0.29
AVIAN			
M. gallisepticum	respiratory	3	0.21
M. gallinarum	respiratory	2	0.14
CANINE			
M. canis	oral, genital	1	0.07
Mycoplasma sp. Serogroup 689	genital	2	0.14
TOTALS		17	1.24

* From Barile et al. (2, 3).

Contamination of primary cell cultures. Table 8 summarizes
our data on mycoplasmas isolated from primary cell cultures. Of
3,200 lots examined, 51 mycoplasmas, about 1 percent, were isolated
from 42 contaminated primary cell culture lots. The lots examined
include primary cell cultures derived from monkey, rabbit and
canine kidneys, as well as from mouse, rat and chick embryos.
Seventy-four percent of the contaminants were either human, bovine
or swine mycoplasmas, indicating that the sources of contamination
for primary cells were similar to those for established continuous
cell lines. However, the probable origin of the *Mycoplasma buccale*
(a simian species of mycoplasma rarely found in humans) and the
murine, avian and canine mycoplasmas, was the original organs or
tissues used to prepare the primary cell culture lot.

Prevalence of mycoplasma contamination. The prevalence of
contamination from human, bovine and swine sources was determined
for the periods 1960 through 1976 (Figure 1). The major source of
contamination in the early 1960's was the human oral mycoplasma
species. In the mid 1960's it was the swine species of mycoplasmas,
and in the early 1970's it was the bovine mycoplasmas. Today, 55
percent of the contaminants are human oral strains, and therefore
the investigators, their environment and quality control procedures

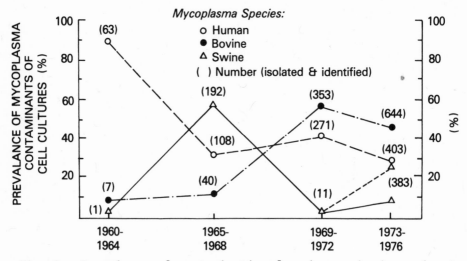

Fig. 1. Prevalence of contamination from human, bovine and swine
sources during period 1960 through 1976. Of 383 strains of *M.
hyorhinis* isolated by cell culture procedures between 1973 and 1976
(---), only 111 grew on artificial agar medium (——); 70 percent
were denoted as "non'cultivable."

TABLE 8

IDENTIFICATION OF MYCOPLASMAS ISOLATED
FROM CONTAMINATED PRIMARY CELL CULTURES

Primary Cell Cultures	Number of lots Contaminated*	Species Identified
Rabbit kidney	12†	*M. orale*, (7)‡; *M. arthritidis* (5) *M. fermentans* (2); *A. laidlawii* (2) *M. hominis* (1).
Monkey kidney	11†	*M. arginini* (5); *M. orale*, (4); *A. laidlawii* (2); *M. hominis* (2); *M. buccali* (2).
Mouse embryo	9	*M. hyorhinis* (9).
Dog kidney	5	*M. arginini* (2); *Mycoplasma* canine serogroup HRC689 (2) *M. canis* (1)
Rat embryo	4	*M. pulmonis* (4)
Chick embryo	1	*M. gallisepticum* (1)
TOTAL	42	51

* Approximately 3200 primary cell culture lots were examined. From Barile et al. (2).
† Five primary rabbit kidney and four primary monkey kidney cell culture lots had two mycoplasmas.
‡ ( ) denotes number of strains isolated.

continue to be the most common source of cell culture contamination. Presently, bovine mycoplasmas cause about 25 percent of the contamination, down from over 50 percent. The reduced rate of contamination is probably due, in part, to better quality control procedures used by the manufacturer in production and by the investigator in preparation of sterile bovine sera.

Prevalence of non-cultivable strains of Mycoplasma hyorhinis. The major source of cell culture contamination in the mid-1960's was from swine origin: 192 strains (60 percent of the contaminants) were identified as *M. hyorhinis*. The rate of swine mycoplasma contamination dropped to 4 percent in the early 1970's, but in recent years it has increased to 27 percent (causing 383 of the contami-

nations) as detected only by our newly developed sensitive cell
culture procedure. By comparison, only one-third of these strains
were detected by use of our direct agar culture procedures. Therefore, more than 70 percent of the strains of *Mycoplasma hyorhinis*
did not grow on agar. Because a cell culture substrate was required
to detect contamination, these strains were designated as "non-cultivable", (10) a subject to be discussed in detail elsewhere in
this monograph.

Spread of mycoplasma contamination. In addition to the original sources which have been discussed, contamination can also be
spread from cell to cell by aerosols of contaminated cell cultures
and media fluids, and by the use of contaminated virus pools, antisera and other materials or cell culture reagents. Another major
means of cross-contamination is due to the use of poor quality control procedures, including the use of contaminated equipment,
apparati, glassware, plastic ware, and other items commonly used
in cell culture studies.

*All cell culture substrates examined were subject to contamina-
tion.* Cell culture substrates derived from all tissues, organs and
animals examined were found to be subject to contamination, including cultures derived from mammalian, avian, reptilian, fish, insect,
and plant origin, and from either normal, infected or neoplastic
tissues, including primary, continuous, diploid, heteroploid, fibroblastic, epithelial cell cultures, and cells grown in monolayer or
suspension. Most mycoplasma contaminants produce titers in most
cell cultures which range from five to nine logs per ml medium
fluids.

CONCLUSION

In summary, primary cell cultures are rarely contaminated while continuous cell cultures are frequently contaminated. The major sources
of contamination are of human origin -- the investigator and other
laboratory personnel, their environment and quality control procedures; of bovine origin - primarily contaminated commercial bovine
sera; and of swine origin. About one percent of the original
organs and tissues used to produce primary cell cultures were also
contaminated. Specimens from man and animals used for virus isolation studies may also contain mycoplasmas, and thereby contaminate
the cell culture. Contamination can also be spread by contaminated
reagents and by use of contaminated materials, equipment, apparati,
and glass and plastic ware commonly used in cell culture studies.
Vigorous quality control procedures used for prevention and elimination of contamination are based on removing the sources and controlling the spread of contamination. In sum, the price of contami-
nation-free cells is eternal vigilance.

REFERENCES

1. Robinson, L. B., R. B. Wichelhausen, and B. Roizman. 1956. Contamination of human cell cultures by pleuropneumonia-like organisms. Science 124: 1147-1148.

2. Barile, M. F., R. A. DelGiudice, H. E. Hopps, M. W. Grabowski, and D. B. Riggs. 1973. Identification of *Mycoplasma* species isolated from contaminated cell cultures and commercial bovine sera. N. Y. Acad. Sci. 225: 251-264.

3. Barile, M. F. 1973. Mycoplasma contamination of cell cultures: Mycoplasma-virus-cell culture interactions. In: J. Fogh (Ed.) *Contamination of Cell Cultures*. Academic Press, New York, NY pp. 131-172.

4. Barile, M. F. 1974. General principles of isolation and detection of mycoplasmas. In: J. M. Bove and J. F. Duplan (Eds.) *Les Mycoplasmes*. Colloques INSERM, Paris 33: pp. 135-142.

5. Barile, M. F. 1977. Mycoplasma contamination of cell cultures: A status report. In: R. Action (Ed.) *Cell Culture and Its Application*. Academic Press, New York, NY.

6. Barile, M. F. 1962. Discussion: Detection and elimination of contaminating organisms. Bethesda, J. Nat. Cancer Institute, Monograph Series #7, pp. 50-53.

7. Barile, M. F., W. F. Malizia, and D. Riggs. 1962. Incidence and detection of pleuropneumonia-like organisms in cell culture by fluorescent antibody and cultural procedures. J. Bacteriol. 84: 130-136.

8. Barile, M. F., and J. Kern. 1971. Isolation of *Mycoplasma arginini* from commercial bovine sera and its implication in contaminated cell cultures. Proc. Soc. Exp. Biol. Med. 138: 432-437.

9. Barile, M. F., and R. A. DelGiudice. 1972. Isolation of mycoplasmas and their rapid identification by plate epi-immunofluorescence. In: Ciba Foundation Symposium. *Pathogenic Mycoplasmas*. Elsevier and North-Holland, Amsterdam. pp. 165-188.

10. Hopps, H. E., B. C. Meyer, M. F. Barile, and R. A. DelGiudice. 1973. Problems concerning "non-cultivable" mycoplasma contaminants in tissue cultures. N. Y. Acad. Sci. 225: 265-276.

CULTURAL AND SEROLOGIC PROCEDURES FOR MYCOPLASMAS IN TISSUE

CULTURE

DAVID TAYLOR-ROBINSON

Clinical Research Centre

Watford Road, Harrow, Middlesex HA1 3UJ, England

CULTURAL PROCEDURES FOR THE DETECTION OF MYCOPLASMAS

Mycoplasmas in cell cultures, or indeed elsewhere, may be detected by both cultural and non-cultural methods (Table 1). The former methods, discussed on several occasions (1-7), are reviewed in this communication.

Table 1.   Methods for Detecting Mycoplasma
             Infection of Cell Cultures

(a) Cultural methods

(b) Non-cultural methods:
   i) Immunofluorescence
   ii) Histological staining:
          Orcein
          Giemsa
          Acridine orange
   iii) Electron microscopy
   iv) Enzyme assays:
          Arginine deiminase activity
          Thymidine degradation
   v) Uridine/uracil ratio
   vi) Genome size
   vii) DNA binding
   viii) Cytopathic effect

Mycoplasma Medium and Cultural Conditions

In the first place, it is necessary to select, mainly by
trial and error, a suitable culture medium. This is based on a
medium that was described by Edward (8) and different workers
have modified it to their own requirements since. Basically, the
medium consists of beef-heart infusion broth supplemented with
serum and yeast extract. It is worth emphasizing that although
horse serum is very frequently used, not all animal sera, nor all
horse sera, have the property of promoting growth and, therefore,
it is necessary to pre-test sera for this ability. Hayflick (1)
described the use of unheated horse serum for the isolation of
M. pneumoniae and this may be important for this mycoplasma and for
certain others, too. However, for the isolation of various other
mycoplasmas, for example M. arginini, heating the serum at 56ºC
for 30 min is helpful. This may be due to the inactivation of
complement components which, even in the absence of specific
antibody, may have a direct killing effect (9).

The type of yeast is important because not all brands are
satisfactory. Although those of Fleischman (USA) and Distillers
Company Ltd. (UK) have consistently given good results, it is
necessary, as in the case of serum, to select and pre-test the
yeast. A 10% (v/v) concentration of a 25% (w/v) extract is usually
used, particularly for M. pneumoniae, but other mycoplasmas may be
isolated in medium containing a lower concentration. DNA and DPN
have been incorporated for the isolation of, for example,
M. synoviae, but it may be less important to supplement medium with
these additives if the yeast is of good quality Incidentally,
neither mycoplasma just mentioned has been found as a tissue culture
contaminant. Glucose, arginine and urea are often added to media,
not primarily as energy sources but because mycoplasmas metabolize
them so that the products may then be used to indicate the presence
of the organisms. However, it must be recognized that too much
arginine inhibits the growth of certain mycoplasmas (10).

Some agar preparations were found, at least a few years ago,
to be extremely toxic for mycoplasmas (11), so that again selection
is important. A final concentration of 1% is usually used and 0.05%
for semi-solid medium. Mycoplasmas grow over a range of pH values
but there are optima. As an example, isolation of ureaplasmas is
best made in medium the pH of which is not more than 6.0. So far
as atmospheric conditions are concerned, the use of 5% carbon
dioxide in nitrogen is better than 5% CO_2 in air for cultivation
of most mycoplasmas (5,12) and the observance of stricter anaerobic
conditions than usual has been an advantage in some hands (13).
Although maximal isolation rates will be obtained when both these
atmospheric conditions are used, from a practical point of view
not much will be lost by using anaerobic conditions alone.

As mentioned throughout, pre-testing of medium and medium components is extremely important, and to do this it is essential to use a mycoplasma which has not had multiple in vitro passes in the laboratory and has been rendered easy to cultivate.

Cultural Techniques

There are several techniques which are summarized in Table 2.

Liquid medium. Specimens may be inoculated directly into liquid medium which is subsequently subcultured on agar medium (1,5,6,7). The volume tested varies from one laboratory to another; our practice is to inoculate a 0.2 ml volume of the specimen into 1.8 ml of medium. It is particularly helpful to use liquid medium as the first step in attempting to isolate mycoplasmas from tissue-culture cells. On subculture to agar medium many of the cells remain behind so that they do not obscure the agar surface and make colony detection difficult, as sometimes occurs following direct inoculation. As mentioned previously, the metabolism of various substrates and the production of a colour change in a pH indicator by the metabolic products can be helpful in indicating when to subculture to agar medium (14). However, it is important to point out that a colour change in the liquid medium of the primary culture may not always take place, several subcultures being required for this to occur. Thus, the absence of a colour change may not necessarily indicate absence of a mycoplasma. In this circumstance, it is necessary to subculture from liquid to agar medium in a routine fashion, and once a week for a period of 3-4 weeks should suffice. Successful isolation may occur much sooner but the essential point is not to discard cultures as negative too early.

Table 2. Cultural Techniques for Detecting Mycoplasmas

(a) Specimen into liquid medium ⟶ agar medium

(b) Specimen directly on agar medium

(c) Semi-solid medium procedure

(d) Feeder-layer technique

(e) Large specimen - liquid culture procedure

Agar medium. Direct inoculation of specimens onto agar medium
(1,5,6,7), in addition to subculture from liquid medium, is an
important procedure. Although it is not a common occurrence,
colonies sometimes may develop when the organisms fail to multiply
in liquid medium. Of course, it must be ruled out that this is
not due to the production of pseudo-colonies(1),a phenomenon that
has received sufficient recognition to not require further
emphasis here.

Semi-solid medium. The incorporation of 0.05% agar into
liquid medium produces a semi-solid medium (5,6,7). In this way
an oxygen gradient is produced so that mycoplasma colonies occur
where the oxygen concentration is optimal for their development.

Feeder-layer technique. This was described by House and
Waddell (15). A monolayer of tissue-culture cells (they used
mouse embryo cells) is covered by mycoplasma agar medium to
which the test inoculum is added. The principle is that nutrients
which are essential for mycoplasma growth and which are not present
in the agar medium, diffuse into it from the monolayer of cells.
The relative value of the technique is largely determined by the
capacity of mycoplasma medium to support growth. As shown by
House and Waddell, the incorporation in mycoplasma medium of
yeast which had been heated to 80°C only (16) produced results
comparable with the feeder-layer technique.

Large specimen - liquid culture procedure. This procedure
(5,6,7,17) is one in which 100 ml of liquid medium are inoculated
with 25 ml of the specimen or, at least, large volumes are used
in about this ratio. This technique has been applied to the
detection of mycoplasmas in serum rather than in tissue cultures
but tissue culture medium containing cells could be inoculated in
the same way. The method is a modification of the liquid medium
technique, the principle being that the larger the volume of
specimen tested, the greater the chance of detecting mycoplasmal
contamination.

Other Important Factors in Isolation

Confluent cell monolayers. These should be examined rather
than sparsely populated cultures, the principle being, as before,
that the more cells tested the greater the chance of mycoplasmal
isolation.

Removal of antibiotics. Many cell cultures contain antibiotics to which the mycoplasmas are completely resistant, so
that it is unnecessary to remove the antibiotics before testing.
However, where attempts have been made to free cell cultures of

mycoplasmal contamination by using antibiotics, it is important at least to remove the antibiotic and preferably to subculture the cells once in its absence before conducting mycoplasma isolation procedures.

Testing cells. Cells should be tested and not just the supernatant media from cell cultures because mycoplasmas are often very much tissue cell associated (4,5). Indeed, there may be more mycoplasmas adherent to the cells than there are in the medium of a culture.

Trypsinization. Cell cultures should be tested before trypsinization and not immediately after because the trypsin can damage the mycoplasma membrane. Obviously, the damage is insufficient to cause elimination of the organisms, but it may make isolation more difficult.

Damage to cells. Freeze-thawing or homogenization of cell cultures may assist in mycoplasmal isolation (18). This suggestion is in obvious conflict with the well-recognized fact that breaking up of tissues deters isolation because mycoplasma inhibitors such as lysolecithin are released from the damaged cells (19,20,21). Although this is true, larger numbers of mycoplasma colonies often may be found if freezing and thawing is carried out only once or the homogenization procedure is gentle. This is probably because these procedures liberate organisms from the cell surface and separate cells rather than causing extensive cell damage.

Overcoming mycoplasma inhibitors. Lysolecithin kills mycoplasmas because it damages the mycoplasma membrane and causes lysis in a similar way to that seen with erythrocytes. However, ammonium reineckate binds lysolecithin and nullifies its effect (21) so that the incorporation of ammonium reineckate (100 µg/ml) into mycoplasma medium, particularly in situations where there has been extensive homogenization of tissues, may be helpful in mycoplasmal isolation. In addition, diluting a specimen at least 10^{-1}, 10^{-2} and 10^{-3} in mycoplasma liquid medium not only dilutes out inhibitors, but also is a useful procedure in helping to determine the number of organisms in the specimen.

SEROLOGIC PROCEDURES

Numerous serological tests have been used for detecting antibody to mycoplasmas. These are listed in Table 3 in decreasing order of sensitivity, the degree of specificity of each also being shown. Several methods are very sensitive and capable of detecting low levels of antibody developed by a host as a result of mycoplasma infection. However, this seems

Table 3.   Relative Sensitivity and Specificity of
Serological Techniques for Mycoplasmas

Serological techniques	Sensitivity	Specificity
Radioimmunoprecipitation	+++++	+++(?)[a]
Complement-dependent cidal	++++	+++(?)
Indirect haemagglutination	+++	++
Metabolism inhibition	+++	+++
Inhibition of growth in liquid medium	+++	+++
CPE inhibition (tissue culture)	+++	+++
Immunofluorescence (colonies on agar)	++	+++
Complement fixation	++	+
Cumulative haemagglutination inhibition (Feldman method)	++	+(?)
Agglutination	++	+
Latex agglutination	++	+(?)
Haemadsorption inhibition	+	+++(?)
Colony inhibition on agar (disc method)	+	+++
Gel diffusion	+	++

a = Insufficient evaluation

irrelevant so far as mycoplasma infection of cell cultures is
concerned. Here the question arises of the areas in which
serological techniques are of value. These are three :
mycoplasmal detection, identification and elimination.

Detection

The only serological method that is applicable for the
detection of mycoplasmas is immunofluorescence (22). This is a
rapid technique and as sensitive as mycoplasma culture methods
when cell cultures are heavily infected but its sensitivity in
comparison with cultural and other methods in minimally infected
cell cultures is not well established. The only other drawback
is that antisera to several possible contaminating mycoplasmas
are required although, as indicated below, their selection is not
usually a difficult problem.

Table 4. Mycoplasmas Isolated from Cell Cultures

HUMAN 44%	M. orale	37.4%
	M. hominis	6.1%
	M. fermentans	0.4%
	M. buccale	0.1%
BOVINE 38%	M. arginini	22.0%
	A. laidlawii	7.0%
	Others	9.0%
SWINE 16%	M. hyorhinis	16.0%
MURINE 0.9%	M. arthritidis	0.5%
	M. pulmonis	0.4%
AVIAN 0.5%	M. gallisepticum	0.3%
	M. gallinarum	0.2%
CANINE 0.3%	M. canis	0.1%
	Others	0.2%

Data compiled from that of Barile and
colleagues (5,8,23,28)

Identification

Many different mycoplasmas have been found as contaminants in cell cultures, so that at first sight identification would seem to be a difficult problem. However, as shown in Table 4, it is possible to identify 90% of the mycoplasmas in tissue cultures by using 5 antisera, namely those to M. orale, M. hominis, M. arginini, A. laidlawii and M. hyorhinis. Thus, from a practical point of view, identification may be seen as follows : during the course of isolation, or subsequently, the ability of the mycoplasma to metabolize arginine, glucose or urea is noted. If it degrades arginine, then antisera to M. orale, M. arginini and M. hominis are used. If glucose is metabolized, then antisera to M. hyorhinis and A. laidlawii may be sufficient to make the identification.

The techniques that are commonly used are agar growth inhibition, metabolism inhibition and immunofluorescence.

Growth inhibition on agar. As shown in Table 3, this is not a sensitive serological technique, but it is specific and simple to perform. The specific antisera are usually incorporated in the discs which are then placed on the agar (24), although placing the antisera in wells in the agar and other modifications increase

the sensitivity of the technique (25). Failure of zones to
develop is seen particularly in the case of M. hyorhinis.
However, with this mycoplasma the antiserum may have a high titer
in the metabolism-inhibition test (26) and, in fact, if there is
a suspicion that M. hyorhinis is present, it is sensible to use
the metabolism-inhibition test initially.

Epi-immunofluorescence. The major attributes of this
technique (27,28) are the speed with which it may be carried out
and the ability to detect a mixture of different mycoplasma
species. Mixtures are far less easily detected by the other
methods, the mycoplasma which grows best being the one most
likely to be identified.

                                   Elimination

Most persons who find a mycoplasma contaminating a cell
culture are not concerned about its identity. They wish only to
eliminate it. Although the best answer to the problem may be to
discard the contaminated culture and start again from a clean
cell stock, there are occasions when preservation of the cells
and elimination of the mycoplasma is desirable. In this case,
knowledge of the identity of the mycoplasma and use of an antiserum directed specifically against it may be helpful.

Pollock and Kenny (29) showed that treatment of mycoplasma-
contaminated cell cultures with specific antiserum which had been
heat-inactivated failed to eliminate the organisms. However, the
use of uninactivated antiserum was successful. This was probably
due to heat labile components of complement in the antiserum which
potentiated the activity of specific antibody. Indeed, damage to
the mycoplasma membrane and lysis are brought about by specific
antibody in the presence of fresh guinea pig serum (30). This is
seen again in the metabolism-inhibition test where an inhibitory
effect may be turned into a mycoplasmacidal one by using fresh
guinea pig serum (31). This is an important principle, insufficiently recognized as a technique for eliminating mycoplasmas
from tissue cultures. Until an effort is made to compare all the
methods that are currently available to rid cell cultures of
mycoplasmas, the best will remain unknown. In the meantime,
however, the combined use of specific antibody and guinea pig
complement should rank high on the list.

REFERENCES

1. Hayflick, L. (1965). Tex. Rep. Biol. Med. 23, Suppl. 1,
        285-303.
2. MacPherson, I. (1966). J. Cell Sci. 1, 145-168.
3. Edward, D.G.ff. (1969). Progr. Immunobiol. Standard. 3, 17-22.
4. Stanbridge, E. (1971). Bacteriol. Rev. 35, 206-227.
5. Barile, M.F. (1973). In: Contamination in Tissue Culture.
        Fogh, J. Ed. Academic Press, New York, pp. 131-172.
6. Barile, M.F. (1974). INSERM 33, 135-142.
7. Barile, M.F., DelGiudice, R.A., Grabowski, M.W. and Hopps,
        H.E. (1974). Develop. Biol. Standard. 23, 128-133,
        Karger, Basel.
8. Edward, D.G.ff. (1947). J. Gen. Microbiol. 1, 238-243.
9. Bredt, W., Wellek, B., Brunner, H. and Loos, M. (1977).
        Infect. Immun. 15, 7-12.
10. Leach, R.H. (1976). J. Appl. Bacteriol. 41, 259-264.
11. Taylor-Robinson (1968). J. Clin. Path. 21. Suppl. 2, 38-51.
12. Barile, M.F. (1962). Nat. Cancer Inst., Monog. 7, 50-53.
13. McGarrity, G.J. and Coriell, L.L. (1973). In Vitro 9, 17-18.
14. Taylor-Robinson, D. and Purcell, R.H. (1966). Proc. Roy. Soc.
        Med. 59, 1112-1116.
15. House, W. and Waddell, A. (1967). J. Path. Bacteriol. 93,
        125-132.
16. Herderscheê, D. (1963). Antonie v. Leeuwenhoek 22, 377-384.
17. Barile, M.F. and Kern, J. (1971). Proc. Soc. Exp. Biol. Med.
        138, 432-437.
18. Mazzali, R. and Taylor-Robinson, D. (1971). J. Med. Microbiol.
        4, 125-138.
19. Tully, J.G. and Rask-Nielson, R. (1967). Ann. N.Y. Acad. Sci,
        143, 345-352.
20. Kaklamanis, E., Thomas, L., Stavropoulos, K., Borman, I.
        and Boshwitz, C. (1969). Nature 221, 860-862.
21. Mårdh, P.-A. and Taylor-Robinson, D. (1973). Med. Mikrobiol.
        Immunol. 158, 259-266.
22. Barile, M.F., Malizia, W.F. and Riggs, D.B. (1962). J.
        Bacteriol. 84, 130-136.
23. Barile, M.F., Hopps, H.E., Grabowski, M.W., Riggs, D.B. and
        DelGiudice, R.A. (1973). Ann. N.Y. Acad. Sci. 225,
        251-264.
24. Clyde, W.A. Jr. (1964). J. Immunol. 92, 958-965.
25. Black, F.T. (1973). Appl. Microbiol. 25, 528-533.
26. Dinter, Z. and Taylor-Robinson, D. (1969). J. Gen. Microbiol.
        57, 263-272.
27. DelGiudice, R.A., Robillard, N.F. and Carski, T.R. (1967)
        J. Bacteriol. 93, 1205-1209.
28. Barile, M.F. and DelGiudice, R.A. (1972). In: Pathogenic
        Mycoplasmas. A Ciba Foundation Symposium. Elsevier,
        Amsterdam. pp. 165-185.

29. Pollock, M.E. and Kenny, G.E. (1963). Proc. Soc. Exp. Biol.
         Med. 112, 176-181.
30. Brunner, H., Kalica, A.R., James, W.D., Horswood, R.L. and
         Chanock, R.M. (1973). Infect. Immun. 7, 259-264.
31. Taylor-Robinson, D., Purcell, R.H., Wong, D.C. and Chanock,
         R.M. (1966). J.Hyg., Camb. 64, 91-104.

MICROBIOLOGICAL METHODS AND FLUORESCENT MICROSCOPY FOR THE DIRECT DEMONSTRATION OF MYCOPLASMA INFECTION OF CELL CULTURES

Richard A. Del Giudice and Hope E. Hopps

NCI Frederick Cancer Research Center, Frederick,
Maryland 21701 and Bureau of Biologics, Food and
Drug Administration, Rockville, Maryland 20852

INTRODUCTION

Our principal experience with immunofluorescence is in its
application to the identification of mycoplasma colonies growing
on agar medium (5). The immunofluorescent identification results
of mycoplasmas isolated from cell cultures over an 11-year period
are summarized herein. Most recently we have used immunofluorescence to identify *M. hyorhinis* in infected cell cultures. These
results will be presented with special reference to auxotrophic
variants of *M. hyorhinis*. The auxotrophs are strains that are
noncultivable on media that support the growth of the type strain
of *M. hyorhinis* (BTS-7) and other similar strains. The term
"noncultivable mycoplasma" (7) is used in this sense to describe
a strain (DBS 1050 = ATCC 29052) that grew in cell cultures but
not on agar medium. This specific connotation is obscured by the
current use of the term in reference to apparent isolation failures.

The possibility that *M. hyorhinis* auxotrophs might be a har-
binger of auxotrophy in other mycoplasma species prompted studies
to evaluate other methods not dependent on axenic media. DNA-
binding fluorochromes were reported by Russel et al. (10) and
Chen (4) as useful to detect mycoplasmas in cell cultures. The
fluorochromes permit direct microscopic demonstration of DNA, a
distinct advantage over indirect biochemical procedures which are
subject to complex and variable physiological interactions between
mycoplasmas and host cells. Fogh (6) has advocated the use of a
cytochemical technique to directly demonstrate mycoplasmas in
infected cell cultures. The Fogh procedure is standardized by
use of indicator cell cultures which provide controls not used by

Russel or Chen. The techniques described here are based on the methodology developed by Fogh combined with the fluorochromes recommended by Russel and Chen.

MATERIALS AND METHODS

Media

The axenic medium is composed of mycoplasma broth base (BBL no. 11458) supplemented with: 10% horse serum, 5% fresh yeast extract, 0.02% deoxyribonucleic acid (calf thymus DNA), 0.002% phenol red, 0.1% glucose, and 0.1% arginine. Except for the serum, the medium components were mixed and autoclaved, after which the horse serum was added aseptically. No bacterial inhibitors were used in the mycoplasma medium. To obtain solid medium, a minimal amount of agar or agarose was added to the broth before autoclaving. The gel strength per gram of different agars was determined by serial dilution of the agar in liquid medium. Until recently we used 0.8% Oxoid Ionagar No. 2; this is no longer marketed so we are now using Sea Plaque Agarose at 1.2% concentration. The major medium components are poorly-defined chemically so that it was necessary to pretest each new lot of material (peptones, horse serum, DNA, yeast extract, and agar) in test batches of media using a selected array of mycoplasma strains. Our minimal acceptance standards required the test medium to support mycoplasma growth in serial passage and permit low density inocula to initiate colony formation on agar.

Indicator Cell Cultures

A variety of cell cultures has been used sucessfully to isolate mycoplasmas from cell culture specimens. The indicator cell culture now in use is 3T6. The 3T6 cells were grown on coverslips contained in 35 mm petri dishes with Eagle's minimum essential medium (EMEM) and no antibiotics. EMEM is without sodium bicarbonate and contains 20 mM of HEPES buffer, permitting the incubation of unsealed dishes in ambient atmosphere. Cells were planted in EMEM containing 5% fetal bovine serum that had been inactivated by heating to 56°C for 30 min. After 2-3 days incubation, the medium was changed and the serum concentration reduced to 2%. The subconfluent cell monolayers thus obtained were the substrate on which to grow mycoplasmas. Test specimens in 0.1 ml amounts were inoculated into the dishes and incubated for an additional 5 days (48 hrs is sufficient for most mycoplasmas) before the coverslips were harvested for immunofluorescent or fluorescent DNA-staining.

Indicator cell cultures are not required and the staining procedures can be applied directly to the test cell culture to be examined for mycoplasma contamination. However, indicator cell cultures are recommended for the following reasons: (1) The system is standardized by employing infected and uninfected control cultures with each group of test specimens; (2) It is possible to test specimens that will not grow on coverslips, such as amniotic fluid, virus preparations, cell extracts, suspension cultures, animal tissues or exudates, etc.; (3) The indicator cell culture serves as an "enrichment medium;" (4) Quantitation of the mycoplasmas is possible by inoculating the indicator cell cultures with serial dilutions of the test specimen; and (5) Time, labor, and materials are saved by avoiding the need to passage each cell culture to be tested. Our laboratory routinely tests 100 specimens per week. Because many of these cell cultures require special media, establishing subcultures can be a formidable problem. We would point out that the above mentioned advantages are no less applicable to biochemical testing procedures, particularly with regard to the use of controls. Fogh has similarly advocated the use of indicator cell cultures to provide a constant base line (6).

Fluorescent DNA Stain

The procedure described by Chen (4) was used with slight modifications. The medium was partially removed from the dish by suction, leaving the coverslip submerged in 1 ml of medium. One ml of Carnoy's fixative (acetic acid-methanol, 1:3) was added to the dish and after 2 min the fixative and medium mixture were aspirated. Carnoy's was reapplied for 5 min, after which the slide was air-dried and stained with Hoechst fluorochrome compound 33258. The stain had been prepared in Hanks' salts solution, as used by Chen (4); however, slides so stained occasionally developed a brown background cast when exposed to UV light. This discoloration was apparently attributable to the Hanks' salt solution.

Stain preparation was modified as follows: 50 µg/ml of fluorochrome was dissolved in water to make a stock; the stock solution was diluted 1000-fold in McIlvaine's phosphate-citric acid buffer, pH 5.5, to make fresh working stain. The final fluorochrome concentration was 0.05 µg/ml. Thimerosal was added to the stain solutions at a concentration of 1:10,000 in order to inhibit microbial growth, and the solutions were stored at 4°C and protected from light. Filter sterilization was not used because the stain apparently binds to membrane filters.

One ml of working stain was applied to a coverslip contained in the original cell culture dish and after 10 min the stain was aspirated. The coverslip was washed twice with distilled water

and mounted (cell side up) on a slide under a second larger coverslip. The mounting medium was McIlvaine's buffer mixed with an
equal volume of glycerol (27.8 ml of 0.2 M disodium phosphate, 22.2
ml of 0.1 M citric acid, and 50 ml of glycerol). The addition of
glycerol to the buffer provided a semi-permanent mounting medium
that was more convenient to use than coverslip cement.

Immunofluorescence

Coverslip cell cultures were removed from the dishes, rinsed
in phosphate buffered saline (PBS, pH 7.4), fixed in acetone for
2 min, rinsed in PBS, and placed in a dish for staining. An optimal conjugate dilution was determined by 2-fold serial dilution.
The *M. hyorhinis*, strain BTS-7, conjugate displayed an extinction
titer of 1:1280 and was used at a 200-fold working dilution. The
diluent was PBS containing 10% fetal bovine serum. The coverslips
were flooded with the working conjugate, incubated for 30 min at
room temperature, and washed in PBS. Buffered glycerol (BBL 40825Y)
was used to sandwich the coverslip between a glass slide and second
larger coverslip. The preparation of antisera, fluorescein conjuga-
tion of globulins, and the staining of mycoplasma colonies on agar
have been described (5).

Microscopy

The same microscope optical arrangement was used to examine
immunofluorescent mycoplasma colonies on agar (5) and immunofluo-
rescent- or DNA-stained mycoplasma-infected coverslips. Specimens
were examined with a Zeiss Universal Microscope equipped with a
high pressure mercury vapor lamp and modified for incident illumination. A UGI exciter filter was used whereas a barrier filter
was not needed because of the filtration by the dichroac mirror in
the incident illuminator. Specimens were examined with a 40X
apochromat oil immersion objective.

RESULTS

Identification of Mycoplasma Colonies

During the 11-year period, 1966 through 1976, microbiological
methods were used to test cell cultures for mycoplasma contamination.
A number of procedural variations and medium modifications were
employed. The one procedural constant was to inoculate the cell
culture suspension, obtained by scraping the monolayer, directly
onto the surface of agar medium and to incubate the agar plate in

an anaerobic atmosphere containing approximately 4-9% carbon dioxide (BBL Gas Pak).   Neither broth enrichment nor aerobic incubation significantly affected the mycoplasma isolation rate from cell cultures in comparison to direct agar inoculation and anerobic incubation.   Thus, the isolation data presented here are, in effect, those derived from direct inoculation and anerobic incubation of a single agar plate. The medium described in the Materials and Methods Section has been in use since the beginning of 1968. Other media have been used with no impact on the isolation data.

From 1966 through 1976, 17,666 cell culture suspensions were inoculated onto agar medium. After approximately 17 days of anerobic incubation, the plates were examined for the presence of mycoplasma colonies. Mycoplasma colonies were discovered on 2,452 (14%) plates and these colonies were serotyped *in situ* by immunofluorescence. A total of 2,775 mycoplasma strains were serotyped. Two or three different mycoplasmas were sometimes isolated in mixed culture from the same specimen, accounting for the disparity between the number of infected cell cultures and the number of mycoplasmas isolated. Table 1 shows the isolation and identification results.

Because aspects of these data are detailed elsewhere in this volume (Barile) our discussion will be brief. Portions of the data from Table 1 are represented graphically in Figure 1. Five mycoplasma species comprised 92% of 2,775 total mycoplasma strains isolated. The single most frequent isolate was *M. orale*, a common inhabitant of the human oral cavity. In contrast, *M. salivarium*, also a common component of the human oral flora, was isolated 4 times, although cell cultures are probably exposed to this mycoplasma as often as to *M. orale*. If the preponderance of *M. orale* over *M. salivarium* cannot be explained by exposure rates, then there may be a difference in cell culture infectivity of the two mycoplasmas (9). *M. hominis* and *M. fermentans* are relatively uncommon in man as well as cell cultures.

Bovine mycoplasmas and the role of commercial serum as a vehicle for their transmission to cell cultures is covered by Barile in this volume. It should be noted that, while the first mycoplasma isolation from commercial bovine serum was in 1971 (2), our data show that mycoplasmas of bovine origin, and *M. arginini* in particular, had become major cell culture contaminants during the preceeding two years. Bovine serum must not have been frequently mycoplasma-contaminated prior to 1969 and contamination since then is usually attributed to changes in serum collecting procedures. Additional factors may influence which mycoplasma species find their way to cell cultures via bovine serum. *M. arginini* was first isolated from cell cultures in 1966 and soon thereafter from sheep and goats (1) and from cattle in 1970 (8). Mycoplasmas of sheep, goats, and cattle have been studied for the past half century so it is difficult to

understand why a ubiquitous organism like *M. arginini* was not recognized until so recently. Improved methodology is the most likely
explanation. However, it is also possible that temporal fluctuation
occurs in the mycoplasma flora of domestic animals and that this is
reflected in the current prevalence of *M. arginini* in bovine serum.

Isolates designated as *Acholeplasma* species (*A. sp*; Table 1)
are strains that were classified as *Acholeplasma* because of their
ability to grow on cholesterol-free medium. None of these 63 isolates reacted with antiserum directed against *A. laidlawii, A.
granularum,* or *A. axanthum*. Antisera were not available for other
Acholeplasma species so the original source of unserotyped isolates
is uncertain.

M. hyorhinis displayed a unique diapause. In the first 3 years
and the last 3 years of the 11-year observation period, the total *M.
hyorhinis* isolations exceeded those of any other single mycoplasma
species. In the intervening 5 years *M. hyorhinis* was quiescent,
with no isolations in 1971, the 11-year midpoint. The decline and
reemergence of *M. hyorhinis* is inexplicable and will remain so until
a channel of infection has been demonstrated. The reemergence of
M. hyorhinis would not have been as pronounced had it not been for
the use of indicator cell cultures and immunofluorescence (Fig. 1).
This procedure was started in 1974 and additional data will be presented in a following section.

Mycoplasma Serogroup 38 is a collection of over 200 strains
that share serologic and cultural properties which separate them
from all other mycoplasmas thus far tested (Del Giudice, unpublished). The first recognized strain of Serogroup 38 was isolated
from a cell culture in 1968. Similar strains now appear with some
regularity, but we have not identified isolates of Serogroup 38
from any other source. (For a different view, see the section by
Barile in this volume.) Fluorescent antibody directed against Serogroup 38, strain 70-159, reacts with strains of *M. bovis*. Three
strains isolated from bovine serum were identified by Barile as
70-159 (Serogroup 38) and by us (RAD) as *M. bovis*. Our laboratory
experience shows the serologic relation between Serogroup 38 and
M. bovis to be a one-way cross by immunofluorescence. In our view,
Serogroup 38 is unique because it is the only mycoplasma thus far
isolated exclusively from cell cultures. All other mycoplasma species that have been isolated from cell cultures are recognized as
flora of man or domestic animals. One of these hosts may prove to
be the natural habitat of Serogroup 38, but this has yet to be
demonstrated.

Eight specimens are listed as unidentified; this is not to
imply that they represent new species. They were not identified
because the strains were lost before serotyping was completed.

TABLE 1

MYCOPLASMA ISOLATION FROM TISSUE CULTURE

Year	1966	1967	1968	1969	1970	1971	1972	1973	1974	1975	1976	Total
No. of Specimens	363	616	271	904	2066	1441	1056	1930	4237	2955	1827	17666
No. of Positives	64	144	94	107	380	209	176	243	413	413	209	2452
No. of Strains	64	147	96	107	393	232	189	265	516	519	247	2775
M. orale	34	21	17	55	172	97	68	83	108	140	26	821
M. hominis	2	6	15	18	1	6	9	1	4	1	1	64
M. salivarium	0	0	0	0	0	1	0	0	1	2	0	4
M. fermentans	0	0	0	0	1	0	0	0	21	6	2	30
M. arginini	1	2	0	30	120	84	41	49	167	114	52	660
A. laidlawii	0	2	0	1	37	19	28	60	53	9	4	233
A. sp.	0	0	0	0	0	18	23	4	9	6	3	63
M. bovis	0	0	3	0	9	0	1	3	2	5	4	27
M. hyorhinis	25	114	47	3	4	0	14	9	116	189	114	635
M. sp. 70-159	0	0	14	0	45	7	4	46	30	42	21	209
Serogroup 38												
M. pulmonis	0	2	0	0	2	0	1	0	0	2	0	7
M. gallisepticum	2	0	0	0	0	0	0	10	0	0	0	12
M. sp. 689	0	0	0	0	2	0	0	0	0	0	0	2
Serogroup 32												
Unidentified	0	0	0	0	0	0	0	0	5	3	0	8

Because of the lack of identification, the classification of these
8 specimens is tentative. They could have been L-forms or artifacts.

Immunofluorescence with Indicator Cell Cultures

The isolation and characterization of the DBS 1050 strain of
M. hyorhinis by use of a cell culture system (7) prompted studies to
determine the incidence of similar strains as contaminants in cell
cultures. Test cell culture specimens were inoculated onto agar medium and into indicator cell cultures and the growth of *M. hyorhinis*
in each system was determined by immunofluorescence. Results comparing the *M. hyorhinis* isolation rate by the two systems are shown
in Table 2. Strains of *M. hyorhinis* were isolated from 394 of 6,974
specimens tested by use of indicator cell cultures in contrast to
150 strains isolated on agar medium. Thus, 244 strains grown in
cell cultures failed to produce colonies on agar medium. None of
the strains which produced growth on agar failed to grow in the indicator cell cultures. Thus, auxotrophic variants of *M. hyorhinis*
appear to be more common in cell cultures than the wild type strains.

No difference in the growth of *M. hyorhinis* strains in the
indicator cell culture could be correlated with the ability of any
particular strain to grow or not grow on agar. With strains of
either group the picture differed with respect to the concentration
of mycoplasma in the inoculum, the state of the cell culture, and
the time after inoculation. As noted by Carski and Shepard (3),
the mycoplasmas were randomly located with regard to cell structure
and showed no tendency to perinuclear location. This is consistent
with our observations and in accord with extracellular mycoplasma
growth.

The general morphologic development cycle of mycoplasmas could
be followed by immunofluorescence. Coccoid elements were randomly
attached to the host cell membrane at the earliest stage of infection. This was usually followed by transient filamentous growth.
The filaments developed periodic constrictions which separated to
form new coccoid mycoplasma cells. At any given time mycoplasma
cells in different stages of development co-existed; however, the
spherical cells were usually predominant.

DNA-Binding Fluorochromes

The general appearance of DNA-stained preparations was similar
to that seen by immunofluorescence. Mycoplasmas were easily seen as
extranuclear fluorescent particles as were other prokaryotic contaminants. Small coccoid bacterial cells resembled mycoplasma and this
was at times a source of confusion. Presumptive recognition of

TABLE 2

ISOLATION OF *M. HYORHINIS* FROM CELL CULTURES BY USE OF
AGAR MEDIUM AND INDICATOR CELL CULTURES WITH IMMUNOFLUORESCENCE

Year	Specimens Tested	Substrate Cell Culture[a]	Agar Medium	Noncultivable on Agar Medium	
1974	2299	100	69	31	31.0%
1975	2955	189	51	138	73.0%
1976	1720	105	30	75	71.4%
Total	6974	394	150	244	61.9%

[a] RK 13, FL, BHK, HeLa, and primary rabbit kidney cell cultures were used in 1974; 3T6 cell cultures were used in 1975 and 1976.

extranuclear agents as mycoplasmas is possible, with practice, on the basis of their small size, shape, and, to a degree, distribution on the host cell membrane. In all cases reported here, the nature of an agent was determined with the aid of serial passage, immuno-fluorescence, gram stain or cultivation on appropriate agar medium. Confusion between mycoplasma and other bacteria was infrequent because antibiotics were not used in the cell culture medium. Bac-terial growth was usually macroscopically evident, but low-level persistent bacterial infection did occur. Interpretation of the DNA-stain is difficult in the presence of antibacterial agents.

DNA-staining results closely agreed with those obtained by agar cultivation and *M. hyorhinis* indicator cell immunofluorescence (Table 3). Mycoplasmas were identified in 204 specimens and 200 of these were judged positive by DNA-staining. False positive results were obtained by DNA-staining in only 9 of the 2,297 specimens tested. These specimens displayed extranuclear fluorescence but a transmissable agent was not demonstrated. There were 13 false negatives, 9 of which were due to bacterial overgrowth of the indi-cator cell culture. Thus, only 4 mycoplasma-infected cell cultures were not detected by DNA-stain when all test conditions were con-sidered satisfactory.

Those mycoplasma species identified and the DNA-staining results are shown in Table 4. The 4 false negative specimens (by DNA-stain) were comprised of 2 strains of Serogroup 38 and one strain each of *M. orale* and *M. arginini*. Only 6 strains of Serogroup 38 were encountered in pure culture, too small a sample to project a fail-ure rate. However, there is reason to suspect that isolation on agar may prove more sensitive than the staining system used here.

TABLE 3

MYCOPLASMA DETECTION BY FLUORESCENT CHROMATIN STAIN OF
3T6 INDICATOR CELL CULTURES AND MYCOPLASMA ISOLATION ON AGAR
AND IN 3T6 CELL CULTURES AS INDICATED BY IMMUNOFLUORESCENCE

Specimens Tested	Mycoplasmas Isolated	Fluorescent Chromatin Stain		
		Positive	False Negative	False Positive
2297[a]	204	200	13[b]	9

[a]Coverslips from 79 specimens were unusable due to bacterial contamination.
[b]9 false negatives were due to bacterial contamination in the specimen.

TABLE 4

MYCOPLASMA DETECTION BY DNA-STAIN OF 3T6 INDICATOR CELLS VS.
IMMUNOFLUORESCENT IDENTIFICATION OF MYCOPLASMAS ISOLATED ON
AGAR MEDIUM AND *M. HYORHINIS* IN 3T6 INDICATOR CELLS

Mycoplasmas Identified	DNA-Stain vs. Culture FA
M. orale	33/34
M. arginini	25/26
Serogroup 38	4/6
M. hyorhinis	77/77
M. salivarium	2/2
M. bovis	3/3
A. laidlawii	9/9
A. sp.	2/2
M. hyorhinis + Serogroup 38	22/22
M. hyorhinis + *M. orale*	10/10
M. hyorhinis + *M. arginini*	1/1
M. hyorhinis + *M. fermentans*	7/7
M. hyorhinis + *A. laidlawii*	1/1
M. hyorhinis + *M. arginini* + *A. laidlawii*	1/1
M. orale + *M. arginini*	1/1
M. bovis + *A. laidlawii*	2/2

Whereas Serogroup 38 obviously grows in cell cultures, the level of
infection is frequently low. When cells are deliberately infected
with high-titered seed and incubated for 5 days, relatively sparse
growth is obtained with some strains of Serogroup 38. This is in
contrast to strains of *M. hyorhinis*, which produce luxuriant growth
within 48 hr.

A combination of agar medium and indicator cell culture was
needed to discern the 22 mixed cultures of *M. hyorhinis* and Serogroup 38. In cell culture, the heavy overgrowth of *M. hyorhinis*
obscured Serogroup 38. Conversely, colonies of Serogroup 38 were
seen easily on agar while *M. hyorhinis* colonies were usually absent.

The correlation between DNA-staining and *M. hyorhinis* immunofluorescence was perfect. The DNA-stain was clearly positive with
all 77 strains of *M. hyorhinis* isolated in pure culture as well as
an additional 42 strains isolated in mixed culture. Thus, all 119
specimens containing *M. hyorhinis* produced a positive DNA-staining
reaction. This is important because the majority of *M. hyorhinis*
strains failed to grow on agar medium.

No mycoplasmas grew in the 3T6 cell cultures but not on agar medium except for strains of *M. hyorhinis*. That is, of 2,297 specimens tested there was no evidence to suggest the presence of other mycoplasma species that are incapable of growth on agar medium.

DISCUSSION

Results have been presented showing the identification of mycoplasma colonies isolated on agar medium over an 11-year period. For the past 3 years, cultivation of mycoplasmas on agar medium was supplemented with cultivation in indicator cell cultures combined with immunofluorescence and a DNA-binding fluorochrome. The microbio-biologic procedures described herein rely on the direct visualization of mycoplasmas. Semantic problems may arise here over the terms "direct procedure" and "indirect procedure". Direct procedure is usually restricted to the demonstration of mycoplasma colonies on agar; indirect refers to all other methods purported to detect mycoplasmas. It is our contention that to see mycoplasmas in cell cultures, particularly when the image is defined by a specific serologic reaction, is no less direct than to see the formation of mycoplasma colonies on agar medium. Indirect procedures detect an activity that may suggest the presence of a mycoplasma. Biochemical mycoplasma tests tend to ignore the fundamental distinction between an activity and an organism.

Direct procedures not relying on the demonstration of colony formation on agar were needed to isolate strains of *M. hyorhinis*. These strains, isolated preferentially in indicator cell cultures, accounted for about 60% of the total *M. hyorhinis* isolations. The ratio of auxotrophic to wild type could have been higher than our data shows. If strains of both types occurred in mixed culture, only the wild type strains would have been detected. Agar medium as used here is selective for wild type strains, but strains of either nutritional type grow in cell cultures.

Studies are in progress on the nutritional requirements of *M. hyorhinis* and its variants. It is not yet clear if all of the strains which fail to grow on agar medium form a homogenous group or if there are different growth requirements among them.

In contrast to *M. hyorhinis*, no other agar noncultivable mycoplasmas were revealed by the DNA-stain of indicator cells. The literature contains oblique implications that noncultivable strains of other mycoplasma species have been detected in cell cultures. We are unaware of any instance where such alleged strains have been serologically identified nor do we know of existence of reference cultures. Noncultivable mycoplasmas, other than *M. hyorhinis*, may well occur in cell culture, but this has not yet been proven.

DNA-binding fluorochromes as used in conjunction with indicator cell cultures should provide a useful ancillary technique to detect mycoplasmas and other microbial contamination. The methodology is broadly similar to the orcein technique used by Fogh. Individual mycoplasma cells are easier to see by fluorescent microscopy than by light microscopy and with low level infection fluorochromes hold an advantage. Unlike biochemical "mycoplasma tests", microscopy offers an opportunity to distinguish mycoplasmas from bacteria. The importance of indicator cells has been discussed and we reiterate that the very concept of a controlled test is at issue. In the context of mycoplasma work these procedures are not commonplace, although they are standard practice in diagnostic virology laboratories.

Immunofluorescence has proved useful in mycoplasma identification. This method was used to serotype 2,775 mycoplasmas isolated from cell culture over an 11-year period. Identification is important in helping to understand the means by which cells become infected and should therefore aid control measures. (See the sections by Barile and McGarrity in this volume.) While the epidemiology of mycoplasma infection of cell cultures is partly understood, some questions remain unanswered. There is no demonstrable explanation for the diapause of *M. hyorhinis*, the origin of Serogroup 38, or how these organisms gain entrance to the cell culture.

REFERENCES

1. Barile, M.F., R.A. Del Giudice, T.R. Carski, C.J. Gibbs and J.A. Morris. 1968. Proc. Soc. Exp. Biol. Med. 129:489.

2. Barile, M.F. and J. Kern. 1971. Proc. Soc. Exp. Biol. Med. 138:432-437.

3. Carski, T.R. and C.C. Shepard. 1961. J. Bacteriol. 81:626-635.

4. Chen, T.R. 1977. Exp. Cell Res. 104:255-262.

5. Del Giudice, R.A., N. Robillard and T.R. Carski. 1966. J. Bacteriol. 93:1205-1209.

6. Fogh, J. 1973. In: Contamination of Cell Cultures (J. Fogh, ed.), Academic Press, New York.

7. Hopps, H.E., B.C. Meyer, M.F. Barile and R.A. Del Giudice. 1973. Ann. N.Y. Acad. Sci. 225:265-276.

8. Leach, R.H. 1970. Vet. Rec. 87:319-320.

9. McGarrity, G.J. 1976. In Vitro 12:643-647.

10. Russel, C.W., C. Newman and D.H. Williamson. 1975. Nature 253:461-462.

PRINCIPLES OF MORPHOLOGICAL AND BIOCHEMICAL METHODS FOR THE DETECTION OF MYCOPLASMA CONTAMINANTS OF CELL CULTURES

Eric J. Stanbridge and Carol Katayama

Department of Medical Microbiology
School of Medicine
University of California, Irvine
Irvine, California 92717

INTRODUCTION

Following the first report of mycoplasmal contamination of cells in culture (1), informed investigators have realized their importance and have instituted routine screening procedures for the detection of mycoplasmas.

The most commonly used procedure to detect mycoplasmas is growth in broth and on agar (2). This method has the advantage of ease of manipulation and visual recognition of characteristic umbonate mycoplasma colonies. In recent years, however, it has become increasingly apparent that not all mycoplasmas can be grown on currently available acellular media (3). Consequently, several noncultural techniques have been developed to aid in the detection of these fastidious microorganisms. Representative methods are outlined in Table 1 and several of these methods are discussed in detail below.

Morphological and Histochemical Techniques

Various light and electron microscopic techniques have been developed to detect mycoplasmas which are either free in the fluid medium or in association with their host cells. Fogh and Fogh devised a method of visual demonstration of mycoplasmas involving hypotonic treatment of the infected cell, fixation and orcein staining, followed by examination by phase microscopy (4). Mycoplasmas are easily recognized as pleomorphic coccobacillary bodies

71

TABLE 1

Indirect Detection Methods for
Mycoplasma Contaminants of Cell Cultures

A. **Morphological**

   Transmission electron microscopy
   Scanning electron microscopy

B. **Histochemical**

   Hypotonic fixation + Orcein or Giesma stain
   Fluorescent DNA binding dyes, e.g. Hoechst 33258 and DAPI
   Fluorescent DNA and RNA binding dyes, e.g. acridine orange

C. **Immunological**

   Specific fluorescein conjugated antibodies. Direct or indirect
   immunofluorescence.

D. **Enzyme assays**

   Citrulline colorimetric assay
   Purine and pyrimidine nucleoside phosphorylase assays

E. **Autoradiography**

   ^{3}H thymidine incorporation into DNA.
   Short pulse ^{3}H uridine incorporation into RNA.

F. **Physical Separation**

   Ammonium sulfate precipitation of ^{3}H-labelled organisms and
   banding in sucrose gradients.

   Separation of extracted mammalian and mycoplasmal ribosomal RNAs
   on polyacrylamide gels.

G. **Alterations in nucleic acid precursor uptake**

   Uridine:uracil ratio method
   Increased uracil incorporation

located primarily at the cell borders, associated with the plasma membrane, and in the intercellular spaces within groups of cells. Modifications of this method have included the use of Giemsa stain and other metachromatic dyes. Possible limitations of this technique for the average cell culturist would include the need for an adequate indicator cell line and the possible interference with interpretation caused by the presence of cell debris attached to the surface of whole cells.

Mycoplasmas have also been studied extensively by electron microscopic techniques. When mycoplasma contaminated cell lines are examined by transmission electron microscopy, the mycoplasmas are seen to reside in a predominantly extracellular location, in close association with the host cell plasma membrane (5,6). Although they are occasionally seen within cytoplasmic vacuoles and free within the cytoplasm of degenerating cells, there is little evidence to suggest that they are capable of penetrating and multiplying inside infected cells. Mycoplasmas can usually be distinguished from viruses due to their size difference, and from bacteria, yeast, rickettsia, and chlamydia by lack of a cell wall. However, mycoplasmas often may be confused with host cell cytoplasmic blebs which are also surrounded by membrane and contain ribosomes. Also, artifacts caused by improper fixations, staining, and embedding have caused considerable difficulties with interpretation, especially when negatively stained preparations are used (7). A recent technique which holds great promise for the detection of mycoplasmas is that of scanning electron microscopy. This relatively new form of microscopy allows one to visualize whole cells and project them in a three dimensional manner. Mycoplasmas are seen as oval bodies with diameters ranging from 350-800 nanometers. Occasional chains of spheres and filamentous forms are also seen (8). The extracellular association between mycoplasma and host cell is particularly striking. An interesting finding is that the mycoplasmas are often polarized on the cell surface, with the organisms located almost exclusively away from the ruffling edges of the cell (8). With this technique, many whole cells may be scanned in a relatively short period of time. This is an important advantage since within any given cell culture it appears that there is considerable heterogeniety with respect to cells which become colonized with mycoplasmas or not. Thus, it should be possible with this technique to detect low level contamination.

Autoradiography

The basis of this test is that uninfected cells incorporate ^{3}H-thymidine into their nuclear DNA such that when cells exposed to this radioisotope are overlayed with emulsion and developed, black grains are seen exclusively over the nuclear area. However, in

cells contaminated by mycoplasmas, ^{3}H-thymidine is incorporated
into extranuclear areas over the cytoplasm, and especially along
the cell margins (9). Characteristic grains are then seen over
these cytoplasmic areas after the cells are overlayed with emulsion
and developed. It has also been noted that when very heavy mycoplasmal contamination occurs, little or no nuclear labeling is seen.
This is due to cleavage of exogenous thymidine to its free base
thymine by mycoplasmal pyrimidine nucleoside phosphorylase activity
(10).

An alternative autoradiographic procedure is to use short term
(approximately 20 minutes) labeling with ^{3}H-uridine, which is
incorporated into RNA. When short labeling periods are used, the
label again is localized predominantly over the nuclear area in
uninfected cells and over the cytoplasm and along the cell borders
in contaminated cells (11).

Fluorescent Techniques

Mycoplasmas may be detected by applying specific fluorescein or
rhodamine conjugated antimycoplasma antibodies to appropriately
fixed coverslip cultures of cells followed by examination with UV
light microscopy. Mycoplasmas are seen as brightly fluorescing
particles on a dark background of the host cell (12). Although
this technique is a simple one it suffers from a number of disadvantages. There have been at least 16 mycoplasma serotypes
which have been reported as contaminants of cell cultures. These
mycoplasma strains exhibit little antigenic cross reactivity;
therefore, polyvalent antisera would be required for their detection. Previously unrecognized serotypes, for which there would
be no available antisera, would obviously not be detected by this
method.

A new rapid fluorescent technique has been described which is
applicable to any DNA containing organism, including DNA viruses
(13,14). Both 4'-6'-diamidino-2-phenylindole (DAPI) and the
benzimidole derivative Hoechst 33258 dye are fluorescent compounds
which specifically bind to DNA. In this method cells are grown on
coverslips and the unfixed populations are either directly stained
with the dye or fixed with Carnoy's fixative (3:1 methanol:glacial
acetic acid) before staining. The unfixed or fixed cells are
stained with the fluorescent compound for approximately 20 minutes,
washed, mounted, and examined using the appropriate exciter and
barrier filter system. In uninfected cells the nuclei fluoresce
brightly but there is little or no cytoplasmic fluorescence
(Fig. 1a). The amount of DNA present in mitochondria is not enough
to cause any interference. Mycoplasma contaminated cells, on the
other hand, in addition to having brightly fluorescing nuclei, also

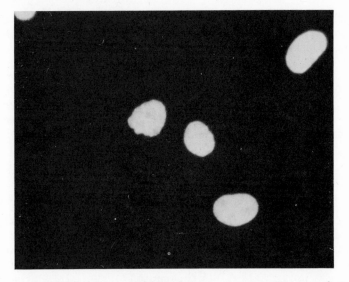

Figure 1A. Uncontaminated HeLa cells stained with 1 µg/ml DAPI. Only nuclear fluorescence can be seen. Magnification 750X. Reduced 30% for reproduction.

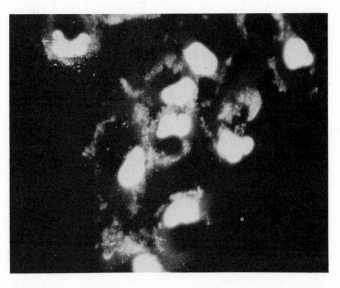

Figure 1B. HeLa cells infected with M. hyorhinis. Distinctive cytoplasmic fluorescence is seen in addition to nuclear fluorescence. Magnification 750X. Reduced 30% for reproduction.

exhibit granular fluorescence over the cytoplasm of the infected
cell (Fig. 1b). This rapid, simple technique is one which is
readily applicable for use in any cell culture laboratory.

Other fluorescent dyes, such as acridine orange, have been used
in the past (15) but they tend to lack the specificity seen with
these newer DNA binding compounds. A possible problem with these
compounds is discussed in a later section dealing with the relative
sensitivities of the various indirect detection methods.

BIOCHEMICAL TECHNIQUES

Enzyme Assays

Several enzyme methods have been developed for the detection of
mycoplasmas. One of the first exploited was the presence of
arginine deiminase activity in mycoplasmas (16). This enzyme
catalyzes the conversion of arginine to citrulline, which can be
measured colorimetrically. Unfortunately, the early promise of
this technique was not realized due to the fact that the majority
of fermentative mycoplasmas lack this enzyme activity and consequently are not detected. Common tissue culture contaminants
include many fermentative mycoplasma species.

A more promising technique, which has been developed by Levine,
is a simple chromatographic procedure for measuring the pyrimidine
nucleoside (uridine) phosphorylase activity in cultured cells (17).
In this method mycoplasma detection involves the measurement of
nucleoside phosphorylase activity by incubation of radioactive
uridine with cultured cell lysates and subsequent chromatographic
separation on Whatman filter paper or thin layer chromatographic
plates. Boric acid, which is present in the solvent, binds with
the sugar moiety of uridine thereby rendering it immobile. Uracil,
however, remains unbound and migrates with the solvent front. The
degree of conversion of uridine to uracil is taken as a measure of
the level of mycoplasmal contamination. In Levine's studies, most
uncontaminated cell lines had conversion values of less than 10%,
whereas mycoplasma contaminated cultures had values ranging from
20-95%. Occasional mycoplasma strains were found to be impermeable
to radioactive uridine and consequently had to be disrupted in
Triton-containing buffer in order to effect the conversion to
uracil. In a few cell lines that were determined to be free of
mycoplasma contamination by cultural methods, nucleoside phosphorylase levels were relatively high. This may represent the
presence of mammalian cell enzyme activity, which would create
problems with this technique. Alternatively, these cell cultures
may have been contaminated with fastidious microorganisms which
were not detected by conventional cultural methods.

Similar enzyme assays, including adenosine phosphorylase activity (18), have been developed. Occasional mycoplasma strains have been found which appear to lack one or other of these enzyme activities, including mycoplasmas which contaminate cell cultures (R. DelGuidice and M. Barile, personal communication).

Physical Separation of Mycoplasmas

During the course of experiments using sucrose gradient sedimentation techniques to identify oncornaviruses in cell cultures, Todaro et al. noted that supernatant fluids from a few of their cell lines incubated with ^{3}H-uridine showed a sharp peak of radioactivity at a density of 1.22 to 1.24 gm/cm^3 after centrifugation in a linear sucrose gradient (19). They then developed this finding into a rapid simple test for the detection of mycoplasma contaminants. After incubation of cell cultures for 18-20 hours with either radioactive uridine or thymidine, the supernatant fluids are concentrated by ammonium sulfate precipitation, layered on to a 15-60% linear sucrose density gradient, and centrifuged at 40,000 rpm for 90 minutes. The gradient is then collected dropwise, the nucleic acids precipiated in TCA, collected on glass filters and counted in a scintillation counter. A sharp peak of radioactivity is seen at 1.22-1.24 gm/cm^3 whereas no radioactive peak is seen in uncontaminated cultures.

Identification of Mycoplasmal RNAs

Levine et al. (20) were the first to demonstrate that mycoplasmal RNAs could be separated from eukaryotic host cell 28S and 18S ribosomal RNAs by sucrose density gradient centrifugation. The introduction of gel electrophoresis has led to an even greater resolution of these RNA species. Markov et al. (21) and Schneider et al. (11,22) have utilized the technique of polyacrylamide gel electrophoresis to detect 23S$_e$ (Svedberg constant by electrophoresis) and 16S$_e$ mycoplasmal RNAs in contaminated cell cultures. Cell lines were incubated with either ^{32}P-orthophosphate or ^{3}H-uridine and the total cellular RNA was phenol extracted. The prokaryotic and eukaryotic ribosomal RNA peaks were readily distinguishable either by disc or slab gel electrophoresis.

Alterations in Nucleic Acid Precursor Uptake

Several investigators have observed marked alterations in the incorporation of free bases and nucleosides into the nucleic acids of mycoplasma infected cells (23-25). Perhaps the most dramatic of these alterations is a marked decrease in uridine incorporation and a corresponding increase in uracil incorporation into total RNA (25). We have utilized these two properties to devise a simple

TABLE 2

Uridine/Uracil Ratios (Urd:U) of Human Diploid Fibroblasts
and HeLa Cells Deliberately Infected with Mycoplasma Species

Cell Culture Designation	Urd:U	Microbiological Culture
HDF * Control 1	830.0	-
HDF Control 2	623.0	-
HDF + A. laidlawii	6.0	+
HDF + A. granularum	3.5	+
HDF + M. hyorhinis	3.2	+
HDF + M. arginini	1.6	+
HDF + M. hominis	13.8	+
HeLa Control	1580.0	-
Hela + A. laidlawii	6.0	+
HeLa + M. hyorhinis	3.5	+
HeLa + M. orale type 1	87.2	+

* human diploid fibroblast cells

technique for the detection of mycoplasma contaminants of cultured cells; the uridine-uracil ratio method (25,26). Cells from the culture to be tested are inoculated at 10^4 cells per cm^2 into 6 plastic 25 cm^2 flasks. The next day parallel cultures are incubated with either ^{3}H-uridine or ^{3}H-uracil for 18 hours. The labeled nucleic acids are then extracted, hydrolyzed, and their radioactivity measured. In developing this technique we have taken advantage of the fact that mammalian cells readily transport and incorporate exogenous pyrimidine nucleosides into their nucleic acids while exogenous pyrimidine bases are incorporated to a negligible extent. Thus, one would expect the ratio of incorporation of uridine to uracil to be very high in axenic cell cultures. This is the case as is outlined in Table 2. Mycoplasmas, by contrast, readily transport and incorporate exogenous bases, as well as nucleosides, into their nucleic acids (3). In addition, by virtue of their possession of pyrimidine nucleoside phosphorylase activity mycoplasmas rapidly convert uridine to its free base uracil, thereby rendering this converted labeled compound unavailable for incorporation into mammalian cell RNA. The consequence of this decreased uridine incorporation and increased uracil incorporation in mycoplasma contaminated cell lines is a significantly lowered uridine: uracil ratio (Table 2). This simple method has been modified so that the whole test procedure can be accomplished within a period of a few hours (27). Using rapid micro methods results comparable to those obtained with the original parallel labeling method are obtained, as illustrated in Table 3. This micro method involves the introduction of ^{3}H uridine and ^{14}C uracil into cell cultures which are actively growing on glass coverslips. After 6 hours of incubation, the nucleic acids are precipitated in TCA, and the coverslips counted in a scintillation counter.

Comparative Studies of Biochemical Detection Methods

It is readily apparent that there are a relatively large number of biochemical methods which have been developed for the detection of mycoplasma contaminants of cell cultures. Several of these methods will be discussed in detail in this workshop and the advantages and disadvantages of each method will hopefully be pointed out. Unfortunately, few comparative studies have been undertaken to determine the relative efficacy of the various biochemical methods. This represents a very important area of research since it is clear that no biochemical or morphological test can be quantitatively as sensitive as microbiological testing, which can theoretically detect a single viable organism, which would replicate and form a colony on agar. Recent studies in our laboratory have been directed toward comparing several of the aforementioned indirect detection methods with regard to their comparative sensitivity with each other and with microbiological testing. In order to quantitate

TABLE 3

Comparison of Uridine:Uracil Ratio Methods using HeLa Cells
Infected with $\underline{M. hyorhinis}$

Surface for Cell Growth	Radio isotope label	Labelling Period (hours)	HeLa Control Urd:U	Mycoplasma infected HeLa Urd:U
T-25 flask (2.5x10^5 cells)	Parallel ^{3}H	18	1034	3.0
T-25	Parallel ^{3}H	5	1220	4.2
T-25	^{3}H/^{14}C double label	18	1074	5.0
T-25	^{3}H/^{14}C	5	1240	23.2
18mm^2 coverslips (2x10^4 cells)	Parallel ^{3}H	18	1124	3.4
Coverslip	Parallel ^{3}H	5	997	6.6
Coverslip	^{3}H/^{14}C	18	1467	1.4
Coverslip	^{3}H/^{14}C	5	879	1.2

TABLE 4

DILUTION OF MYCOPLASMA	DNA BINDING STAIN (DAPI)	IMMUNO-FLUORESCENCE	URIDINE:URACIL INCORPORATION	SUCROSE DENSITY GRADIENT	NUCLEOSIDE PHOSPHORYLASE ACTIVITY	CULTURAL (MYCOPLASMA PER CELL)
10^0	+	+	+ (16)[c]	+	+	60
10^{-1}	+	+	+ (18)	+	+	60
10^{-2}	+	+	+ (19)	+	+	60
10^{-3}	+	+	+ (26)	+	+	40
10^{-4}	+	+	+ (41)	+	-	15
10^{-5}	+[a]	+	+ (463)	-	-	3
10^{-6}	-	+[b]	- (760)	-	-	0.2
10^{-7}	-	-	- (1135)	-	-	0.05
10^{-8}	-	-	- (963)	-	-	0.00
CONTROL	-	-	- (854)	-	-	0.00

a. Cytoplasmic fluorescence seen only in approximately 20% of the cells.

b. Fluorescence seen in 1-10% of the cells, and often confined to the perinuclear or nuclear area of the cell.

c. Numbers in parentheses represent uridine:uracil ratios.

the sensitivity of these various methods, it is necessary to establish graded infections of cultured cell lines. This is not an easy
task since it is well known that, almost paradoxically, mycoplasmas
often fail to establish a successful infection of their host cells
in a short period (3,28). We found it necessary to adapt a strain
of Mycoplasma hyorhinis to rapid colonization of HeLa cells by
repeated passage in vitro. We then used these mycoplasmas, which
had been adapted to a cellular environment, as our test organisms.
HeLa cells were seeded into flasks or petri dishes at a concentration
of 1×10^4 cells/cm^2. Twenty-four hours later they were infected
with serial tenfold dilutions of M. hyorhinis. The highest input
number of organisms was usually 10^6 colony forming units/culture.
The organisms were incubated with the HeLa cells for a 48 hour
period in order to establish infection and then the infected cells
were subjected to testing by a number of methods outlined in Table
4. Several interesting observations were noted in these experiments.
Firstly, as suspected, the most sensitive method of detection is the
cultural method. Secondly, the indirect procedures examined varied
considerably with respect to their relative sensitivity in detecting
mycoplasma contaminants. Interestingly, the most sensitive method
from a quantitative standpoint appeared to be that of specific
immunofluorescence. Specifically, its sensitivity compared to that
of the DNA binding stain (DAPI) was seen to be due to the distribution
of the mycoplasmas over the surface of the cells at low levels of
contamination. When mycoplasmas were present in low numbers they
appeared to localize predominantly over the nuclear area of the
infected cells. Consequently, these mycoplasmas were not detected
by DAPI staining because of the masking effect of the nuclear fluorescence. This localizing effect is presumably associated with
polarization due to ruffling of the host cell membranes as described
by Brown et al. (8). These comparative tests should be regarded as
preliminary only but they do point up the necessity for the comparison and standardization of these indirect detection methods.

Concluding Remarks

The hazards that mycoplasma contaminants present to cell culturists are well documented (3). Because of the problems in interpreting data derived from mycoplasma contaminated cells, most cell
biologists routinely screen cell cultures for the presence of these
microorganisms. Currently, the most widely used technique for mycoplasma detection involves the growth of these organisms in specially
prepared broth and on solid agar. Positive identification of mycoplasmas requires the appearance of characteristic "fried egg"
colonies on agar. Limitations of this standard microbiological
testing for mycoplasmas have become increasingly apparent. It is
now recognized that there are fastidious mycoplasmas that are extremely difficult, if not impossible, to grow on currently available

acellular media (3,25,29). These extremely fastidious mycoplasmas are not necessarily heretofore unrecognized species. Hopps
et al. have described several cases of contamination of cell cultures
with an agent which grew luxuriantly in tissue culture producing a
cytopathic effect but could not be cultivated on cell free mycoplasma media (30). The agent was finally identified as Mycoplasma
hyorhinis by specific immunofluorescent techniques. This mycoplasma
species is a common contaminant of cell cultures and usually can be
readily propagated on mycoplasma media (3). The enormity of this
problem has only recently been appreciated. It has been found, in
a recent survey, that mycoplasmas could not be cultivated on agar
from greater than 50% of cell cultures which were contaminated with
Mycoplasma hyorhinis, as determined by specific immunofluorescence
(Barile and Del Giudice, personal communication).

Thus, there is an obvious need for the development of improved
growth media for detection of mycoplasmas. It is equally important
to realize that probably no one medium will support the growth of
all mycoplasma species. Until a universal medium can be developed
for the detection of mycoplasmas it is imperative that biochemical
detection methods be used in conjunction with cultural methods in
order to minimize the possibility of a false negative result when
cell lines are contaminated with these very fastidious mycoplasmas.

Can the same problem exist with noncultural detection methods?
By their very nature biochemical or morphological methods are inherently insensitive. They cannot be quantitatively as sensitive
as microbiological methods, which should theoretically detect a
single viable organism. Thus, a certain minimum number of organisms
must be present in any given sample before they can be detected by
any of the noncultural methods. The second problem is that with
the exception of immunofluorescent techniques, none of the non-
cultural methods described above specifically detect mycoplasmas.
The techniques are merely capable of indicating contamination but
in general they do not determine whether it is a viral, bacterial,
mycoplasmal, or other microbial agent (27,29). Nevertheless, to
the cell culturist, the chief concern is whether the culture is
free from contamination, rather than specific identification of the
contaminant. In fact, methods are becoming available whereby the
specific identification of noncultivable mycoplasmas may be possible
(31,32).

In closing we strongly recommend that both biochemical and
microbiological detection methods be used in order to provide the
maximum opportunity for detecting mycoplasmal contamination of
cultured cells. The choice of biochemical technique depends upon
the equipment and expertise of the laboratory. At this time sufficient data are not available to allow one to determine which is
the most sensitive noncultural detection method.

Acknowledgements

Supported, in part, by a grant from the U. S. Public Health Service (CA 19401-01) and University of California Institutional Grant NO. 7617. Eric J. Stanbridge is a Leukemia Society of America Special Fellow.

References

1. Robinson, L.B., R.H. Wichelbrausen, and B. Razinan. 1956. Contamination of human cell cultures by pleuropneumonia organisms. Science 124:1147.

2. Edward, D.G. ff. 1947. A selective medium for pleuro-pneumonia-like organisms. J. Gen. Microbiol. 1:238-243.

3. Stanbridge, E. 1971. Mycoplasmas and cell cultures. Bacteriol. Rev. 35:206-227.

4. Fogh, J. and H. Fogh. 1964. A method for direct demonstration of pleuropneumonia-like organisms in cultured cells. Proc. Soc. Exp. Biol. Med. 117:899-901.

5. Anderson, D.R., H.E. Hopps, M.F. Barile and B.C. Bernheim. 1965. Comparison of the ultrastructure of several rickettsiae, ornithosis virus and Mycoplasma in tissue culture. J. Bacteriol. 90:1387-1404.

6. Hummeler, K., D. Armstrong and N. Tomassini. 1965. Cyto-pathogenic mycoplasmas associated with two human tumors. II. Morphological aspects. J. Bacteriol. 90:511-516.

7. Wolanski, B. and K. Maramorosch. 1970. Negatively stained mycoplasmas: fact or antifact? Virology 42:319-327.

8. Brown, S., M. Teplitz and J.P. Revel. 1974. Interaction of mycoplasmas with cell cultures, as visualized by electron microscopy. Proc. Nat. Acad. Sci. USA 71:464-468.

9. Studzinski, G.P., J.F. Gierthy and J.J. Cholon. 1973. An autoradiographic screening test for mycoplasmal contamination of mammalian cell cultures. In Vitro 8:466-472.

10. Hakala, M.T., J.F. Holland and J.S. Horoszewicz. 1963. Change in pyrimidine deoxyribonucleoside metabolism in cell culture caused by mycoplasma (PPLO) contamination. Biochem. Biophys. Res. Commun. 11:466-471.

11. Schneider, E.L., C.J. Epstein, W.L. Epstein, M. Betlach and G. Abbo-Halbasch. 1973. Detection of mycoplasma contamination in cultured human fibroblasts - comparison of biochemical and microbiological techniques. Exp. Cell Rev. 79:343-349.

12. Barile, M.F., W.F. Malizia, and D.P. Riggs. 1962. Incidence and detection of pleuropneumonia-like organisms in cell cultures by fluorescent antibody and cultural procedures. J. Bacteriol. 84:130-136.

13. Russell, W.C., C. Newman, and D.H. Williamson. 1975. A simple cytochemical technique for demonstration of DNA in cells infected with mycoplasmas and viruses. Nature 253:461-462.

14. Chen, R.R. 1977. In situ detection of mycoplasma contamination in cell cultures by fluorescent Hoechst 33258 stain. Exp. Cell Res. 104:255-262.

15. Ebke, J. and E. Kuwert. 1972. Detection of Mycoplasma orale type 1 in tissue cultures by means of the acridine orange stain. Zentr. Bakteriol. (Orig. A) 221:87-93.

16. Barile, M.F. and R.T. Schimke. 1963. A rapid chemical method for detecting PPLO contamination of tissue cultures. Proc. Soc. Exp. Biol. Med. 114:676-679.

17. Levine, E.M. 1972. Mycoplasma contamination of animal cell cultures: a simple rapid detection method. Exp. Cell Res. 74:99-109.

18. Hatanaka, M., R. DelGiudice, and C. Long. 1975. Adenine formation from adenosine by mycoplasmas: adenosine phosphorylase activity. Proc. Nat. Acad. Sci. USA 72:1401-1405.

19. Todaro, G.J., S.A. Aaronson and E. Rands. 1971. Rapid detection of mycoplasma-infected cell cultures. Exp. Cell Res. 65:256-257.

20. Levine, E.M., I.G. Burleigh, C.W. Boone and H. Eagle. 1967. An altered pattern of RNA synthesis in serially propagated human diploid cells. Proc. Nat. Acad. Sci. USA 57:431-438.

21. Markov, G.G., I. Bradvarova, A. Mintcheva, P. Petrov, N. Shishkov and R.G. Tsanev. 1969. Mycoplasma contamination of cell cultures: interference with ^{32}P-labelling pattern of RNA. Exp. Cell Res. 57:374-384.

22. Schneider, E.L., E.J. Stanbridge, C.J. Epstein, M. Golbus, G.
     Abbo-Halbasch and G. Rodgers. 1974. Mycoplasma contamination
     of cultured amniotic fluid cells: a potential hazard to
     prenatal chromosomal diagnosis. Science 184:477-480.

23. Perez, A.G., J.H. Kim, A.S. Gelbard and B. Djordjevic. 1972.
     Altered incorporation of nucleic acid precursors by myco-
     plasma-infected mammalian cells in culture. Exp. Cell Res.
     70:301-310.

24. Harley, E.H., K.R. Rees and A. Cohen. 1970. HeLa cell nucleic
     acid metabolism, the effect of mycoplasma contamination.
     Biochim. Biophys. Acta. 213:171-182

25. Schneider, E.L., E.J. Stanbridge and C.J. Epstein. 1976. Incor-
     poration of ^{3}H-uridine and ^{3}H-uracil into RNA: a simple
     technique for the detection of mycoplasma contamination of
     cultured cells. Exp. Cell Res. 84:311-318.

26. Schneider, E.L. and E.J. Stanbridge. 1975. A simple biochemical
     technique for the detection of mycoplasma contamination of
     cultured cells. Methods in Cell Biol.X:278-290.

27. Stanbridge, E.J. and E.L. Schneider. 1976. A simple biochem-
     ical method for the detection of mycoplasmas and other
     microbial contaminants of cell cultures. Tissue Culture
     Association Manual 2:371-374.

28. Brautbar, C., E.J. Stanbridge, M.A. Pellegrino, R.A. Reisfeld
     and L. Hayflick. 1973. Expression of HL-A antigens on cul-
     tured human fibroblasts infected with mycoplasmas. J.
     Immunol. 111:1783-1789.

29. Schneider, E.L. and E.J. Stanbridge. 1975. Comparison of meth-
     ods for the detection of mycoplasmal contamination of cell
     cultures: a review. In Vitro 11:20-34.

30. Hopps, H.E., B.C. Meyer, M.F. Barile, et al. 1973. Problems
     concerning "non-cultivable" mycoplasma contaminants in tissue
     cultures. Ann. N.Y. Acad. Sci. 222:265-276.

31. Stanbridge, E.J. 1976. A re-evaluation of the role of mycoplas-
     mas in human disease. Ann. Rev. Microbiol. 30: 169-187.

32. Reff, M.E., E.J. Stanbridge and E.L. Schneider. 1977. Phylo-
     genetic relationships between mycoplasmas and other prokary-
     otes based upon the electrophoretic behavior of their
     ribosomal RNAs. Int. J. Syst. Bacteriol. (in press).

BIOCHEMICAL METHODS FOR DETECTING MYCOPLASMA CONTAMINATION

Elliot M. Levine and Barbara G. Becker

The Wistar Institute of Anatomy and Biology

36th Street at Spruce, Philadelphia, PA

INTRODUCTION

"If I am not for myself
   Who will be?
But if I am for myself only,
   What am I?
And if not now, when?   Hillel, 1st Century

The above quotation is relevant to the theme of this presentation, since we intend to discuss the biochemical procedures for mycoplasma detection developed by others, as well as presenting our own uridine phosphorylase method in somewhat greater detail.

Other participants in this workshop have or will make you aware of the drastic effects mycoplasma contamination can have on mammalian cell metabolism. For those of us developing biochemical detection procedures this has been an inspiration in two ways. First, the devastation produced by mycoplasma contamination made it imperative to devise simple rapid screening techniques so that suspect cultures could be discarded or at least quarantined as soon as possible. Of course, rapid screening techniques should be combined with the classic methods of isolation and identification which require much longer times for incubation and analysis. But, one cannot overemphasize the importance of quickly identifying contaminated cultures to guard against cross contamination. The profound effects of mycoplasma on cultured cells provided inspiration in another way. In many cases the very changes produced in cultured cells, such as the alterations in arginine, purine, and pyrimidine metabolism are so characteristic that they form the basis of various detection methods.

Some of the important microscopic procedures such as electron-microscopy, fluorescent antibody, and DNA staining will be considered by other Workshop participants. In addition, Dr. Stanbridge (1,21) has already described the uridine/uracil ratio method. We arbitrarily have divided the remaining biochemical detection procedures into three categories: non-isotopic enzymatic methods, autoradiographic techniques and those procedures utilizing radioactive tracers. The last category includes various sedimentation, electrophoretic, incorporation and enzymatic methods.

NON-ISOTOPIC ENZYMATIC METHODS

Under the heading of non-isotopic enzymatic methods, there are two major procedures which have been developed: the arginase procedure of Schimke, Barile, and their colleagues (2, 19) and the colorimetric nucleoside phosphorylase procedure of Horoszewics and Holland and their colleagues (3, 20). Arginase (or arginine deiminase) is an enzyme typical of most bacteria and mycoplasma. The assay is based on the conversion of arginine to citrulline (2, 19) and the colorimetric measurement of the latter amino acid. Unfortunatunately, as documented by Barile and Schimke (4), the usefulness of the assay is limited by the fact that two common cell culture contaminants M. hyorhinis and A. laidlawii are among those mycoplasma species which do not ferment arginine via citrulline.

The colorimetric determination of nucleoside phosphorylase activity forms the basis for a second assay procedure (3). This procedure was later modified in our laboratory by using radioactive substrates to improve its sensitivity, reliability and speed. The original assay is based on the phosphorolytic cleavage of the nucleoside thymidine to its pyrimidine base thymine and ribose phosphate. Ribose phosphate, or more accurately ribose, then is measured colorimetrically after reaction with diphenylamine reagent. Possibly because of the insensitivity inherent in colorimetric procedures, false negatives were reported by House and Waddel (5) using this detection method.

AUTORADIOGRAPHY

Autoradiography is a rather commonly used detection method, in part because many laboratories are using autoradiographic procedures to study various aspects of mammalian cell metabolism (6, 22). The difference between contaminated and uncontaminated cultures as revealed by autoradiography can be quite dramatic.

Nardone and co-workers (7) were the first to recognize that
autoradiographs of mycoplasma contaminated cell cultures labeled
with thymidine showed apparent cytoplasmic instead of nuclear
localization of silver grains. As we demonstrated subsequently,
this alteration results from the presence of high levels of
nucleoside phosphorylase in contaminated cultures (8). As a
result of this enzymatic activity, radioactive thymidine is cleaved
to thymine. As is the case for most nucleoside bases, thymine is
rapidly incorporated into mycoplasma, but only very slowly if at
all, into mammalian cells. The result is the shift from nuclear
incorporation to apparent cytoplasmic (but actually extracellular)
incorporation. In addition to thymidine labeling, short,twenty
minute pulses of radioactive uridine can be employed to produce
nuclear labeling in uncontaminated cultures and extracellular
incorporation in infected cells. Labeling with radioactive uracil
can also be used and in this case only infected cultures will
exhibit significant incorporation. Depending on the particular
laboratory set-up, autoradiography can be a convenient detection
method, but there is a significant time delay before assay results
are known and there can be ambiguities in interpretation. A
serious drawback to this method is that certain mycoplasma strains
are impermeable (9) to nucleic acid precursors and thus cannot be
detected by this procedure (see Table 8).

SEDIMENTATION AND ELECTROPHORETIC TECHNIQUES

The changes in radioactive tracer incorporation into contaminated cultures revealed on a cellular level by autoradiography also
can be detected by other radioactive tracer techniques. In general,
these tracer techniques have greatly increased sensitivity over
other indirect detection methods. The radioactive tracer can be
used to label the mycoplasma particle itself (as in the method
developed by Todaro, et al (10)) which is then separated by ultra-
centrifugation or to label the mycoplasma nucleic acids. As
observed in our laboratory several years ago (8), and subsequently
confirmed by others (11, 23, 24), mycoplasma ribosomal RNA can be
distinguished from mammalian ribosomal RNA on the basis of
sedimentation properties or electrophoretic mobilities. In mycoplasma contaminated cell cultures labeled with radioactive uridine
the presence of mycoplasma RNA is further accentuated because it
if preferentially labeled due to the high uridine phosphorylase
activity (Table 1). All the electrophoretic and sedimentation
analysis, however, involve the use of specialized equipment and
techniques and rather lengthy times for separation and analysis.

TABLE 1

Uridine + PO_4 → Uracil + Ribose -P

Thymidine + PO_4 → Thymine + Ribose -P

Flurodeoxyuridine + PO_4 → Flurodeoxyuracil + Ribose -P

Adenosine + PO_4 → Adenine + Ribose -P

In addition, the failure of some mycoplasma strains to incorporate tracer uridine leads to false negative results just as in the case of autoradiography.

ISOTOPIC ENZYMATIC METHODS

Nucleoside phosphorylase activity as well as differential uptake of uracil form the basis of the incorporation ratio method described by Drs. Schneider and Stanbridge (1, 21). The ratio method is a simple rapid procedure which measures precursor incorporation into living intact cells. The method of Perez, et al (12) also indirectly measures nucleoside phosphorylase activity by determining the ability of living cultures to convert labeled nucleosides added to their culture fluids to the corresponding purine or pyrimidine bases. A method recently described by Hatanaka, Del Guidice and Long (13) similarly measures the conversion of labeled adenosine in the culture fluid to labeled adenine.

The method developed in our laboratory for measuring nucleoside (i.e., uridine) phosphorylase activity differs from those described above. Our assay depends on the presence of enzyme activity in cell lysates, not supernatant fluids or intact cells. By directly measuring activity in the cells and the mycoplasma which adhere to them, we have avoided the complications introduced by cell and mycoplasma permeability, and continued cellular growth during the assay. An outline of our detection procedure is shown in Table 2. A detailed description of the procedure has been published (4, 14, 15), and as can be seen the method is inherently quite simple. Although assays are usually performed on 2 x 10^7 cells lysed in 3 ml, as little as 3 x 10^6 cells in 0.5 ml can be handled conveniently. ^{14}C-uridine is used as the nucleoside substrate, since we have found that tritiated nucleosides deteriorate rapidly in storage. Depending on the level of enzyme activity incubation times as short as 30 minutes can be used, but most lysates are sampled at both 30 and 180 minutes.

TABLE 2

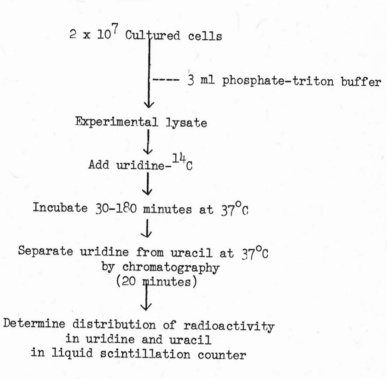

2×10^7 Cultured cells

---- 3 ml phosphate-triton buffer

Experimental lysate

Add uridine-^{14}C

Incubate 30-180 minutes at 37°C

Separate uridine from uracil at 37°C
by chromatography
(20 minutes)

Determine distribution of radioactivity
in uridine and uracil
in liquid scintillation counter

Total time for procedure: 4 hours

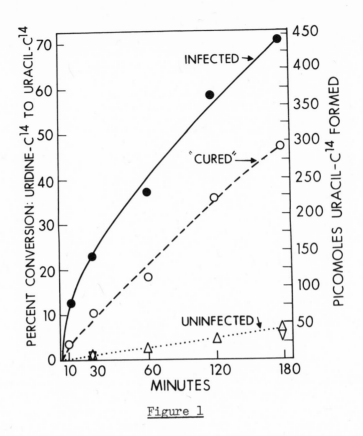

Uridine phosphorylase activity in infected and uninfected cell cultures. Abscissa: min; ordinate: (left) % conversion ^{14}C-uridine to ^{14}C-uracil; (right) pmoles ^{14}C-uracil formed. Lysates were prepared from the following monolayer cultures: ●--● infected, 'RA' cells, contaminated with M. hyorhinis detected by agar plate cultivation; o--o "cured", a sister culture of RA cells treated with aureomycin, tylocine, and kanamycin for 4 days and negative by agar plate and broth cultivation; ∇···∇, uninfected, KL-2 cells, uncontaminated as demonstrated by the above methods; △···△, uninfected HeLa cells uncontaminated as demonstrated by the above methods and electronmicroscopy. Reprinted with permission of Academic Press In New York, N.Y. from Figure 3 (page 103), "Mycoplasma Contamination Animal Cell Cultures: A Simple Rapid Detection Method" by E.M. Lev Experimental Cell Research, Volume 74 (1972).

TABLE 3

COMPOSITION OF CHROMATOGRAPHY SOLVENT

1. 70 ml boric acid (4%, ca 0.65M)

2. 1 ml concentrated ammonium hydroxide

3. 430 ml n-(1)-butanol

Add reagents in the above sequence. N.B. At room
temperature some separation of phases occurs in this
solvent. A homogeneous solution is obtained by
warming to $37^{\circ}C$ in tightly stoppered bottles and
shaking.

Chromatographic separation of the ^{14}C-uridine substrate from
the ^{14}C-uracil product is accomplished at $37^{\circ}C$ using a borate-
containing solvent (Table 3). Chromatography at room temperature
is slower and requires a solvent with a greater proportion of
butanol. Errors in preparation of the chromatography solvent are
the most common source of questionable results (see 14, 15 for
details). The borate chelates the nucleoside sugar moiety and
as a result, uridine remains at the origin, while uracil migrates
with an Rf of 0.4. The uridine and uracil spots are located on the
developed chromatogram using a short wave UV light, and the radioactivity in those areas is determined. Results are expressed as
the percent conversion of radioactive uridine to uracil; Figure 1
illustrates uridine phosphorylase activity determined by this method
in several types of cell cultures. In a lysate from a representative contaminated culture approximately 70% of the ^{14}C-uridine was
converted to uracil, while in lysates from uninfected cells only 5%
conversion was detected. Treatment of contaminated cultures with
tetracycline, tylocine, and kanomycin reduces but by no means
eliminates uridine phosphorylase activity even though agar plate and
broth cultivation from such cultivations are negative. Since no
one detection method can be used as an absolute standard of actual
mycoplasma titer it is difficult to establish the relative sensitivity of different methods. However, our previous work indicates
that RNA labeling patterns dependent on nucleoside phosphorylase can
be detected (8) in cell cultures containing approximately ten
mycoplasma per cell. Consistent with this, Table 4 indicates that
mycoplasma have a much higher specific activity of the enzyme activity than normal mammalian tissue or cultured cells.

TABLE 4

SPECIFIC ACTIVITIES OF URIDINE PHOSPHORYLASE
FROM VARIOUS SOURCES

Tissue, cell culture, or mycoplasma	% Uridine → uracil conversion in 180 min. per mg. protein
Mouse liver	10.3
Mouse kidney	37.6
Mouse lung	54.5
Uncontaminated 3T3	6.1
Contaminated 3T3	28.6
Uncontaminated WI-38	5.5
M. arginini	1006.3

All the mycoplasma species we have tested contain uridine phosphorylase activity including those reported as common cell culture contaminants (Table 5). In addition to those strains listed, Mycoplasma species HRC 70-159, a cell culture contaminant isolated by Hatanaka, et al (18) and reported not to contain adenosine phosphorylase did exhibit uridine phosphorylase activity. In contrast, in repeated tests of over 30 different uncontaminated normal, tumor-derived, and virally transformed cell cultures from a variety of animal species and tissues none showed significant increments in uridine phosphorylase activity (Table 6). Furthermore suspension monolayer cultures at any growth stage can be assayed without complication.

TABLE 5

URIDINE PHOSPHORYLASE ACTIVITY IN REPRESENTATIVE MYCOPLASMA SPECIES

Mycoplasma species	Presumed origin	Relative frequency as tissue culture contaminant[a]	Percent conversion to uracil at 30min.	180min.	Relative uridine phosphorylase activity[b]
M. hyorhinis(GDL)	Porcine	4+	43	90	100
A. laidlawii	Bovine,saprophytic	4+	89	90	313
M. arginini	Ovine, caprine	4+	88	89	312
M. hominis 1	Human	4	12	31	15
M. orale 1	Human	4	19	38	19
M. salivarium	Human	2	28	80	55
M. gallisepticum	Avian	1	13	20	6
M. neurolyticum	Rat	0	30	76	53
M. arthriditis	Rat	0	23	79	49
M. fermentans	Human	0	84	93	280

a   An approximation derived from frequencies of contamination previously reported by several authors (14). In this laboratory, M. hyorhinis has been the most commonly detected contaminant.

b   Calculated from the reciprocal of the time required for a 50% conversion to uracil by lysates from 48-hour broth cultures containing 10^7 to 10^9 colony-forming units per milliliter. Lysates were prepared by centrifuging 9.5 ml of broth culture at 1000g for 10 minutes and resuspending the pellet in 3 ml of incubation medium. The value for M. hyorhinis has been set arbitrarily at 100; this culture effected a 50% conversion of uridine to uracil in 50 minutes. Cultures of M. hominis 1 and M. orale 1 effected 31% and 40% conversions, respectively, in 180 minutes.

TABLE 6

URIDINE PHOSPHORYLASE ACTIVITY IN UNCONTAMINATED[a] CELL CULTURES

| Cell cultures[b] | Origin[c] | | Increment[d] in uridine phosphorylase activity (%) |
	Species	Tissue or Cell type	
HeLa	Human	Cervical carcinoma	4.1[e]
HeLa S3	Human	Cervical carcinoma	4.0
MS-2	Human	Diploid skin fibroblast	0.8
KL-2	Human	Diploid lung fibroblast	6.9
WI-38	Human	Diploid fetal lung fibroblast	2.4
MRC-5	Human	Diploid fetal lung fibroblast	2.1
IMR-90	Human	Diploid fetal lung fibroblast	4.1
Chang Liver	Human	Liver	6.9
J-111	Human	Monocytic leukemia	3.7
MA 160	Human	Prostate[f]	8.8
WI-26-VA	Human	SV-40 trans. lung fibroblast	6.4
PICK	Human	Fetal brain SV-40 trans.	1.4
S-1002	Human	MS	
HEP-2	Human	Epithelial	7.9
Neuro	Human	Neuroblastoma	6.4
3T3	Mouse	Embryo	3.9
3T3/Balbc	Mouse	Embryo[g]	0.2
NTG-2	Mouse	3T3/Balbc Thioguanine resist.	0.1
C57	Mouse	Embryo[h]	0.4
45.6	Mouse	Myeloma	1.6
V9	Mouse	Bone Marrow	5.3
V10	Mouse	Rauscher-virus infected	5.9

TABLE 6 (cont'd)

| Cell cultures[b] | Origin[c] | | Increment[d] in uridine phosphorylase activity (%) |
	Species	Tissue or Cell type	
Neuro	Mouse	Neuroblastoma	4.3
HTC	Rat	Hepatoma	7.8
E-3	Rat	Liver[i]	3.3
WIRL	Rat	Liver	4.1
NIL-2	Hamster	Embryo	6.8
B-1	Hamster	BudR-resistant BHK-21/13[j]	2.3
RPMI-3460	Hamster	Skin melanoma	1.5
CHO	Hamster	Skin melanoma	1.5
Lens	Rabbit	Lens	9.1
2VH	Viper	Viper heart epithelial	3.8
TH-1	Turtle	Turtle heart epithelial	4.9
NVSW	Viper	Viper spleen	0.3

[a] As adjudged by aerobic agar plate cultivation in a 5% CO_2 atmosphere; for other criteria, see footnote e.

[b] All cells were grown as monolayer cultures except HeLa S3, which was grown in suspension with mechanical agitation, and the mouse myeloma lines, which were cultured as non-adherent cells in plastic petri dishes.

[c] Unless otherwise indicated, origins of cell lines are given in reference 14.

[d] Increase in percentage conversion to uracil between 30 and 180 minutes. With low levels of activity this is a more meaningful value than absolute conversion at a single time point.

[e] Negative by electron microscopic examination, sucrose density gradient analysis (8), agar plate and broth cultivation with cultured cell feeder layers (16), and agar plates incubated anaerobically.

TABLE 7

CORRELATION BETWEEN ELEVATED URIDINE PHOSPHORYLASE ACTIVITY AND
MYCOPLASMA IN CONTAMINATED CULTURES

Cell Designation	Results of agar plate cultivation	Elevated uridine phosphorylase activity (% in 180 min.
HeLa	+	56
HeLa S3	+	59
L-929	+	74
CV-1	+	44
R. Glia	+	85

For lysates of mycoplasma contaminated cultures, on the other
hand, conversion ranged from 20-90% with an average of approximately
60%. Most cultures with high enzymatic activity were also positive
by agar plate cultivation (Table 7), and more importantly, we have
not yet encountered a culture with cultivable mycoplasma and a
negative result from the uridine phsophorylase method. As would
be expected, cultures deliberately infected with several mycoplasma
species exhibit elevated enzyme activities.

Although most mycoplasma-infected cultures were able to convert
uridine to uracil even when intact cells and organisms were tested
in their original growth medium, contaminated RA cultures did not
unless disrupted in Triton-containing buffer (Table 8). Consistent
with this indication that the mycoplasma present in RA cultures are
"cryptic strains" (i.e., impermeable to nucleosides) is the observation that such cultures are pulse labeled with ^{14}C uridine and
analyzed by sucrose density gradient analysis did not contain labele
mycoplasma RNA (8). Furthermore, autoradiographs of RA cultures
pulse labeled with ^{3}H-thymidine did not indicate any cytoplasmic
incorporation of the type usually observed in mycoplasma-infected
cell cultures.

Data for cultures in group Table 9 illustrates the effect of
antibiotic treatment on mycoplasma-infected cultures. In agreement
with the results presented previously "cured" cultures are negative
by agar plate assay, but retain an appreciable measure of phosphorylase activity. In addition, as illustrated by SV 3T3, high levels
of enzyme activity may reappear in subsequent subcultures even in
the presence of antibiotics.

TABLE 8

DETECTION OF URIDINE PHOSPHORYLASE ACTIVITY IN A "CRYPTIC" STRAIN OF MYCOPLASMA

	Time of incubation (min.)	Uracil cpm	Uridine cpm	Total cpm	% conversion to uracil
RA: Supernatant fluid nondisrupted cells	30	829	23,339	25,770	3.2%
	180	1,085	19,322	20,407	5.3%
RA: Triton lysate of cells	30	5,921	18,876	24,797	22.2%
	180	9,905	12,539	22,444	40.0%

TABLE 9

ANTIBIOTIC TREATMENT

Cell Designation	Results of agar plate cultivation	Elevated uridine phosphorylase activity (% in 180 min.)
RA	+	22
RA + anti	-	7
3T3	+	21
3T3 + anti	-	9
SV 3T3	+	
SV 3T3 + anti-1	-	16
SV 3T3 + anti-2	-	72

In some cases, we were unable to grow mycoplasma on agar (17) from cell cultures which possess elevated levels of uridine phosphorylase activity. We have grouped these cultures into two categories: "false positives" and "quasi-negatives" (Table 10). False positives illustrate a limitation of the uridine phosphorylase method in that several other detection methods (i.e., cultivation, microscopic, or autoradiographic) did not give positive results for these cultures. Only a very few cell types which apparently have high endogenous levels of mammalian uridine phosphorylase fall into this category. As mentioned previously, false positives have never been encountered in HeLa, 3T3, CHO, or human diploid fibroblasts. Quasi-negative cultures illustrate that the uridine phosphorylase assay can detect mycoplasma-like organisms which we were unable to cultivate on agar plates (17) (Table 11).

TABLE 10

COMPLICATIONS OF THE URIDINE PHOSPHORYLASE METHOD

	Agar Cultivation	Uridine Phosphorylase	Other tests
False positives	-	+	-
Quasi-negatives			
Cell line A[1]	-	+	±
Cell line A[2]	-	-	-

N.B.: False positives have never been obtained with HeLa, 3T3, CHO, and all the human diploid fibroblasts tested thus far.

TABLE 11

QUASI NEGATIVE CULTURES

Cell Designation	Results of agar plate cultivation	Elevated uridine phosphorylase activity(% in 180 min.)
HeLa S3-"A"	–	4
HeLa S3-"B"	–	37
Neuro-"A"	–	5
Neuro-"B"	–	60
V9-"A"	–	5
V9-"B"	–	30
V-10-"A"	–	6
V-10-"B"	–	95
3T3-"A"	–	4
3T3-"B"	–	46

When tested initially, most of these cultures (3T3-"A", HeLa-S3-"A", etc.) exhibited low levels of uridine phosphorylase. Subsequently, when cells of the same cell line (derived from these initial stocks or obtained from different sources) were tested, some exhibited high levels of uridine phosphorylase in the absence of cultivable mycoplasma (3T3-"B", HeLa S3-"B", etc.); i.e., agar plates were "negative". In all of the above cases enzyme activity was depressed in sister cultures treated with antibiotics. Therefore, one may conclude that the enzyme levels in quasi negative cultures are not inherent in those mammalian cell lines, but derive from an extracellular agent, such as a mycoplasma.

In conclusion, I hope I have presented a somewhat balanced overview of various biochemical methods available for mycoplasma detection although I have an obvious bias towards one of these methods, I cannot put too strong an emphasis on my belief that (provided one is aware of its limitation) any detection method is better than none at all.

Finally, I want to end with a paraphrase of my beginning quotation:
    "If you are not worried about mycoplasma contamination of
        your cell cultures,
        Who will be?
    And, if you are not testing for contamination now,
        When will you be?"

REFERENCES

1. Stanbridge, E.J., and E.L. Schneider. 1976. A simple bio-
    chemical method for the detection of mycoplasmas and other
    microbial contaminants of cell cultures. TCA Manual 2:
    3 371-374.

2. Schimke, R.T., and M.F. Barile. 1963a. Arginine breakdown
    in mammalian cell culture contaminated with pleuropneumonia-
    like organisms (PPLO). Exp. Cell Res. 30: 593-596.

3. Horoszewics, J.S., and J.T. Grace. 1964. PPLO detection
    in cell culture by thymidine cleavage. Bacteriol. Proc.
    64: 131.

4. Barile, M.F., R.T. Schimke, and D.B. Riggs. 1966. Presence
    of the arginine dehydrolase pathway in Mycoplasma. J.
    Bacteriol. 91: 189-192.

5. House, W., and A. Waddell. 1967. Detection of mycoplasma in
    cell cultures. J. Pathol. Bacteriol. 93: 125.

6. Levine, E.M., I.G. Burleigh, C.W. Boone, and H. Eagle. 1967.
    An altered pattern of RNA synthesis in serially propagated
    human diploid cells. Proc. Nat. Acad. Sci., U.S. 57: 431-4.

7. Nardone, R.M., G. Todd, P. Gonzalez, and E.V. Gaffney. 1965.
    Nucleoside incorporation into strain L cells: inhibition by
    pleuropneumonia-like organisms. Science 149: 1100-1101.

8. Levine, E.M., L. Thomas, D. McGregor, L. Hayflick, and H. Eagl
    1968. Altered nucleic acid metabolism in human cell culture
    infected with mycoplasma. Proc. Nat. Acad. Sci., U.S. 60:
    583-589.

9. Levine, E.M. 1972. Mycoplasma contamination of animal cell
    cultures: a simple, rapid detection method. Exp. Cell Res.
    74: 99-109.

10. Todaro, G.J., S.A. Aaronson, and E. Rands. 1971. Rapid
    detection of mycoplasma-infected cell cultures. Exp. Cell
    Res. 65: 256-257.

11. Schneider, E.L., C.J. Epstein, W.B. Epstein, M. Betlach, and
    G. Abbo-Halbasch. 1973a. Detection of mycoplasma contamina-
    tion in cultured human fibroblasts. Exp. Cell Res. 79:
    343-349.

12. Perez, A.G., J.H. Kim, A.S. Gelbard, and B. Djordjevic. 1972.
     Altered incorporation of nucleic acid precursors by mycoplasma-
     infected mammalian cells in culture. Exp. Cell Res. 70:
     301-310.

13. Hatanaka, M., R. delGiudice, and E. Long. 1976. A new quick
     screening of mycoplasma contamination in cell culture by
     adenine detection. TCA Manual 2: 437-438.

14. Levine, E.M. 1974. A simplified method for the detection of
     mycoplasma. In: D.M. Prescott (ed.), Methods in Cell
     Biology. Volume 8. Academic Press, London and New York,
     pp. 229-248.

15. Becker, B.G., and E.M. Levine. 1976. A simple, rapid method
     for detecting mycoplasma contamination. TCA Manual 2: 305-308.

16. Zgorniak-Nowosielska, I., W.G. Sedwick, K. Hummler, and H.
     Koprowski. 1967. New assay procedure for separation of
     mycoplasmas from virus pools and tissue culture systems.
     J. Virol. 1: 1227-1239.

17. Hayflick, L. 1965. Tissue cultures and mycoplasmas. Tex.
     Rep. Biol. Med. 23: 285-303.

18. Hatanaka, M., R. delGuidice, and C. Long. 1975. Adenine
     formation from adenosine by mycoplasmas: adenosine phos-
     phorylase activity. Proc. Nat. Acad. Sci., U.S. 72:
     1401-1405.

19. Schimke, R.T., and J.F. Barile. 1963b. Arginine metabolism in
     pleuropneumonia-like organisms isolated from mammalian
     cell cultures. J. Bacteriol. 86: 195-206.

20. Holland, J.F., R. Korn, J.O. O'Malley, H.J. Minnemeter, and
     H. Tieckelmann. 1967. 5-Allyl-2'-deoxyuridine inhibition
     of nucleoside phosphorylase in HeLa cells containing
     mycoplasma. Cancer Res. 27: 1867-1873.

21. Schneider, E.L., E.J. Stanbridge, and C.J. Epstein. 1974.
     Incorporation of ^{3}H-uridine and ^{3}H-uracil into RNA: A
     simple technique for the detection of mycoplasma contamination
     of cultured cells. Exp. Cell Res. 84: 311-318.

22. Studzinski, G.P., J.R. Gierthy, and J.J. Cholon. 1973. An
     autoradiographic screening test for mycoplasmal contamina-
     tion of mammalian cell cultures. In Vitro 8: 466-472.

23.   Markov. G.G., I. Bradvarova, A. Mintcheva, P. Petrov. N.
      Shishkov, and R.G. Tsanev. 1969. Mycoplasma contamination
      of cell cultures: interference with ^{32}P-labelling patterns
      of RNA. Exp. Cell Res. 57: 374-384.

24.   Harley, E.H., K.R. Rees, and A. Cohen. 1970. HeLa cell nuclei
      acid metabolism: The effect of mycoplasma contamination.
      Biochim. Biophys. Acta 213: 171-182.

DETECTION OF MYCOPLASMA CONTAMINATION OF CELL CULTURES BY

ELECTRON MICROSCOPY

David M. Phillips

The Population Council

Rockefeller University, New York, N.Y. 10021

INTRODUCTION

Since mycoplasma infections of cell cultures are a frequent and serious problem, it behooves the cell culturist to find reliable and reasonably easy methods for the detection of mycoplasma contamination. In this chapter we will discuss the electron microscope as a tool for the detection of mycoplasma infections of cultured cells. We will describe how mycoplasma infections appear in the scanning and transmission electron microscope and will discuss the advantages and disadvantages of electron microscopy in terms of reliability, sensitivity and practicality. The reader is referred to other chapters of this book for thorough discussions of various methods of detection and for discussions of the particular ways which mycoplasma alter the physiology, chemistry and morphology of cell cultures. It is often necessary to employ more than one technique to detect mycoplasma or to be reasonably certain that a culture is mycoplasma free. Each method has its advantages and disadvantages. Different techniques for detecting mycoplasma, therefore, often complement each other.

MATERIALS AND METHODS

Cultures

The cultures we have examined came from a variety of sources. In many cases we have examined A9 cells, a cell line derived from

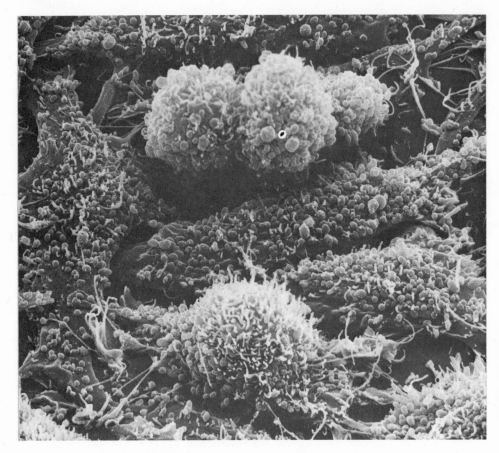

Fig. 1.   A9 cells (mouse L-cell derived) deliberately infected
           with Mycoplasma hyorhinis. In heavily infected cul-
           tures each fibroblast is generally associated with
           several hundred cells. Mycoplasma are associated with
           both interphase and mitotic cells. X 2,500.

mouse L-cells (Littlefield, '64). A9 cultures were deliberately
infected with Mycoplasma hyorhinis or Acholeplasma laidlawii. We
have also examined cultures of L929-cells (mouse), RAG cells
(mouse), KB cells (human), primary human cultures (started from
testis or semen), and human-mouse hybrid cell lines. Since at
the time we examined the cultures we were generally interested
only in determining whether or not a particular culture was contaminated, we made no effort to determine the species of mycoplasma
that had infected the culture.

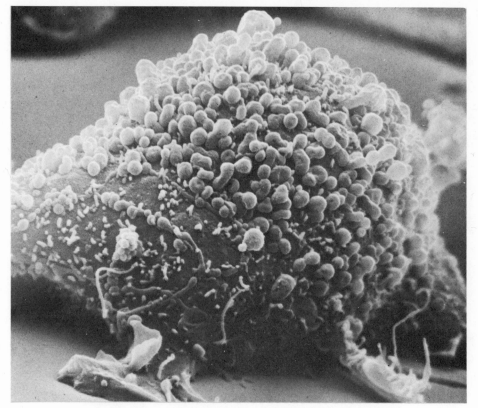

Fig. 2.   Mycoplasma associated with RAG cell (mouse kidney
           derived). Mycoplasma always display pleomorphic
           morphology. Sometimes they occur in long filaments
           with intermittent bulges. X 6,000.

Electron Microscopy

For scanning microscopy, cells were grown on glass coverslips. Cells were fixed in either 2.5% glutaraldehyde buffered
at pH 7.4 with 0.2 M Collidine or a modified glutaraldehyde-Colli-
dine fixative (Phillips and Phillips, '71). Cells were dehydrated
in ethanol series to absolute alcohol and transferred to acetone.
Coverslips were critical point dried with liquid CO_2 in a Sorvall
Critical Point Drying System, coated with gold using an Edwards
306 coater, and viewed with an ETEC autoscan.

For transmission microscopy cells were grown on Falcon or
Lux plastic Petri dishes. Cells were fixed in the same glutaraldehyde fixative used for SEM. Cells were subsequently rinsed in
collidine and postfixed in 1% OsO_4 buffered with 0.2 M Collidine.

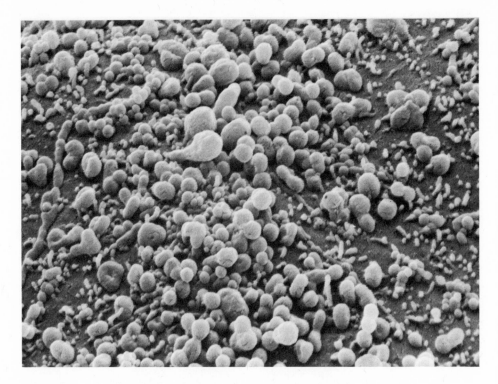

Fig. 3.   Surface of a human X mouse hybrid cell accidentally
           contaminated with mycoplasma showing pleomorphic
           morphology. X 9,000.

After postfixation, cells were dehydrated through alcohol and embedded in Epon as described (Phillips and Phillips, '71). Sections
were viewed with a Philips 300 Microscope.

RESULTS AND DISCUSSION

Scanning Electron Microscope (SEM)

     Cultures being evaluated for accidental mycoplasma infection
are often so heavily infected that the majority of cells are
covered with mycoplasma, and thus contamination is obvious in the
SEM. When mycoplasma are not immediately obvious in a culture,
we generally do not find mycoplasma at all, even after close examination. This suggests that when a culture becomes contaminated,
the mycoplasma generally spread rapidly.

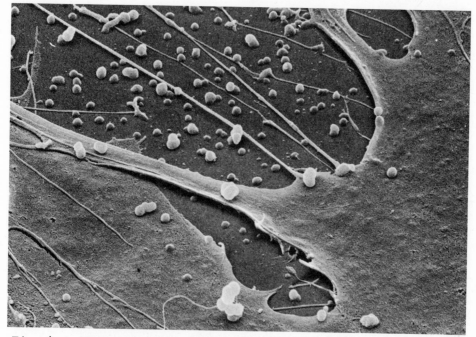

Fig. 4.   Mouse A9 cells deliberately infected with <u>Acholeplasma</u>
<u>laidlawii</u>. Although this species of mycoplasma is
generally not cell-associated, it is easily detected
with SEM because mycoplasma are found on the surface
of the glass coverslip. X 5,000.

We have examined accidentally contaminated cultures from
different laboratories and grown under different culture conditions. We have examined primary cultures and early passages.
With some notable exceptions the morphology of the mycoplasma is
generally similar in different cultures and resembles <u>Mycoplasma</u>
<u>hyorhinis</u>. This is due, to some extent, to the fact that all
mycoplasma species are pleomorphic. Nevertheless, we feel that
species of mycoplasma which infect cell cultures tend to be
similar in appearance.

In micrographs taken with the scanning electron microscope,
infected cells in monolayer are generally associated with several
hundred mycoplasma (Fig. 1). Mycoplasma always vary in size and
shape. Some are small spheres only 0.3 micron in diameter whereas
other spherical forms can be as large as 1 micron. Mycoplasma
occur in many shapes besides spheres (Figs. 2 and 3). Often they
have a dimple, giving them an appearance reminiscent of a mammalian
erythrocyte. They are frequently dumbbell-shaped. They can be
oblong, irregularly shaped, or long and thin -- sometimes 1 or 3

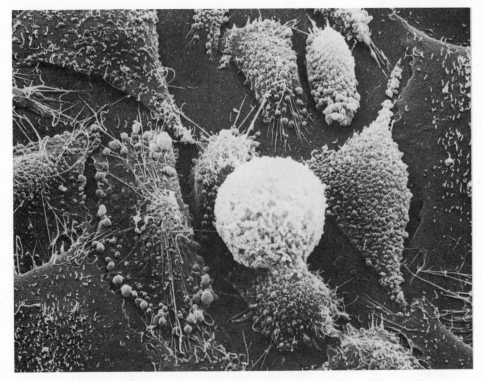

Fig. 5.   Mycoplasma often associated with some cells preferen-
           tially. Here the surface of some A9 cells are covered
           with mycoplasma while other cells are mostly myco-
           plasma free. X 1,200.

micron long and only 0.3 micron wide. Elongate forms generally
have swellings (Figs. 2 and 3). The contours of mycoplasma
always appear smooth in the SEM. The pleomorphic morphology we
observe in accidental infections is generally similar to morphology of M. hyorhinis infected A9 cells (Fig. 1) and M. hyorhinis
infections of other cell types (Brown et al, '74) and consistent
with the appearance that mycoplasma generally have when cultured
by themselves (Anderson and Barile, '65; Black et al, '72; Hummeler
et al, '65; Smith, '71). Long thin forms with swellings are
particularly prevalent in cultures of Mycoplasma pneumonie grown
on agar (Kammer et al, '70; Klainer and Pollack, '73). Although
mycoplasma in accidentally contaminated cultures are preferentially observed on cell surfaces rather than on the coverslip,
occasionally mycoplasma occur in higher density on the coverslip
than on the cells. We found this to be true when we infected A9
cells with Acholeplasma laidlawii (Fig. 4).

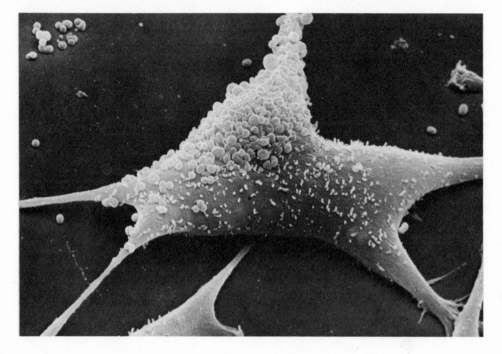

Fig. 6.   In cultures which are not heavily infected, we fre-
          quently find mycoplasma localized to one area of a
          cell. This facilitates detection because one can
          spot such clusters of mycoplasma easily on the SEM
          screen. RAG cell, accidentally infected, X 3,500.

     Although mycoplasma are generally distributed uniformly on
cultured cells (Fig. 1), it is not uncommon to find cells where
some regions of the cell surface are covered with mycoplasma
while other regions of the same cell are completely devoid of
mycoplasma (Fig. 5). Brown et al ('74) found this to be common
in their monolayer cultures infected with M. hyorhinis. We have
also frequently observed cultures where some cells are covered
with hundreds of mycoplasma and other cells appear mycoplasma
free (Fig. 6). Heavily infected and apparently uninfected cells
are sometimes situated adjacent to each other.

Transmission Electron Microscope (TEM)

     One sees relatively few mycoplasma associated with a cell
in thin sections as compared to SEM micrographs because the majority of the mycoplasma associated with a cell will be missed by
any single section. Nevertheless, in transmission electron micro-

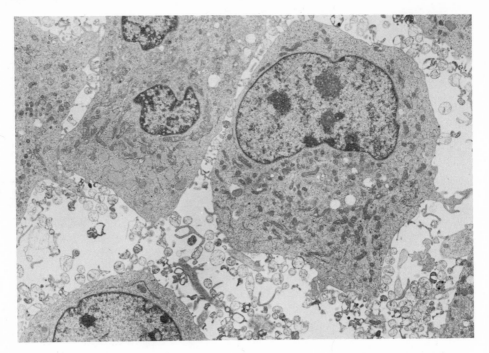

Fig. 7.   In a typical section of a heavily contaminated culture
           we observe from 10 to 50 mycoplasma associated with
           each cell.   Therefore heavily infected cultures can
           be easily detected with the transmission EM.   A9 cells
           deliberately infected with M. hyorhinis.   X 4,000.

graphs of heavily infected cultures, mycoplasma are very obvious.
It is not uncommon to find sections of cells where one can count
10 to 50 mycoplasma associated with the surface of a single cell
(Fig. 7).   Although we see fewer mycoplasma in micrographs of
sectioned material than in scanning electron micrographs, mycoplasma are easier to identify positively in thin-sectioned material.
That is to say, if one observes a few spheres associated with the
surface of a cultured cell in SEM, it may be impossible to be sure
that the structures are mycoplasma.   They might represent blebb-
ing or debris from a dead cell that was in the culture and which
had become cell-associated.   In the TEM, however, mycoplasma have
a very distinctive morphology.   The most marked characteristic is
the chromatin which, in the usual glutaraldehyde-OsO_4 preparation,
is composed of delicate branching structures (Figs. 8 and 9).
Ribosomes of mycoplasma appear smaller and less clearly defined
than ribosomes seen in the cytoplasm of the mammalian cells with
which they are associated (Figs. 8 and 9).   This is not surprising
since ribosomes of mycoplasma are smaller (70S rather than 80S)

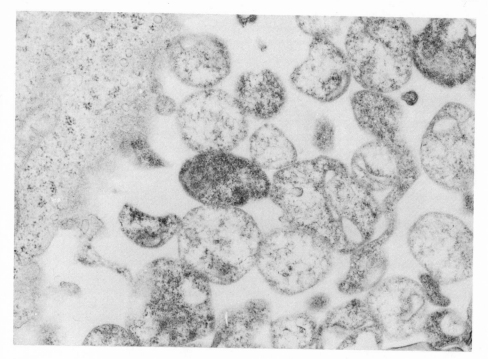

Fig. 8.   Mycoplasma can easily be distinguished from cytoplasm
           of cultured cells by the chromatin filaments and
           smaller more irregular shaped ribosomes. X 31,000.

than ribosomes of mammalian cells (Maniloff et al, '62, '65a,
'65b; Maniloff, '72). A space of about 50A containing fibrous
material separates the cultured cell from associated mycoplasm.
Generally, the plasma membrane of the cultured cell is involuted
slightly to fit the contour of the mycoplasm and appears slightly
more electron dense in the region where the plasmalemma is indented.

We have on several occasions observed virus-like particles
near the surface and in the cytoplasm of cells which have accidentally become infected with mycoplasma (Fig. 10). Several types
of peculiar looking bodies reminiscent of mycoplasma are also
frequently found within the cytoplasm of such cells. Virus-like
particles have been observed associated with mycoplasma isolated
from human leukemia (Hummeler et al, '65) and mycoplasma are virus-
like in some respects (Hayflick and Chanock, '65). Therefore, the
association of virus-like particles and mycoplasma may be more
than coincidental.

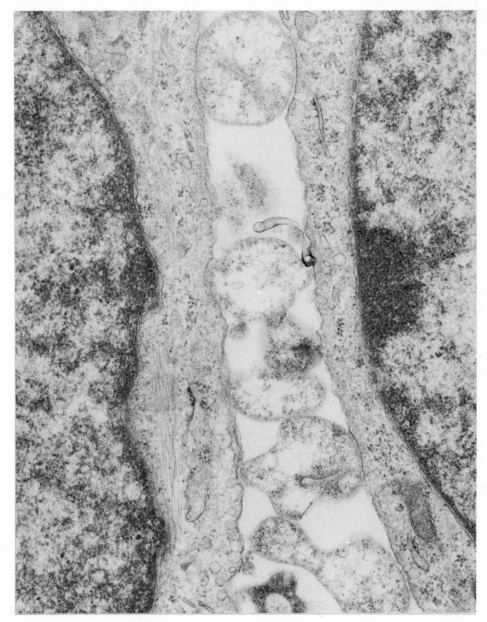

Fig. 9.   A space of about 50A containing some amorphous material
          separates mycoplasma from cultured cells. The plasma-
          lemma of cultured cells appears to be indented and
          slightly more electron dense where the cell surface is
          associated with a cycoplasma. A9 cell deliberately
          infected with M. hyorhinis. X 44,000.

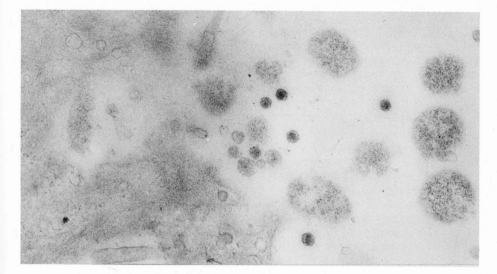

Fig. 10. Virus-like particles are sometimes observed near the
surface of mycoplasma contaminated cells. X 26,000.

Suspension Cultures

Cells grown in suspension can be examined with SEM or TEM
for the presence of contaminating mycoplasma. For SEM, suspension
cultures are fixed and centrifuged into a pellet. Cells are then
resuspended in distilled water and repelleted. The cells are
then suspended in about 1 ml of water, placed on a poly-L-lysine-
coated coverslip and left 15-30 minutes to settle and attach.
(The poly-L-lysine coated coverslip is previously prepared by
placing a coverslip in a solution of 2 mg/ml poly-L-lysine Sigma
for a few minutes and washing the coverslip in water.) The
coverslip is then dehydrated, critical-point dried and coated with
gold. For transmission microscopy cells are pelleted prior to
fixation; the fixative will crosslink associated cells and give
the pellet integrity so it can be dehydrated and embedded. A drop
of collagen or agar solution can be added to tiny pellets to make
them large enough to see.

Scanning Microscopy - Advantages and Disadvantages

In order to detect mycoplasma with the scanning electron
microscope one needs a scanning electron microscope. Obviously,
most tissue culture laboratories do not have a scanning electron
microscope and most tissue culturists are not trained in the use
of the SEM. Some may have friends with a SEM or may find a good
microscopist to collaborate with. It is easy to fix cells and

after fixation they can be sent through the mail. Concerning
effectiveness, I do not think we know at this point how effective
SEM is. Certainly SEM can detect non-cultivatable strains of M.
hyorhinis even when they are present in small numbers. We have
detected mycoplasma contamination in cultures which contain only
an average of one or two mycoplasma associated with each cell.
We feel that SEM may be very effective; however, until the method
is compared to other detection methods in a blind study employing
a large number of cultures, we will not know for sure.

Preparation of samples for the SEM is reasonably quick and
easy. One can prepare samples and view the same day if necessary.
In our laboratory, it requires perhaps 2-3 hours work to prepare
a dozen samples. Viewing the samples takes longer. In about an
hour an experienced microscopist can examine perhaps a hundred
cells from a number of areas of a culture. Since one sees the
entire upper surface of each cell and, in cultures with low levels
of contamination the mycoplasma tend to be found close together
on the same cell, very low mycoplasma concentrations can be
detected. Although one mycoplasma could be mistaken for a bleb,
a group of a dozen mycoplasma would not be confused with anything
else by an experienced worker. Heavily contaminated cultures
can be spotted immediately and do not require looking beyond the
first cell.

It would be very difficult to standardize SEM as a detection
method. Detection, for example, is dependent on the morphological
characteristics of the cells. Mycoplasma are much more difficult
to see on cells which are covered with microvilli than on cells
with smooth surfaces. The morphology of cells depends on a number
of factors such as the particular cell line, the substrate, and
the culture conditions. The same cell line grown in different
laboratories may look different. Although the success of any
technique depends on the skill of the investigator, the success
of SEM is particularly sensitive to differences among investigators.
Microscopy is somewhat of an art, and micrographs of similar
material taken in different laboratories employing the same
techniques often look very different. In addition, unless a
culture is heavily contaminated, identifications of mycoplasma on
the SEM screen takes a great deal of skill and experience, because
the image on the SEM screen is not as good as in a printed photo-
graph and dark-room work is very time-consuming. Viewing in the
SEM, therefore, should be done by a highly skilled worker who is
experienced at looking for mycoplasma contamination.

Transmission Microscopy

Transmission microscopy is more available to most tissue culturists than scanning microscopy. The preparation of samples is more tedious and time consuming as one must embed the material and cut sections. In a section one examines only one plane through a cell. Sampling of different areas of a culture requires that the investigator section different areas of culture independently. Therefore, although it is probably not possible to be sure that culture is not contaminated with transmission EM, one can be sure that a culture is contaminated. The probability of detecting mycoplasma contamination can be increased by sectioning a pellet of trypsinized cells, since in the pellet one looks at cells from different regions of the culture. One can alternatively section the "mitochondrial fraction" as mycoplasma sediment with mitochondria.

A disadvantage of both scanning and transmission microscopy as compared to culture or serological techniques is that they allow only the detection of cell-associated or substrate-associated mycoplasma. Although the species and strains of mycoplasma which commonly infect cell cultures are cell-associated, there may be infections where mycoplasma do not associate with cells or substrate. Our experience with Acholeplasm laidlawii, which is found on the substrate, and generally not on cells, suggests that even mycoplasma which do not associate with cells may settle down and associate with substrate in numbers sufficient for detection.

Acknowledgment

The author wishes to thank Ms. Susan Mahler for her excellent technical assistance.

References

Anderson, D.R., Barile, M.F. (1965) J. Bacteriol. 90:180
Black, F.T., Birch, A.A., Freund, E.A. (1972) J. Bacteriol. 111:254
Brown, S., Teplitz, M. and Revel, J.P. (1974) Pro. Nat. Acad. Sci. 71:464
Hayflick, L. and Chanock, R.M. (1965) Bacteriol. Rev. 29:185
Hummeler, K., Tomassini, N., and Hayflick, L. (1965) J. Bacteriol. 90:517
Kammer, G.M., Pollack, J.D. and Klainer, A.S. (1970) J. Bacteriol. 104:499
Klainer, A.S. and Pollack, J.D. (1973) Ann. N.Y. Acad. Sci. 225:236

Littlefield, J.W. (1964) Nature 12:1142
Maniloff, J., Morowitz, H.J. and Barrnett, R.J. (1965a) J. Cell
    Biol. 25:139
Maniloff, J., Morowitz, H.J. and Barrnett, R.J. (1965b) J. Bact-
    eriol. 90:193
Maniloff, J. (1972) In: Pathogenic mycoplasma. (ed.) E.K. Birch,
    Amsterdam Assoc. Sci. Publ.
Morowitz, H.J., Tourtellotte, M.E., Guild, W.R., Castro, E. and
    Wiese, C. (1962) J. Mol. Biol. 4:93
Phillips, S.C. and Phillips, D.M. (1971) J. Cell Biol. 49:785
Smith, P.F (1971) Academic Press, N.Y.

SOME EFFECTS THAT MYCOPLASMAS HAVE UPON THEIR INFECTED HOST

Eric J. Stanbridge[1] and Claus-Jens Doersen[2]

[1]California College of Medicine
University of California, Irvine, Irvine, California

[2]Stanford University School of Medicine, Stanford,
California

Mycoplasma contamination of cultured cells was first reported
in 1956 (1). A multitude of reports have followed this original
observation, illustrating the frequent occurrence of these contaminants (reviewed in 2). Although mycoplasmas are common contaminants of tissue cultures many investigators regard them merely as
a nuisance and have ignored their presence in experimental procedures since these organisms often exert no obvious effect upon
the well-being of the infected cell population.

In this session we will review the evidence that shows mycoplasmas constitute a real hazard to the cell culturist in terms of
the interpretation of data derived from contaminated cells. Some
of the effects that mycoplasmas have upon cultured cells are outlined in Table 1; a number of which will be dealt with in more
detail below. In addition to outlining their actual effect on host
cell physiology we shall also point out areas where the interpretation of data pertinent to host cell metabolism can be influenced
by the presence of contaminating mycoplasmas.

MYCOPLASMA-CELL ASSOCIATION

Mycoplasmas reside predominantly in an extracellular environment in close association with the host cell plasma membrane (3).
When examined by electron microscopy they occasionally appear to be
free in the cytoplasm of degenerating cells, or within cytoplasmic
vacuoles. The apparent vacuolar location may be due, however, to
fortuitous cross sectioning of cell surface invaginations. Recently the technique of scanning electron microscopy, which allows for

Table 1.   Some Effects That Mycoplasmas Have Upon Cells in Culture

Interference with the growth rate of cells

Inhibition or stimulation of lymphocyte transformation

Induction of morphologic alterations, including cytopathology

Alteration of host cell metabolism

Alteration of ribosomal RNA profiles

Alteration of enzyme patterns

Induction of chromosomal aberrations

Depletion of the essential amino acid arginine from cell
    culture growth medium

Inhibition or enhancement of virus yields

Possible modulation of host cell plasma membranes

Apparent reduction in the tumorigenic potential of malignant
    cells

---

the study of whole cell mounts, has conclusively demonstrated that
mycoplasmas reside in a predominantly extracellular environment
closely associated with the host cell plasma membrane (4).

The predilection for host cell surface membranes may be explained by the fact that there appears to be specific cell receptor
sites for mycoplasmas (5,6).   These receptor sites are chemically
heterogeneous and vary with both mycoplasma and host cell species.
Both carbohydrate and protein receptors have been described.   It
is possible that there are multiple receptor sites on both mycoplasmas and participating host cells.

The few studies that have been directed at an examination of
the kinetics of mycoplasma-host cell associations have produced
some very interesting results (7,8).   At low multiplicity of infection, mycoplasmas preferentially associate with the host cell
plasma membranes and very few, if any, organisms are found free in
the surrounding medium.   If a high multiplicity of infection is
used there is a rapid equilibration (which takes approximately 30
minutes) between cell associated and free, extracellular mycoplasmas
However, even after maximum adsorption there are very few mycoplasmas attached to each cell.   In contrast, the mycoplasma-cell

ratio in the same cells after several days or weeks of infection
is 10-100 fold greater. This suggests that there has been some
modulation of the host cell membrane during the course of chronic
infection that allows many more mycoplasmas to attach. The relationship, if any, of this phenomenon to the effects that mycoplasmas have upon cultured cells is unknown.

EFFECTS ON THE GROWTH OF MAMMALIAN CELLS

The presence of mycoplasmas in cell cultures often leads to
deleterious changes in the growth potential of the infected cells.
However, the effects of mycoplasmas on cell growth encompass the
full spectrum from stimulation to complete lysis of the cell
culture. Mycoplasma-induced stimulation of growth is, in a sense,
a rather special event since it has been adequately documented
only in short-term lymphocyte cultures. Non-specific mitogenic
effects of M. pulmonis and M. pneumoniae on lymphocytes have been
reported. The chemical nature of the mitogens is unknown but,
interestingly, M. pneumoniae induces polyclonal antibody formation
in mouse B cell (9), a property also shared by bacterial lipopoly-
saccharide and a purified protein derivative (PPD) of tuberculin.

Mycoplasmas have also been shown to inhibit lymphocyte mitosis
in vitro (10-12). This inhibitory effect is confined to non-
fermentative mycoplasma species and appears to be due to the depletion of arginine as a consequence of mycoplasmal arginine
deiminase activity.

Long term cell cultures infected with mycoplasmas often grow
more slowly and to lower final population densities than uninfected
cells of the same origin. Although slower growth may often be
accompanied by cell cytopathology covert infection is also encountered, where the only obvious effect is a slower growth rate.
However, total lysis of cultured lymphoma cells following mycoplasma infection has been reported (13). This drastic effect
could be prevented by the addition of arginine, an essential amino
acid for the growth of mammalian cells. Initially, it was thought
that all cases of growth retardation were due to depletion of
arginine in the cell culture growth medium (as a result of mycoplasmal arginine deiminase activity) and that this inhibition
could be reversed by the addition of large amounts of arginine.
However, later reports indicated that fermentative mycoplasmas,
which lack arginine deiminase activity, were also capable of causing growth retardation and cytopathogenicity (14). In these cases,
the addition of excess arginine did not prevent or reverse the
changes. The deleterious effects of fermentative mycoplasmas has
been ascribed to adverse acid pH conditions and to a competitive
utilization of nucleic acid precursors, a property which will be
discussed in detail later.

MORPHOLOGIC CHANGES IN MYCOPLASMA-INFECTED CELLS

As noted with the influence of mycoplasmas on the growth rate
of infected cells, morphologic changes may range from the undetectable to complete lysis of the culture. The most readily apparent
morphologic change is cytopathology. The cytopathic effect (CPE)
may be focal or systemic, and bears many similarities to virally
induced cytopathology. The effects of mycoplasmas on the morphology of cells in culture vary according to the strain of mycoplasma,
the cell type, and the environment of the cell culture. The
studies of Kraemer et al (15) are a good illustration of such
variations. They found that when they infected the mouse lymphoma
line L5178Y with non-fermentative mycoplasmas, for example
M. hominis, total lysis of the culture occurred. However, infection
of the same cell line with fermentative mycoplasmas produced no
readily apparent cytopathology.

In addition to producing CPE of graded severity in infected
cells, mycoplasmas may also induce more subtle changes which can
be detected only in fixed and stained preparations, or ultrastruc-
turally. One of the characteristic features of mycoplasma contamination which has been observed in a number of cell lines infected
with a variety of fermentative and nonfermentative mycoplasmas is
the so-called "leopard-cell effect" (16). The nuclei of these
cells contain numerous areas of condensed chromatin, which are
stained by basophilic dyes. These areas of heterochromatin are
readily distinguished from nucleoli, which tend to segregate into
large masses in the infected cells. It has been suggested that
these nuclear changes are due to the inhibition of host cell DNA
synthesis, mediated by the depletion of the essential amino acid
arginine and/or by competitive utilization of the host cell's soluble pool of purine and pyrimidine nucleotides which would affect
the delicate balance in concentrations of these compounds needed
to complete DNA synthesis. This latter suggestion has been tendered
in part, because of the known absolute requirement of mycoplasmas
for nucleic acid precursors, which are usually not present in the
cell culture growth medium and must be supplied by the host cells
(2) and also because similar nuclear effects are seen when uninfected cells are treated with cytosine arabinoside, an analogue of
deoxycytidine and cytidine, which inhibits DNA synthesis.

Another morphologic change often noted in mycoplasma-infected
cells is the segregation of nucleolar components into large,
aggregated masses. This segregation is often accompanied by a halo
around the nucleolus which resists staining with metachromatic
dyes (16,17). Segregation of nucleolar components can also be
produced by a variety of chemical and physical agents, and also by
viruses. It appears to be a general distress reaction by cells
in culture, and various mechanisms, including inhibition of DNA

synthesis and alterations in RNA and protein metabolism, have been invoked to explain the phenomenon. The mechanism whereby myco- plasmas induce nucleolar changes in unknown.

EFFECTS ON HOST CELL METABOLISM

Many of the host cell changes wrought by mycoplasma contamin- ation are inextricably linked to what has been called the arginine effect. Depletion of essential amino acids has profound conse- quences for mammalian cell metabolism. Removal of any one of the essential amino acids leads to the demise and eventual death of the deprived cell culture. One of the major precipitating events would presumably be the shutdown of protein synthesis, which would in turn orchestrate a cascade of deleterious changes in the cell's metabolic machinery, including cessation of DNA synthesis, ribosomal and messenger RNA synthesis, etc.

Non-fermentative mycoplasmas use arginine as a major energy source (19) and large amounts are consumed fairly rapidly via the arginine dihydrolase pathway. In cell cultures contaminated with these organisms arginine is converted to ornithine via citrul- line. Neither of these compounds will substitute for arginine as growth promoters. Thus, it would be expected that cells infected with these mycoplasmas would cease to divide and finally die unless their arginine source were replenished by adding fresh medium. It is certainly true of cell lines such as L5178Y which are exquisite- ly sensitive to the depletion of arginine. Other cell lines sur- vive and propagate, albeit at a much diminished rate. This variation in response could be due to a variety of reasons. To name but a few: (i) non-fermentative mycoplasmas vary in their ability to degrade arginine; (ii) intracellular protein turnover may contribute sufficient available arginine for survival; and (iii) host cell and mycoplasmal proteolytic enzymes may act upon serum proteins in the growth medium releasing free amino acids.

Since depletion of arginine leads to profound alterations in the metabolism of mammalian cells it is pertinent to ask if other essential amino acids are utilized in excess by non-fermentative or fermentative mycoplasmas, especially since it has been suggested that glutamine, another essential amino acid, serves as an energy source for certain mycoplasmas (20). We have studied the amino acid metabolism of a number of mycoplasma species when grown in tissue culture medium in the absence of mammalian cells (21). The only amino acid that was totally depleted was arginine by non- fermentative mycoplasmas, with a concomitant increase in citrulline and ornithine. Glutamine levels were reduced, accompanied by a corresponding rise in the concentration of glutamic acid. However, the decrease in glutamine did not approach a level that would be

critical for the well-being of the mammalian cells. Several amino
acids actually increased in concentration, a possible indication
of serum or mycoplasmal proteolytic activity. A similar result
was found when human fibroblasts were infected with fermentative
or non-fermentative mycoplasmas (Table 2). Preliminary studies
of ureaplasma metabolism also indicate no excessive utilization of
amino acids (Stanbridge, unpublished).

From a biochemical standpoint, perhaps the most interesting
effects observable in mycoplasma-infected cells are the alterations in nucleic acid metabolism. Radioisotopically labeled
nucleic acid precursors are the usual means by which transport,
incorporation and degradation of nucleic acids are measured.
Mycoplasmas have their most drastic effects upon the incorporation
of precursors into DNA and RNA. Mammalian cells readily incorporate nucleosides into their nucleic acids but incorporate free
bases only to a negligible extent. This is not due to a lack of
transport of the free bases but to the lack of adequate phosphoribosyl transferase activity (22). Mycoplasmas and other prokaryotes, on the other hand, incorporate free bases and nucleosides
equally efficiently. Another property of mycoplasmas which will
affect incorporation studies is that many strains possess nucleoside phosphorylases which catalyse the conversion of nucleosides
to their respective free bases. It has been calculated that some
mycoplasmas are capable of converting as much as 95% of exogenously
added labeled nucleoside within 60 minutes (23). Not surprisingly,
these properties have profound effects on the measurement of DNA
and RNA synthesis in mycoplasma-infected mammalian cells in culture.
These measurements are usually accomplished by adding radioisotopically labeled thymidine or uridine to the growth medium and
measuring the rate of incorporation into acid precipitable material
over an appropriate time period. When mycoplasmas are present there
is rapid conversion of thymidine to thymine or uridine to uracil
(23-25), neither of which will be incorporated into host cell
nucleic acids. Interestingly, although the now converted free
bases are not incorporated nucleic acid synthesis per se is unaffected, because mammalian cells are capable of de novo synthesis
of nucleic acid precursors. However, erroneous conclusions as to
the rate of nucleic acid synthesis, as measured by radioactive
precursor incorporation, will undoubtedly occur.

Mycoplasmas contribute non-specifically to the degradation
of host cell nucleic acids, presumably due to the release of
deoxyribonucleases and ribonucleases. Randall et al (27) reported
the lability of host cell DNA in mycoplasma-infected HeLa cells
as measured by release of acid-soluble oligonucleotides into the
growth medium and subsequently demonstrated the presence of mycoplasmal deoxyribonuclease activity in the infected cells.
Elevated levels of deoxyribonuclease and ribonuclease activity
have also been reported in infected BHK21 cells (28).

Table 2. Amino Acid Changes in the Growth Medium of Control and Mycoplasma-Infected WI-38 cells. Amino Acid Concentrations are Calculated as μmoles per ml.

Amino Acid	Fresh Control	Incubated Control 4 days at 37°C	WI-38 Control 8 days at 37°C	M. hyorhinis-infected WI-38 cultures		M. hominis-infected WI-38 cultures	
				4 days at 37°C	8 days at 37°C	5 days at 37°C	10 days at 37°C
Aspartic acid	0.003	-	0.015	0.021	0.015	0.010	0.019
Threonine	0.106	0.139	0.091	0.076	0.096	0.099	0.117
Glutamine	1.08	0.875	0.292	0.388	0.099	0.625	0.825
Proline	0.022	0.021	0.160	0.087	0.151	0.081	0.207
Glutamic acid	0.072	0.153	0.264	0.252	0.259	0.183	0.369
Glycine	0.043	0.046	0.072	0.048	0.111	0.088	0.172
Alanine	0.031	0.031	0.334	0.235	0.502	0.195	0.255
Valine	0.150	0.169	0.082	0.097	0.108	0.133	0.150
Cystine	0.015	0.013	0.002	0.004	0.004	0.010	0.009
Methionine	0.031	0.028	0.016	0.016	0.019	0.025	0.031
Isoleucine	0.136	0.147	0.049	0.043	0.061	0.094	0.096
Leucine	0.193	0.228	0.077	0.067	0.105	0.169	0.180
Tyrosine	0.060	0.088	0.054	0.043	0.049	0.049	0.060
Phenylalanine	0.057	0.096	0.067	0.040	0.061	0.057	0.073
Histidine	0.045	0.051	0.037	0.030	0.031	0.034	0.046
Ornithine	0.003	0.004	0.010	0.007	0.007	0.039	0.045
Lysine	0.145	0.140	0.100	0.097	0.097	0.126	0.120
Ammonia	N.R.	N.R.	N.R.	N.R.	N.R.	N.R.	N.R.
Tryptophan	Trace	0.003	0.003	0.003	0.002	0.003	0.004
Arginine	0.078	0.072	0.055	0.048	0.049	Trace	-
Citrulline	-	0.001	-	-	-	0.052	0.075

Spurious alterations in RNA patterns have been reported by
several investigators, notably changes in the sedimentation
velocity and electrophoretic profiles of ribosomal RNA (29-32).
The electrophoretic profile of ribosomal RNA (rRNA) extracted
from mycoplasma-free cells consists of two main peaks, corresponding to 28S and 18S mammalian rRNA, and a minor 4-5 S peak.   When
RNA from mycoplasma-infected cells was examined two unusual peaks
were observed which corresponded to prokaryotic 23S and 16S rRNA.
When ^{3}H-uridine label was used the radioactive profiles showed a
high level of incorporation into the 23S and 16S peaks and smaller
peaks of 28S and 18S radioactivity than that seen in uninfected
cultures.   When the same gels were stained and scanned for optical
density, however, no differences in the sizes of the 28S and 18S
peaks from either infected or uninfected cultures were observed,
and the 23S and 16S peaks were undetectable (31,32).   A reasonable
interpretation of these data is that: (a) label is rapidly incorporated into mycoplasmal RNA owing to their high turnover rate;
(b) decreased incorporation of labeled uridine into host cell RNA
is due to the cleavage of this nucleoside exogenously by mycoplasmal pyrimidine nucleoside phosphorylase activity; and (c) no
difference was seen in the actual amount of host RNA, as measured
by optical scanning, because the host cells were able to synthesize
their RNA de novo, and this function was apparently unaffected by
the presence of mycoplasmas.   Mycoplasmal RNA was not detected
optically because it represented a very small fraction of the
total RNA measured.

The profound effect that mycoplasmas have upon the nucleic
acid metabolism of host cells can be explained by their absolute
requirement for nucleic acid precursors.   In many instances the
tissue culture growth medium does not contain the necessary purines
and pyrimidines required for mycoplasma growth (21).   The host
mammalian cells, therefore, act as the major repository of these
precursors in a form available to the mycoplasmas.   The parasitic
mycoplasmas scavenge for nucleic acid precursors, either by competitive utilization of the soluble pool of nucleotides in the
host cell, or by actual breakdown of host cell nucleic acids.

MODULATION OF ENZYME PATTERNS

A correlate to the parasitic nature of mycoplasmas and their
close association with host cells is the apparent alteration in
host cell enzyme patterns.   These alterations probably reflect a
contribution of mycoplasmal enzyme activities rather than drastic
alterations in host cell enzymes.

An adequate illustration is the finding by Stanbridge et al
(33) that mycoplasmal infection of HeLa cells lacking hypoxanthine
guanine phosphoribosyl transferase (HGPRT) activity resulted in the

appearance of levels of HGPRT activity approaching those of wild-
type HeLa cells. Characterization of the newly emerged activity
by slab gel electrophoresis showed that the HGPRT enzyme was derived from mycoplasmas (Figure 1) rather than by reactivation of
a repressed host cell enzyme.

We have encountered a similar phenomenon in cells which lack
thymidine kinase (TK⁻) activity. When these TK⁻ cells were infected with mycoplasmas thymidine kinase activity was measurable in
the cell-free extracts (Stanbridge, unpublished observations).

More recently there have been reports of the detection of
mycoplasmal DNA polymerase activity in infected cells (34). We
have been characterizing DNA polymerases from mycoplasma and
acholeplasma species (35)(L.B. Mills et al, unpublished) and have
found that they have properties which are somewhat similar to
those reported for mitochondrial DNA polymerase from HeLa cells
(36). Obviously, given the rather primitive state of the characterization of mammalian DNA polymerases, those investigators who
rely upon cultured cells for their source material run the risk of
erroneously assigning a mammalian origin for mycoplasmal polymerases.

Similar risks apply in the identification of isoenzyme patterns and in prenatal diagnosis, especially now that techniques are
becoming available whereby single cells can be screened for enzyme
activity (37).

MYCOPLASMA-INDUCED CHROMOSOMAL ABERRATIONS

Fogh (38) and Paton et al (39) were the first to report the
induction of chromosomal aberrations in mycoplasma contaminated
cells. The latter workers reported that the infection of human
diploid fibroblasts with M. orale type 1 led to an increased frequency of chromosomal breakage and chromosome rearrangements. The
most common damage observed was the appearance of achromatic gaps
and true breaks. However, dicentrics, ring chromosomes, and
other bizarre forms were observed. Fogh et al reported the appearance of chromosomal aberrations in a heteroploid human amnion cell
line, deisgnated FL, following contamination by a mycoplasma later
identified as M. fermentans. These reports were quickly confirmed
by other investigators (40).

In these earlier studies the contaminating mycoplasmas were
all identified as species which contained the arginine dihydrolase
enzyme complex and rapidly depleted the cell culture medium of
arginine. In all cases where arginine levels were examined the
appearance of chromosomal abnormalities was associated with depletion of this specific amino acid from the cell culture growth

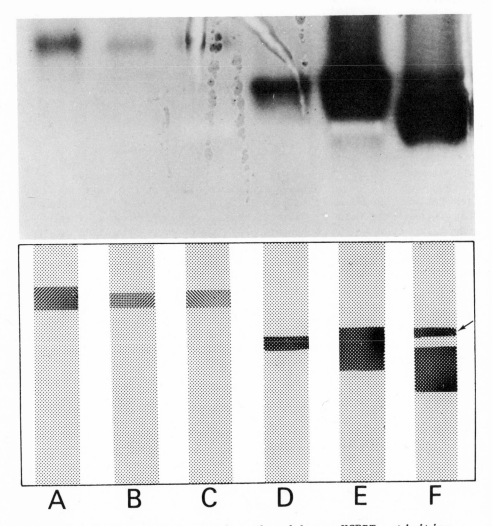

Figure 1. Separation of mycoplasmal and human HGPRT activities.
Electrophoretic analysis was done according to the method of
Rischfield et al.[9] The technique involves slab get electrophoresis
followed by lanthanum precipitation of the charged, labelled product
and autoradiography of the dried gel. A, M. hyorhinis; B and C,
D98/AH-2 and A. laidlawii mixed just before electrophoresis; F, HeLa
control for human HGPRT. Note the extra band (arrowed) which may
be due to accidental mycoplasma contamination (see text). See E.J.
Stanbridge et al. (ref. 33). Reproduced by permission of Nature.

medium.   This correlation led to the suggestion that damage to chromosomes as a consequence of mycoplasma infection was due primarily to the depletion of arginine.

Further studies by Stanbridge et al (16), however, showed that both non-fermentative and fermentative mycoplasmas (which lack the arginine dihydrolase pathway) induce comparable chromosomal damage when they colonize human diploid fibroblasts.   These authors have offered an additional hypothesis to the arginine effect, in which they suggest that chromosomal damage is due to an interference with host cell DNA synthesis, either by a competitive utilization of the acid soluble pool of nucleotide DNA precursors or by actual degradation of host cell DNA by mycoplasmal nucleases.

EFFECT OF MYCOPLASMAS ON CELL-FREE PROTEIN SYNTHESIS

During an investigation involving the selection and characterization of HeLa cells which exhibited resistance to drugs that inhibit mitochondrial protein synthesis we found that mycoplasma contamination drastically altered our experimental results (C. Doersen and E.J. Stanbridge, in preparation).   HeLa cells were mutagenized with ethyl methane sulfonate and then were selected for resistance to erythromycin (an inhibitor of mitochondrial protein synthesis) by supplementing the growth medium with 200-300 µg/ml of this drug.   The selection process took between 6-12 weeks, after which time clones of cells grew which appeared to have acquired a heritable resistance to erythromycin.   We attempted to acquire proof of this resistance by measuring the degree of mitochondrial protein synthesis in cell-free extracts in the presence and absence of erythromycin.   Mitochondrial isolation and protein synthesis assays were performed according to Spolsky and Eisenstadt (41).   The degree of contamination by cytoplasmic ribosomes was measured by incorporating cycloheximide into the reaction mixture.   Our initial experiments indicated that control HeLa cells were sensitive to both chloramphenicol and erythromycin whereas the mutagenized HeLa were resistant to 300 µg/ml of erythromycin, but still sensitive to chloramphenicol.   However, in later experiments we found that our control cells also showed erythromycin resistant mitochondrial protein synthesis although they had never been exposed to the drug (Table 3).   This mystery was resolved when we found that during the selection for erythromycin resistant HeLa cells those same cells at some stage had become contaminated with mycoplasmas which, presumably by selection, had also become totally resistant to 300 µg/ml erythromycin, but were sensitive to chloramphenicol.   At some later stage the control HeLa population had become cross contaminated with the erythromycin resistant mycoplasmas.   We further determined that the contaminating mycoplasmas co-purified with mitochondria.   The bulk of amino acid incorporation

Table 3. Effect of Mycoplasma Contamination on Mitochondrial
          Protein Synthesis in a Cell-free System

	Mean Specific Activity[a]			
Cell Line	Control	300 µg/ml Cycloheximide	200 µg/ml Chloramphenicol	400 µg/ml Erythromycin
HeLa	1.59 ± 0.01[a]	1.06 ± 0.12 (67%)[b]	0.40 ± 0.24 (25%)	0.06 ± 0.00 (4%)
HeLa infected with mycoplasma	1.70 ± 0.59	1.49 ± 0.46 (88%)	0.10 ± 0.06 (6%)	1.16 ± 0.44 (68%)

a. Mean Specific Activity = picomoles ^{3}H leucine incorporated per 30 minutes

    per mg. mitochondrial protein.

b. Percent of control value.

    See text for details of the experiment.

seen in the presence of erythromycin is, therefore, probably due
to the protein synthesizing components of the contaminating mycoplasmas. These preliminary results indicate the potential hazard
of contaminating mycoplasmas in the interpretation of cell-free
protein synthesis assays, especially those involving putative
drug resistant mutants.

                        CONCLUDING REMARKS

     We have presented evidence that mycoplasmas can have profound
effects upon the metabolism of infected host cells. As indicated
in Table 1 their influence is felt in other areas, including
effects on virus yields, transformation assays, modulation of host
cell membranes, etc. These effects are discussed in detail elsewhere in this workshop.

     It is clear from the preceding remarks that virtually any
study of mammalian cell physiology can be influenced by mycoplasma
contamination. Interpretation of data derived from mycoplasma-
infected cells is likely to be erroneous if the presence of these
contaminating organisms is not taken into account. Every effort

should be made to prevent infection and cross-contamination of cell cultures. Safety procedures have been outlined by McGarrity and Coriell (42,43). It is equally important that cell cultures be routinely screened for the presence of these fastidious micro-organisms. Mycoplasma detection methods have been reviewed extensively elsewhere (2,24).

Acknowledgements

Supported, in part, by a grant from the U.S. Public Health Service (CA 19401-01) and University of California Institutional Grant No. 7617. Eric J. Stanbridge is a Leukemia Society of America Special Fellow.

REFERENCES

1. Robinson, L.B., R.H. Wichelbrausen, and B. Razinan. 1956. Contamination of human cell cultures by pleuropneumonia organisms. Science 124:1147.

2. Stanbridge, E. 1971. Mycoplasmas and Cell Cultures. Bacteriol. Rev. 35:206-227.

3. Anderson, D.R., H.E. Hopps, M.F. Barile and B.C. Bernheim. 1965. Comparison of the ultrastructure of several rickettsiae, ornithosis virus, and mycoplasma in tissue culture. J. Bacteriol. 90:1387-1404.

4. Brown, S., M. Teplitz, and J.-P Revel. 1974. Interaction of mycoplasmas with cell cultures as visualized by electron microscopy. Proc. Nat. Acad. Sci. USA 71:464-468.

5. Manchee, R., and D. Taylor-Robinson. 1969. Studies on the nature of receptors involved in attachment of tissue culture cells to mycoplasmas. Brit. J. Exp. Pathol. 50:66-75

6. Sobeslavsky, O., B. Prescott, and R.M. Chanock. 1968. Adsorption of Mycoplasma pneumoniae to neuraminic acid receptors of various cells and possible role in virulence. J. Bacteriol. 96: 695-705.

7. Larin, N.M., N.V. Saxby, and D. Buggey. 1969. Quantitative aspects of Mycoplasma pneumoniae - cell relationships in cultures of lung diploid fibroblasts. J. Hyg. 67:375-385.

8. Fogh, J., and H. Fogh. 1967. Morphological and quantitative
    aspects of mycoplasma-human cell relationships. Proc. Soc.
    Exp. Biol. Med. 125:423-430.

9. Biberfeld, G. and E. Gronowicz. 1967. Mycoplasma pneumoniae
    is a polyclonal B-cell activator. Nature 261:238-239.

10. Callewaert, D.M., J. Kaplan, W.D. Peterson and J.W. Lightbody.
    1975. Suppression of lymphocyte activation by a factor pro-
    duced by Mycoplasma arginine. J. Immunol. 115:1662-1664.

11. Simberkoff, M.S., G.J. Thorbecke, and L. Thomas. 1969. Studies
    of PPLO infection. V. Inhibitors of lymphocyte mitosis and
    antibody formation by mycoplasmal extracts. J. Exp. Med. 129:
    1163-1181.

12. Barile, M.F., and B.G. Levinthal. 1968. Possible mechanism for
    mycoplasma inhibition of lymphocyte transformation induced by
    phytohaemagglutinin. Nature 219:751-752.

13. Kraemer, P.M. 1964. Interaction of mycoplasma (PPLO) and murine
    lymphoma cell cultures. Prevention of cell lysis by arginine.
    Proc. Soc. Exp. Biol. Med. 115:206-212.

14. Butler, M. and R.H. Leach. 1964. A mycoplasma which induces
    acidity and cytopathic effect in tissue culture. J. Gen.
    Microbiol. 34:285-294.

15. Kraemer, P.M., V. Defendi, L. Hayflick, and L. Manson. 1963.
    Mycoplasma (PPLO) strains with lytic activity for murine lym-
    phoma cells in vitro. Proc. Soc. Exp. Biol. Med. 112:381-387.

16. Stanbridge, E., M. Önen, F.T. Perkins, and L. Hayflick. 1969.
    Karyological and morphological characteristics of human
    diploid cell strain WI-38 infected with mycoplasmas. Exp. Cell
    Res. 57:397-410.

17. Jezequel, A.-M, M.M. Shreeve, and J.W. Steiner. 1967. Segregat-
    ion of nucleolar components in mycoplasma-infected cells. Lab
    Invest. 16:287-304.

18. Kenny, G. 1973. Contamination of mammalian cells in culture by
    mycoplasmata. In: Contamination in Tissue Culture (J. Fogh, Ed.)
    Academic Press, New York, pp. 108-131.

19. Schimke, R.T., C.M. Berlin, E.W. Sweeney and W.R. Carroll.
    1966. The generation of energy by the arginine dihydrolase
    pathway in M. hominis. J. Biol. Chem. 241:2228-2236.

20. Smith, P.F. 1960. Amino acid metabolism of PPLO. Ann. N.Y. Acad. Sci. 79:543-550.

21. Stanbridge, E.J., L. Hayflick, and F.T. Perkins. 1971. Modification of amino acid concentrations induced by mycoplasmas in cell culture medium. Nature New Biol. 232:242-244.

22. Plagemann, P.G., and D.P. Richeyn. 1974. Transport of nucleosides, nucleic acid bases, choline and glucose by animal cells in culture. Biochem. Biophys. Acta. 344:263-305.

23. Perez, A.G., J.H. Kin, A.S. Gelbard, and B. Djordjevic. 1972. Altered incorporation of nucleic acid precursors by mycoplasma-infected mammalian cells in culture. Exp. Cell Res. 70:301-310.

24. Schneider, E.L., and E.J. Stanbridge. 1975. Comparison of methods for the detection of mycoplasmal contamination of cell cultures: A review. In Vitro 11:20-34.

25. Hellung-Larsen, P., and S. Frederiksen. 1976. Influence of mycoplasma infection on the incorporation of different precursors into RNA components of tissue culture cells. Exp. Cell Res. 99:295-300.

26. Levine, E.M. 1972. Mycoplasma contamination of animal cell cultures: a simple rapid detection method. Exp. Cell Res. 74:99-109.

27. Randall, C.C., L.G. Gafford, G.A. Gentry, and L.A. Lawson. 1965. Lability of host-cell DNA in growing cell cultures due to mycoplasma. Science 149:1098-1099.

28. Russell, W.C. 1966. Alterations in the nucleic acid metabolism of tissue culture cells infected by mycoplasmas. Nature 212:1537-1540.

29. Levine, E.M., I.G. Burleigh, C.W. Boone, and H. Eagle. 1967. An altered pattern of RNA synthesis in serially propagated human diploid cells. Proc. Nat. Acad. Sci. USA 57:431-438.

30. Markov, G.G., I. Bradvarova, A. Mintcheva, P. Petrov, N. Shiskov and R.G. Tsanev. 1969. Mycoplasma contamination of cell cultures: interference with ^{32}P-labeling pattern of RNA. Exp. Cell REs. 57:374-384.

31. Schneider, E.L., C.J. Epstein, W.L. Epstein, M. Betlach, and G. Abbo Halbasch. 1973. Detection of mycoplasma contamination in cultured human fibroblasts - comparison of biochemical and microbiological techniques. Exp. Cell Res. 79:343-349.

32. Schneider, E.L., E.J. Stanbridge, and C.J. Epstein. 1974. In-
    corporation of ^{3}H-uridine and ^{3}H-uracil into RNA: a simple
    technique for the detection of mycoplasma contamination of cul-
    tured cells. Exp. Cell Res. 84:311-318.

33. Stanbridge, E.J., J.A. Tischfield, and E.L. Schneider. 1975.
    Appearance of hypoxanthine guanine phosphoribosyl transferase
    activity as a consequence of mycoplasma contamination.
    Nature: 256:329-331.

34. Miller, R.L. and F. Rapp. 1976. Distinguishing cytomegalovirus,
    mycoplasma, and cellular DNA polymerases. J. Virol. 20:564-569.

35. Mills, L.B., E.J. Stanbridge, D. Korn, and D. Sedwick. 1976
    DNA polymerase from mycoplasmatales. Fed. Proc. 35:1590.

36. Fry, M. and A. Weissbach. 1973. A new DNA dependent DNA poly-
    merase from HeLa cell mitochondria. Biochem. 12:3602-3608.

37. Milunsky, A. and J.W. Littlefield. 1972. The prenatal diagnosis
    of inborn errors of metabolism. Ann. Rev. Med. 23:57-76.

38. Fogh, J. and H. Fogh. 1965. Chromosome changes in PPLO-infected
    FL human amnion cells. Proc. Soc. Exp. Biol. Med. 119:233-238.

39. Paton, G.R., J.P. Jacobs and F.T. Perkins. 1965. Chromosome
    changes in human diploid cell cultures infected with mycoplasma.
    Nature 207:43-45.

40. Aula, P. and W.W. Nichols. 1967. The cytogenetic effects of
    mycoplasma in human leucocyte cultures. J. Cell Physiol. 70:
    281-290.

41. Spolsky, C.M., and J.M. Eisenstadt. 1972. Chloramphenicol re-
    sistant mutants of human HeLa cells. Febs Letters 25:319-324.

42. McGarrity, G.J. and L.L. Coriell. 1971. Procedures to reduce
    contamination of cell cultures. In Vitro 6:257-265.

43. McGarrity, G.J. 1976. Spread and control of mycoplasmal infec-
    tion of cell cultures. In Vitro 12:643-647.

MYCOPLASMA-CELL CULTURE-VIRUS INTERACTIONS: A BRIEF REVIEW

Michael F. Barile and Marion W. Grabowski

Bureau of Biologics, FDA, Bethesda, Maryland 20014

It has been established that certain mycoplasmas can alter the activity and function of contaminated cell cultures and thereby markedly affect the results of study. Some of these effects have been reviewed elsewhere (1, 2). This presentation will briefly discuss three general aspects of mycoplasma-cell-virus interaction including: a) the cytopathic effects (CPE) produced by the mycoplasma fermenters; b) the inhibitory effect produced by the arginine utilizing mycoplasmas on lymphocyte blastformation; and c) the effects of mycoplasmas on virus propagation.

Mycoplasma-cell interactions. We might begin by asking: How do mycoplasmas injure host tissue cells? Although the factors responsible for virulence and pathogenicity have not been well established, they surely are related to the events which follow the interactions between the mycoplasma pathogens and host tissue cells. These events include: a) hemadsorption, hemagglutination and hemolysis; b) spermadsorption and spermagglutination; c) attachment to epithelial and fibroblastic cell cultures grown in suspension or monolayer with the resulting changes in cell morphology, including severe CPE; d) attachment to ciliated tracheal and fallopian cells causing damage to the mucosal epithelial tissues, and e) the development of autoantibodies, e.g. cold (anti-I) agglutinin and agglutinins to lung, brain and liver tissues in patients with *Mycoplasma pneumoniae* pneumonia. A more detailed discussion of these interactions follows.

Hemolysis. Many pathogenic mycoplasmas produce hemolysis, including *M. gallisepticum* (5, 6), *M. mycoides* var. *mycoides* (5), and *M. mycoides* var. *capri* (7), and others (see Aluotto et al (8).

135

The only human species that produces hemolysins is *M. pneumoniae*, the cause of primary atypical pneumonia, and therefore, production of hemolysis has been used as a diagnostic tool for the presumptive identification of *M. pneumoniae* (9, 10). The production of hemolysis has been associated with virulence and the ability to produce disease (11). Some of the mycoplasma hemolysins have been shown to be peroxides (7, 12, 13).

Hemadsorption. Mycoplasmas can hemadsorb (14), including *M. pneumoniae* (15), *M. gallisepticum* (16), *M. pulmonis* (1), and others [see Tully and Razin (17)]. Guinea pig erythrocytes can hemadsorb to mycoplasma infected or contaminated cell cultures as demonstrated by the same procedure used to establish virus hemagglutination (18). Thus, the investigator isolating or characterizing viruses must rule out mycoplasma contamination in order to properly interpret the results of hemadsorption studies. In addition to hemadsorption, mycoplasmas have other properties in common with viruses. They are filterable, produce cytopathic effects, are ether- and chloroform-sensitive, and are neutralized by antiserum.

Hemagglutination. Some mycoplasmas can agglutinate erythrocytes, and the hemagglutination inhibition test has been used for the sero-identification of certain pathogenic mycoplasmas (16). The attachment or binding site of some mycoplasmas is probably sialic acid because prior treatment of cells with neuraminidase can inhibit hemagglutination by *M. gallisepticum* (19), *M. pneumoniae* and *M. synoviae* (20, 21). However, neuraminiadase does not inhibit hemagglutination by all Mycoplasma species (20, 21). Therefore, the attachment moiety can vary with the species of *Mycoplasma*, and there are at least two or more receptor sites for this group of organisms (20, 21, 22-26).

Mycoplasma attachment to other host tissues. Mycoplasmas can adsorb to many tissues as demonstrated by various microscopic procedures, including ordinary light [standard histologic (Giemsa) staining], ultraviolet (immunofluorescence and DNA-fluorochrome staining) and electron microscopy. Most of our information on attachment has been obtained with studies on mycoplasmas in infected (27-31) and contaminated cell cultures (1, 32-35), or in infected tracheal organ cultures (25, 26, 37-40), in lungs of infected developing chick embryos (41), and in bronchial tissues of experimentally infected hamsters (26). Because some mycoplasmas initiate infection by attachment, cytadsorption has been associated with virulence and the ability to produce disease. The degree of cytadsorption varies with the species and strain of mycoplasma as well as the host cell tissue substrate. In general: a) the pathogenic species (especially the fermenters) are better cytadsorbing agents than are nonpathogenic species; b) strains isolated from infected animals and from chronically infected or contaminated cell cultures show a greater degree of cytadsorption than do laboratory strains maintained in continuous broth and agar subculture; c) continuous passage in cell cultures or in animals can increase cytadsorbability; and d) continuous passage in broth and agar medium can decrease ability to cytadsorb. Thus, in general, the degree of cytadsorption can be a reflection of the history and passage of a particular strain. In our studies, we have examined the ability of mycoplasmas to cytadsorb to VERO cell cultures as determined by specific immunofluorescence. The highest degree of cytadsorption (100 to 1000 mycoplasmas per infected VERO cell) was seen among strains of *M. hyorhinis* (especially the "non-cultivable" strains), *M. pulmonis* (ASH), and *M. fermentans*, (PG18). Strains 1184 and 1185 of *M. hominis*, isolated from chronically contaminated cell cultures showed a far greater degree of cytadsorption than did the high passage broth and agar cultures of strain PG21 of *M. hominis*. A moderate degree of cytadsorption (10 to 100 mycoplasmas per infected VERO cell) was seen with *M. gallisepticum*, (PG31), *A. laidlawii*, (PG8), *A. axanthum*, (S743), *M. arginini*, (G230), *M. arthritidis*, (PG27), and *M. orale*, (CH19299). Minimum cytadsorption (1 to 10 mycoplasmas per infected VERO cell) was seen with *M. gallinarum*, (PG16), *M. faucium*, (DC333), *M. pneumoniae*, (FH), and *M. buccale*, (CH20247). The site and pattern of cytadsorption varied with the mycoplasma species and the cell culture substrate, but, in general, two common patterns were seen: a) a cluster of mycoplasmas in microcolony formation, and b) a generalized infection of the entire cell with mycoplasma attachment seen primarily along the periphery of the tissue cell membrane.

Three of the respiratory pathogens have organized terminal apparati, e.g. *M. gallisepticum* (22, 23) and *M. pulmonis* (42) have a terminal bleb, and *M. pneumoniae* has a terminal spike (24-26). Because the terminal apparati of *M. pulmonis* and *M. pneumoniae* have been seen positioned at the point of cell attachment, some workers consider these tips to be attachment apparati. Some mycoplasmas (*M. pneumoniae*, *M. gallisepticum* and *M. mycoides* var. *mycoides*) initiate respiratory disease by first attaching to and then colonizing the bronchial ciliated cells causing ciliostatis, ciliolysis, followed by erosion of the entire mucosal epithelial lining. Much of our knowledge regarding infection has been obtained using tracheal (25, 26, 37-40) and fallopian (43) organ cultures. These studies have shown that the hemolysin of certain mycoplasmas (e.g. *M. mycoides* var. *mycoides*) but not all (*M. gallisepticum*) may be responsible for the ciliary damage.

Spermadsorption and spermagglutination. Some mycoplasmas attach to spermatozoa and spermadsorption and spermagglutination are dependent on the particular species of mycoplasma and on the host sperm (44, 45). Some workers (45, 46) contend that spermadsorption may be responsible for the development of sperm autoantibodies (analogous to cold agglutinins) and may play a role in the

development of infertility, but these contentions lack the support
of definitive data.

Autoantibodies and mycoplasma disease. Patients with mycoplasma pneumonia produce antibodies against their own erythrocytes
(cold and anti-I agglutinins) (47, 48), lung tissue, the site of
infection, and brain tissue in cases with or without complicating
central nervous system disease (49-51). These same patients may
also produce agglutinins to *Streptococcus* MG (52, 53), and to
Wassermann cardiolipins (54). The development of heterogenetic
agglutinins is probably due to the presence of commonly shared,
cross-reacting, membrane-associated glycolipid antigens because
adsorption of sera with the glycolipid fraction of *M. pneumoniae*
can drastically reduce or remove the agglutinin titers to human
lung, brain, or liver tissues (55). However, adsorption with
glycolipids of *M. pneumoniae* does not reduce the cold agglutinin
titer, and therefore the cold agglutinins are produced by a
different mechanism. Cold agglutinins are probably produced as a
result of the interaction between the human red blood cell and
M. pneumoniae, causing an alteration of the antigen-I component
of the erythrocytes (56). The altered erythrocyte becomes immuno-
logically foreign, causing the development of cold (anti-I)
agglutinins (71).

Covert mycoplasma contamination. To the unsuspecting observer,
mycoplasma contamination may appear insidious and may go undetected
because: a) even large numbers of mycoplasmas, i.e. gross contamination, do not produce overt, turbid growth in cell cultures
commonly associated with bacterial and fungal contamination; b) some
mycoplasma contaminants, and especially the arginine users, do not
necessarily alter cell morphology, or the initial cytopathic effects
may be minimal or inapparent, and c) many of the mycoplasma contaminants compete with the cell culture for amino acids, sugars, and
precursors, and remove or deplete an essential nutrient, causing
"toxic" or "nutritional" cellular effects. Because changing the
media (replenishing essential nutrients) can reverse these
"nutritional" effects temporarily, the investigator may not suspect
contamination. To a large extent, the biochemical activity of the
mycoplasma contaminant predetermines the type of cytopathic effect.
For example, the cellular changes produced may depend on whether
the mycoplasma contaminant utilizes arginine or glucose for energy.
The arginine utilizing contaminants can consume large amounts of
arginine and may deplete the medium of this essential amino acid,
causing a dysfunction in cell activity, such as inhibition of
lymphocyte blastformation (57) or a decrease in virus yields (58).
However, arginine depletion does not always cause destructive
cellular changes. On the other hand, the fermenting mycoplasma
contaminants can release large amounts of acid metabolites, causing
a rapid acid shift in pH, resulting in severe cytopathic effects,

including the complete destruction of the cell culture monolayer.
In addition, many of the mycoplasma fermenters are excellent cytadsorbing agents. Cell attachment produces an intimate interaction
between the pathogen and host cell and permits the contaminant to
release its toxic metabolites in close proximity to the tissue cell
membrane, facilitating severe cytopathic effects. Changing the
media removes the toxic metabolites and reverses, temporarily, the
severe destructive cytopathic effects, providing the investigator
with a false sense of security. In brief, *the investigator should
suspect contamination whenever changes occur in the appearance or
activity of the cell culture.*

   *Principles of indirect procedures for detecting mycoplasma
contamination.* The indirect, non-culture procedures are reviewed
elsewhere (1, 2). In brief, these procedures detect contamination
by exploiting a basic biological, biochemical, or antigenic property
of mycoplasma contaminants, such as: a) cytadsorption, i.e. because
mycoplasmas attach to the membranes of cultured cells, producing a
typical pattern of infection, and because they can be visualized by
orginary microscopy at high magnifications, a variety of specific and
non-specific staining procedures have been developed and used to detect mycoplasma contamination, including: i) the use of acridine
orange (59), orcein (60), hematoxylin and eosin, and Giemsa stains
(1, 2, 6); ii) specific conjugated antisera (62); and iii) the DNA
binding fluorochrome stains commonly used for chromosome banding
(2, 52), such as bisbenzimidazole; b) the presence of a particular
enzymatic pathway in mycoplasmas, but not in tissue culture cells,
such as arginine deiminase (63) or uracil phosphoribosyl transferase
activity (64) detected by using biochemical procedures; and c) the
presence of mycoplasmal RNA (65) in contaminated cell cultures
detected by using physical-chemical procedures.

   Usefulness of indirect procedures. The usefulness of any detection procedure is dependent upon at least three basic factors: a)
the sensitivity of the procedure, i.e. what is the minimal number of
mycoplasmas detectable? (It has been our experience that the minimum
number of mycoplasmas detected by most indirect procedures is approximately 7 logs of mycoplasmas or greater); b) *the specificity of the
procedure,* i.e. do all mycoplasma contaminants possess the basic
property or activity under examination? For example, not all mycoplasma contaminants have arginine deiminase activity, and some do not
have uracil phosphoribosyl transferase activity. Therefore, these
procedures have limitations. Moreover, some mycoplasma contaminants
are poor cytadsorbing agents and reside mainly in the medium fluids.
The poor cytadsorbing mycoplasmas are not detected as readily and,
therefore, the ability of the contaminant to cytadsorb can affect
the sensitivity of the staining procedures; c) *the presence and
amount of non-specific background activity.* Many transformed cells
may contain excessive amounts of DNA material scattered throughout
the cytoplasm. This DNA material produces background activity which

can pose difficulties with interpretation of results obtained with
DNA staining and auto-radiography procedures. In order to minimize
background activity, we inoculated the test-cell culture-specimen
into an indicator cell culture. An indicator cell culture procedure
can be standardized and includes positive and negative controls to
determine the sensitivity and validity of each test. The uninoculated negative control cells can also be used to monitor for absence
of mycoplasma contamination in each weekly passage of the indicator
cell culture.

Selecting the most convenient or suitable indirect procedure
depends in part on the reagents, equipment, apparati and procedures
available to the investigator. For example, some laboratories
routinely perform biochemical enzyme assays, while others may con-
duct routine radiolabeling studies, or may examine cell cultures by
electron microscopy, etc. The investigator is well-advised to use
such convenient reagents, equipment or procedures routinely available to him, but he must also be aware of the limitation of the
indirect procedures. The advantage of the staining procedures
using an indicator cell culture is that they are very sensitive for
detecting the "non-cultivable" mycoplasma contaminants, they are
inexpensive, and they are available to every investigator.

Staining procedures for detecting mycoplasma contamination.
Histologic staining procedures. Because most cell cultures become
heavily contaminated, the ordinary histologic staining procedures
provide a simple, effective indirect method for detecting mycoplasma
contamination. The staining procedures are particularly effective
for detecting contamination by the "non-cultivable" strains of *M.*
hyorhinis, i.e. for detecting strains that do not grow on agar-broth
media (61). These strains of *M. hyorhinis* are the only mycoplasmas
known to require cell cultures for growth. The mycoplasmas in contaminated cell cultures appear as small, dense, pleomorphic bodies
attached or in close proximity to the membranes (1, 2).

Immunofluorescence. The fluorescent antibody procedure has
been extremely effective for detecting and speciating the mycoplasma
contaminants of cell cultures (1, 2, 32, 33, 69). It has been
especially effective for detecting the "non-cultivable" strains of
M. hyorhinis (61). We have used immunofluorescence to detect cells
experimentally infected or naturally contaminated with the following
species of mycoplasmas and acholeplasmas: *A. laidlawii, A. axanthum,*
A. granularum, A. modicum, M. arginini, M. arthritidis, M. buccale,
M. conjunctivae, M. faucium, M. fermentans, M. gallinarum, M.
gallisepticum, M. hominis, M. orale, M. pneumoniae, M. pulmonis,
M. salivarium, M. bovis, M. bovoculi, M. alkalescans, M. canis,
M. maculosum, M. neurolyticum, M. spumans, and *M. primatum.* Immunofluorescence has also been used by other workers to study a wide
range of other mycoplasmas.

Sensitivity of the immunofluorescence procedure. The sensitivity of the fluorescent-antibody procedure for detecting mycoplasmas in contaminated cell cultures is dependent upon several
factors, including: a) the contaminated tissue cell culture substrate; b) the strain and species of mycoplasma contaminants; c)
the severity of mycoplasma infection; d) the ability and the degree
of cytadsorption, i.e. the cytadsorbing contaminants are concentrated on the membrane of the cell culture and, therefore, the mycoplasma antigen is more readily visualized; e) the potency and specificity of the conjugated mycoplasma antisera (69); f) the intensity
of the ultraviolet beam; and g) the microscope. We have used a
C. Zeiss Universal microscope with an epi-illuminator. Because the
ultraviolet beam is not transmitted through the mounting glass or
specimen, epi-illumination directs a larger amount of incident
ultraviolet light onto the surface of the specimen. In addition,
new power supply sources and improved ultraviolet bulbs are available which generate a greater amount of useable ultraviolet light.
The new direct current-power supply produces a constant beam of
high ultraviolet energy (indirect current produces an intermittent
pulse of energy), and the short arc bulb (Orsam HBO-50-W3-D.C.)
emits a narrow, concentrated beam of ultraviolet light. The narrow
beam permits all of the ultraviolet light to reach the specimen,
whereas the older bulbs (with broader arcs) permitted only a portion
of the light to reach the specimen.

An appraisal of the immunofluorescence procedure. Immunofluorescence is the only procedure available to us for identifying the
"non-cultivable" strains of *M. hyorhinis* in contaminated cell
cultures and, therefore, it should be included in each test.
Because most cell cultures become heavily contaminated, the immunofluorescence procedure has been a very effective method for detection and speciation of all the mycoplasma contaminants of cell
cultures. Moreover, the use of an indicator cell culture increases
the sensitivity of the immunofluorescence procedure because: a) it
amplifies the mycoplasma titer in a given specimen, i.e. small
numbers of mycoplasmas inoculated into cell cultures reach high
titers within a few days; and b) it can be standardized to include
negative (uninoculated) and positive (*M. hyorhinis*-infected)
controls.

DNA fluorochrome staining procedure. The fluorochrome stains,
such as 4'-6-diamidino-2-phenylindole (66) and bisbenzimidazole
(Hoechst 33258) (2, 62), which bind specifically to DNA, have been
used effectively for the detection of mycoplasmas in contaminated
cell cultures. The procedure routinely used in our laboratory is
as follows: a) a stock concentrate (50 µg/ml) of the DNA-fluorochrome stain [bisbenzimidazole (No. 33258), Hoechst Pharmaceuticals,
Somerville, NJ] is prepared in Hank's balanced salt solution (without sodium bicarbonate or phenol red) and with 1:10,000 parts

thimerosal added and stored at 2-8°C in the dark in an opaque bottle
wrapped in aluminum foil; b) a 3 to 4 ml suspension of the indicator
VERO (African green monkey) cell culture [containing 10^5 cells/ml
in Basal Medium No. 2 (Eagle) with 2 to 5 ml of fetal bovine serum
and 100 U/ml of penicillin] is added to and grown on a glass coverslip placed in a small plastic non-toxic dish and incubated at
36 ± 1°C in 5% carbon dioxide in air; c) the indicator VERO cell
culture is inoculated, in duplicate, with 0.05 to 0.1 ml of each
test cell culture specimen within 24 hr or when the cells reach 30
to 40% confluence. A positive (M. hyorhinis-infected) and negative
(non-inoculated) cell culture control is included in each test;
d) the cell culture specimens are examined 4 to 6 days following
inoculation. The medium fluids are aspirated and the specimen is
fixed with two ml of a 1:3 parts glacial acetic acid and methanol
fixative for 5 min. The fixative is removed; fixation is repeated
a second time for 10 min and the specimen is air-dried for 1 to 2
hr at room temperature (R.T.°); e) a fresh working concentration
(0.05 µg/ml) of the staining solution is prepared for each test
from the stock concentrate and diluted in Hanks' balanced salt
solution. The stain is mixed thoroughly with a magnetic stirrer
for 30 min before use. Two ml of stain is placed to cover the
entire cell culture specimen and the stained preparation is incubated at R. T.° for 30 min. The stain is removed and the specimen
is rinsed three times with deionized water. Excess water is removed
with a Pasteur pipet. Unused stain is discarded; f) the specimen
coverslips are mounted on a large microscope slide (2" x 3");
mounting fluid is placed above and below the specimen, covered with
a large coverslip (18 x 75 mm) and examined by ultraviolet microscopy, using the procedure described in an earlier section for immunofluorescence. The mounting fluid consists of 22.2 ml of 0.1 $\underline{M}$
citric acid, 27.8 ml of 0.2 $\underline{M}$ disodium phosphate, and 50 ml glycerol
at pH 5.5 and stored refrigerated at 2-8°C.

Cytopathic effects. Severe cell destruction can be produced
by many mycoplasmas (1, 2), and especially the fermenters, including *A. laidlawii, A. granularum, A. axanthum, M. hyorhinis, M.
pulmonis, M. conjunctivae, M. mycoides* var. *mycoides, M. mycoides*
var. *capri, M. fermentans, M. neurolyticum,* and *M. capricolum.* Some
of the arginine utilizing mycoplasmas can also produce CPE, including strains of *M. hominis, M. orale,* and *M. arginini.* Mycoplasmas
produce cellular damage by either producing large amounts of acid
metabolites (e.g. *M. hyorhinis* and other mycoplasma fermenters), or
toxic metabolites (e.g. hemolysins), or by releasing potent proteolytic enzymes, e.g. by strain 14 of *M. capricolum.* Some of the
mycoplasma contaminants produce gross macroscopic cytopathic effects
characterized by an inverted V-shaped destruction of the entire
cell culture monolayer when grown in test tubes (1). The macroscopic CPE is so characteristic that it can be used for the presumptive identification of mycoplasma contamination (1, 2). In brief,

tenfold dilutions of the test-cell culture-specimen ("pour-off" or spent tissue culture medium) are inoculated into a series of test tubes containing primary rabbit or monkey kidney cell cultures. The cultures are incubated for 2 to 3 weeks without feeding and observed for macroscopic CPE. Uninoculated cell cultures serve as negative controls. Most mycoplasma fermenters will produce massive destruction of the cell culture monolayer (1) within two weeks.

The type and severity of CPE varies with the strain and species of the mycoplasma contaminant, and with the cell culture substrate (1), e.g. *A. laidlawii* (in WI-38) and *M. pulmonis* (in primary rabbit kidney cell culture) produce micro-colonies, followed by micro-lesions with small multiple foci of necrosis (1). Some contaminants, such as *M. gallisepticum* (6) produce plaque formation, a property commonly associated with viruses. *M. hyorhinis* (in WI-38, HEp-2, VERO, 3T6, or primary rabbit kidney cell cultures) and *M. pulmonis* (in HEp-2 cultures) produce a more generalized infection involving every cell in the entire monolayer; these mycoplasmas attach to the cell membranes, multiply rapidly to a peak population of up to 1000 mycoplasmas per infected tissue cell and cause cell lysis with destruction of the entire cell culture (1).

Effects of mycoplasma contamination. In addition to producing severe cytopathic effects, mycoplasmas can also affect cell function and activity [see (1) and (2) for references]. For example, some mycoplasmas can inhibit lymphocyte blastformation, cause chromosomal aberrations and increase or decrease virus yields. Others deplete nutrients from medium and affect protein and nucleic acid synthesis (67). Some mycoplasmas alter the antigenicity of cell membranes, causing the production of autoantibodies, such as cold (anti-I) agglutinins. A discussion of these effects follows.

Effect on lymphocyte blastformation. The arginine-utilizing mycoplasma contaminants can inhibit lymphocyte blastformation. In our studies (57), lymphocyte cultures were infected with either mycoplasma fermenters or with arginine users. Whereas arginine-using mycoplasmas markedly inhibited the stimulatory effect of phytohemagglutinin (PHA), the mycoplasma fermenters (which do not utilize arginine for energy) had either no effect or a stimulatory effect. In subsequent studies we showed that arginine depletion by the arginine-utilizing mycoplasmas was responsible for the inhibitory effect. Whereas *M. hominis* inhibited PHA stimulation, adding fresh medium to the culture or supplementing the spent medium with additional arginine reversed the inhibitory effect. Freshly prepared arginine-free medium did not reverse the effect (57). Thus, mycoplasma can affect lymphocyte function *in vitro*. Mycoplasma infection can also alter the immune response *in vivo*. For example, infecting rabbits with mycoplasmas can suppress their antibody response to certain bacteriophage known to be mediated by T-cells (70).

Effect of mycoplasmas on virus yields. Mycoplasmas can affect virus propagation (58), and the effect is dependent upon the species of mycoplasmas, the virus and the cell culture substrate. Whereas some mycoplasmas have no detectable effect, others can either increase or decrease virus yields. Several mechanisms have been established: a) the arginine-using mycoplasmas can decrease yields of arginine requiring DNA viruses by depleting arginine from the medium, and b) some mycoplasmas can increase virus yields by inhibiting interferon induction and/or activity (1, 2, 58).

Decreased vaccinia virus yields by arginine depletion. Cell cultures contaminated with arginine-utilizing mycoplasmas can decrease the titer of vaccinia virus (an arginine-requiring DNA virus) ten to one-hundredfold (58). Addition of arginine reversed the effect. *M. hyorhinis* (a fermenter which does not require arginine for energy) had no effect.

Decreased herpesvirus yields by arginine depletion. Cell cultures infected or contaminated with arginine-utilizing mycoplasmas can decrease the titers of *Herpes simplex virus* (HSV), another arginine-requiring DNA virus (68). The titers of virus grown in cells contaminated with *M. arginini* were 100 to 1000 times lower than titers obtained with mycoplasma-free cell cultures. *M. hyorhinis*, a fermenter, had no effect. Addition of arginine reversed the effect. We have suggested that the arginine depletion effect by mycoplasmas may provide a simple procedure to establish the arginine requirement for other DNA viruses (1, 2).

Reduction of viral plaques. Mycoplasma contamination can reduce the size and morphology of plaques, as well as the titers produced by *Semliki forest virus* (58) and *Herpes simplex virus*. The reduction of *herpesvirus* plaques was reversed by the addition of arginine. *A. laidlawii*, a non-arginine-utilizing mycoplasma, had no effect. To summarize, the arginine-utilizing mycoplasmas can reduce the size and titer of plaques produced by certain arginine-requiring DNA viruses, and the addition of arginine to the medium can reverse the effect.

Increasing virus yields by inhibiting interferon induction. Mycoplasmas can also increase virus yields by inhibiting the induction of interferon. These studies were undertaken because the same cell cultures, maintained in parallel, gave different titers for *Semliki forest virus* (SFV). Subsequent studies showed that the cell culture producing the higher titers was contaminated with *M. hyorhinis*. Increased SFV titers were obtained only when low virus input was used. With low input, a smaller number of cells are infected, leaving most of the non-infected cell cultures available to accept the interferon generated, and to develop resistance to viral infection. Thus, several cycles of virus multiplication were required to achieve amplification and show a significant increase in virus yield. With high virus input, most or all of the cells are infected initially, and the effect of mycoplasmas on interferon inhibition and on cell resistance cannot be demonstrated [see (58) for references].

Inhibiting virus induction of interferon. Although mycoplasmas do not induce interferon in cell culture monolayers, they can inhibit interferon activity induced either by viruses, such as *Vesicular Stomatis Virus* (VSV), or by synthetic RNA co-polymers. In our studies, mycoplasma-free and mycoplasma-infected cells were inoculated with high input of VSV and then assayed for both virus and interferon titers. Whereas mycoplasma did not affect the virus titers, they did inhibit induction of interferon, reducing titers from a high of 1:256 to less than 1:4. Additional arginine had no effect [see (58) for references].

Inhibiting poly I·C induction of interferon. Similar effects were reported with the synthetic double-stranded Poly I·C, a potent inducer of interferon (58). The addition of Poly I·C stimulated interferon production and produced cell resistance with a significant decrease in virus yields. When cell cultures were infected with mycoplasmas, interferon production was inhibited, nullifying the Poly I·C effect and resulting in titers similar to the control cell cultures without Poly I·C.

Effect on interferon activity. Mycoplasmas can also affect interferon activity. In these studies, a standard preparation of hamster interferon was assayed for activity in mycoplasma-free and mycoplasma-contaminated hamster cell cultures. Mycoplasma contamination decreased interferon activity four to eightfold, and rendered cell cultures less sensitive to exogenously supplied interferon. Therefore, mycoplasma contamination can affect the results of standard interferon assays.

Mycoplasma contamination might be used to advantage. Inhibition of interferon production and activity by mycoplasmas may be used to enhance virus yields and may play a useful role in the detection of latent viruses.

Conclusions. Several features of mycoplasma-cell interactions have been reviewed. The findings discussed indicate that mycoplasma contamination can alter a number of functions and activities of cell cultures. Consequently, the investigator must be aware of mycoplasma contamination and its effects on cell activity, and must maintain vigilant surveillance to detect mycoplasma contamination of cell cultures under investigation. Moreover, the investigator must provide information in published reports on procedures used and data obtained on the presence or absence of mycoplasmas in cell cultures used during the study in order that the reader might be able to properly interpret the results of study.

REFERENCES

1. Barile, M. F. 1973. Mycoplasma contamination of cell cultures: Mycoplasma-virus-cell culture interactions. In: J. Fogh (Ed.) *Contamination of Cell Cultures*. Academic Press, New York, NY, pp. 131-172.

2. Barile, M. F. 1977. Mycoplasma contamination of cell cultures: A status report. In: R. Action (Ed.) *Cell Culture and Its Application*. Academic Press, New York, NY.

3. Warren, J. 1942. Observations on some biological characteristics of organisms of the pleuropneumonia group. J. Bacteriol. 43: 211-228.

4. Edward, D. G. ff. 1950. An investigation of the biological properties of organisms of the pleuropneumonia group, with suggestions regarding the identification of strains. J. Gen. Microbiol. 4: 311-329.

5. Adler, H. E. 1964. A comparison of some characteristics of *Mycoplasma mycoides* var. *mycoides* and *Mycoplasma gallisepticum*. Amer. J. Vet. Res. 25: 243-245.

6. O'Malley, J. P., Z. A. McGee, M. F. Barile and L. F. Barker. 1966. Identification of the A-1 agent as *Mycoplasma gallisepticum*. Proc. Nat. Acad. Sci. U. S. 56: 895-901.

7. Cherry, J. D. and D. Taylor-Robinson. 1970. Peroxide production by mycoplasmas in chicken tracheal organ cultures. Nature 228: 1099-1100.

8. Aluotto, B. B., R. B. Wittler, C. O. Williams and J. E. Faber. 1970. Standardized bacteriological techniques for the characterization of mycoplasma species. Int. J. Syst. Bact. 20: 35-58.

9. Somerson, N. L., D. Taylor-Robinson, and R. M. Chanock. 1963. Hemolysin production as an aid in the identification and quantitation of Eaton agent (*Mycoplasma pneumoniae*). Amer. J. Hyg. 77: 122-128.

10. Clyde, W. A., Jr. 1963. Hemolysis in identifying Eaton's PPLO. Science. 139: 55.

11. Cohen, G., and N. L. Somerson. 1967. *Mycoplasma pneumoniae*: Hydrogen peroxide secretion and its possible role in virulence. Ann. N. Y. Acad. Sci. 143: 85-87.

12. Somerson, N. L., R. H. Purcell, D. Taylor-Robinson, and R. M. Chanock. 1965. Hemolysin of *Mycoplasma pneumoniae*. J. Bacteriol. 89: 813-818.

13. Cole, B. D., J. R. Ward, and C. H. Martin. 1968. Hemolysin and peroxide activity of *Mycoplasma* species. J. Bacteriol. 95: 2022-2030.

14. Manchee, R. J., and D. Taylor-Robinson. 1968. Hemadsorption and hemagglutination by mycoplasmas. J. Gen. Microbiol. 50: 465-478.

15. DelGuidice, R. A., and R. Pavia. 1964. Hemadsorption by *Mycoplasma pneumoniae* and its inhibition with sera from patients with atypical pneumonia. Bact. Proc. p. 71.

16. Van Herick, W., and M. D. Eaton. 1945. An unidentified pleuro-pneumonia-like organism isolated during passages in chick embryos. J. Bacteriol. 50: 47-55.

17. Tully, J. G., and S. Razin. 1977. "Mycoplasmas and ureaplasmas", in *Handbook of Microbiology*, Chemical Rubber Co., Cleveland, Ohio.

18. Lennette, E. H., and N. H. Schmidt. 1969. (Ed.). In *Diagnostic Procedures* for Viral and Rickettsial Infections. American Public Health Assoc., Inc. N.Y.

19. Gesner, B., and L. Thomas. 1966. Sialic acid binding sites: role in hemagglutination by *Mycoplasma gallisepticum*. Science 151: 590-591.

20. Manchee, R. J., and D. Taylor-Robinson. 1969. Utilization of neuraminic acid receptors by mycoplasmas. J. Bacteriol. 98: 914-919.

21. Manchee, R. J., and D. Taylor-Robinson. 1969. Studies on the nature of receptors involved in attachment of tissue culture cells to mycoplasmas. Brit. J. Exp. Pathol. 50: 66-75.

22. Zucker-Franklin, D., M. Davidson, and L. Thomas. 1966. The interaction of mycoplasmas with mammalian cells. I. HeLa cells, neutrophils and eosinophils. J. Exp. Med. 124: 521-532.

23. Zucker-Franklin, D., M. Davidson, and L. Thomas. 1966. The interaction of mycoplasmas with mammalian cells. II. Mono-cytes and lymphocytes. J. Exp. Med. 124: 533-542.

24. Biberfeld, G., and P. Biberfeld. 1970. Ultrastructural features of *Mycoplasma pneumoniae*. J. Bacteriol. 102: 855-861.

25. Collier, Am. M., and W. A. Clyde, Jr. 1971. Relationship between *M. pneumoniae* and human respiratory epithelium. Infec. Immunity 3: 694-701.

26. Collier, A. M. 1972. Pathogenesis of *M. pneumoniae* infection as studied in the human fetal trachea in organ culture. In: *A Ciba Foundation Symposium on Pathogenic Mycoplasma*. Elsevier, Amsterdam.

27. Clyde, W. A., Jr. 1961. Demonstration of Eaton's agent in tissue culture. Proc. Soc. Exp. Biol. Med. 107: 715-718.

28. Clyde, W. A., Jr. 1963. Studies on growth of Eaton's agent in tissue culture. Proc. Soc. Exp. Biol. Med. 112: 905-909.

29. Marmion, B. P., and G. M. Goodburn. 1961. Effect of organic gold salts on Eaton's primary atypical pneumonia agent and other observations. Nature 189: 247-248.

30. Goodburn, G. M., and B. P. Marmion. 1962. A study of the properties of Eaton's primary atypical pneumonia organism. J. Gen. Microbiol. 29: 271-290.

31. Eaton, M. D., A. E. Farnham, J. D. Levinthal, and A. R. Scala. 1962. Cytopathic effect of the atypical pneumonia organism in cultures of human tissues. J. Bacteriol. 84: 1330-1337.

32. Carski, T. R., and M. C. Shepard. 1961. Pleuropneumonia-like (mycoplasma) infections of tissue cultures. J. Bacteriol. 81: 626-635.

33. Barile, M. F., W. F. Malizia, and D. B. Riggs. 1962. Incidence and detection of pleuropneumonia-like organisms in cell cultures by fluorescent antibody and culture procedures. J. Bacteriol. 84: 130-136.

34. Fogh, J., N. B. Holmgren, and P. O. Ludovici. 1971. A review of cell culture contamination. In Vitro 7: 26-41.

35. Anderson, D. R. 1969. Ultrastructural Studies of Mycoplasmas and the L-Phase of Bacteria. In: L. Hayflick (Ed.) *The Mycoplasmatales and the L-Phase of Bacteria*. Appleton, NY pp. 365-402.

36. Collier, A. M., W. A. Clyde, Jr., and F. W. Denny. 1969. Biologic effects of *Mycoplasma pneumoniae* and other mycoplasmas from man on hamster tracheal organ culture. Proc. Soc. Exp. Biol. Med. 132: 1153-1158.

37. Collier, A. M., W. A. Clyde, Jr., and F. W. Denny. 1971. *Mycoplasma pneumoniae* in hamster tracheal organ culture: Immunofluorescent and electron microscopic studies. Proc. Soc. Exp. Biol. Med. 136: 569-573.

38. Cherry, J. D., and D. Taylor-Robinson. 1970. Large quantity production of chicken embryo tracheal organ cultures and use in virus and mycoplasma studies. Appl. Microbiol. 19: 658-662.

39. Cherry, J. D., and D. Taylor-Robinson. 1970. Growth and pathogenesis of *M. mycoides* var. *capri* in chicken embryo tracheal organ cultures. Infec. Immunity 2: 431-438.

40. Butler, M., and W. J. Ellaway. 1971. Growth and cytopathogenicity of mycoplasmas in human and chicken tracheal explants. J. Comp. Pathol. 81: 359-364.

41. Liu, C. 1957. Studies on primary atypical pneumonia. 1. Localization, isolation and cultivation of virus in chick embryos. J. Exp. Med. 106: 455.

42. Richter, C. B. 1970. Application of infectious agents to the study of lung cancer: Studies on the etiology and morphogenesis of metaplastic lung lesions in mice. In: P. Nellesheim, M. G. Hanna, Jr., and J. W. Deatherage, Jr. (Eds.) *Morphology of Experimental Respiratory Carcinogenesis*. USAEC Symposium Series 21. pp. 365-382.

43. Taylor-Robinson, D., and F. E. Carney. 1974. Growth and effect of mycoplasmas in fallopian tube organ cultures. Brit. J. Vener. Dis. 50: 212-216.

44. Taylor-Robinson, D., and R. J. Manchee. 1967. Spermadsorption and spermagglutination by mycoplasmas. Nature 215: 484-487.

45. Gnarpe, H., and J. Friberg. 1973. T-mycoplasmas as possible cause for reproductive failure. Nature 242: 120-121.

46. Gnarpe, H., and J. Friberg. 1972. Mycoplasmas and human reproductive failures. Amer. J. Obstet. Gyn. 114: 727-731.

47. Peterson, O. L., T. H. Ham, and M. Finland. 1943. Cold agglutinins (autohemagglutinins) in primary atypical pneumonia. Science 97: 167-168.

48. Finland, M., O. L. Peterson, H. E. Samper, and M. W. Barnes. 1945. Cold agglutinins. II. Cold isohemagglutinins in primary atypical pneumonia of unknown etiology with a note on the occurrence of hemolytic anemia in these cases. J. Clin. Invest. 24: 454-473.

49. Thomas, L., E. C. Curnen, G. S. Mirick, J. E. Ziegler, and F. L. Horsefall. 1943. Complement fixation with dissimilar antigens in primary atypical pneumonia. Proc. Soc. Exp. Biol. Med. 52: 121-125.

50. Thomas, L. 1964. Circulating autoantibodies and human disease. With a note on primary atypical pneumonia. New Engl. J. Med. 270: 1157-1159.

51. Biberfeld, G. 1971. Antibodies to brain and other tissues in cases of *Mycoplasma pneumoniae* infection. Clin. Exp. Immunol. 8: 319-333.

52. Finland, M., B. A. Samper, and M. W. Barnes. 1945. Cold agglutinins. VI. Agglutinins for an indifferent streptococcus in primary atypical pneumonia and in other conditions and their relation to cold isohemagglutinins. J. Clin. Invest. 24: 497-502.

53. Thomas, L., G. S. Mirick, E. C. Curnen, J. E. Ziegler, and F. L. Horsefall. 1945. Studies on primary atypical pneumonia. II. Observations concerning the relationship of a non-hemolytic streptococcus to the disease. J. Clin. Invest. 24: 227-240.

54. Marmion, B. P. 1967. The Mycoplasmas. New information on their properties and their pathogenicity for man. In: Waterson, A. P. (Ed.) *Recent Advances in Medical Microbiology.* J. and A. Churchill Ltd. London. pp. 170-250.

55. Biberfeld, G. 1971. Immunological, epidemiological and ultrastructural studies of *Mycoplasma pneumoniae.* Tryckeri Balder AB, Stockholm.

56. Feize, T., D. Taylor-Robinson, M. D. Shields, and R. A. Carter. 1969. Production of cold agglutinins in rabbits immunized with human erythrocytes treated with *Mycoplasma pneumoniae.* Nature 222: 1253-1256.

57. Barile, M. F., and B. G. Leventhal. 1968. Possible mechanism for mycoplasma inhibition of lymphocyte transformation induced by phytohemagglutinin. Nature 219: 751.

58. Singer, S. M., M. F. Barile, and R. L. Kirschstein. 1973.
    Mixed mycoplasma-virus infections in cell cultures. Ann.
    N. Y. Acad. Sci. 225: 304-310.
59. Ebke, J., and E. Kuwert. 1972. Nachweis von Mykoplasma orale
    Typ 1 in Gewebekulturen mit der Akridinorange-Farbüng.
    [detection of *Mycoplasma orale* type 1 in tissue cultures by
    means of acridine orange.] Zentralbl. Bakt. Parasit. Infekt.
    221: 87-93.
60. Fogh, J., and H. Fogh. 1964. A method for direct demonstration
    of pleuropneumonia-like organisms in cultured (human amnion)
    cells. Proc. Soc. Exp. Biol. Med. 119: 233-238.
61. Hopps, H. E., B. C. Meyer, M. F. Barile, and R. A. DelGiudice.
    1973. Problems concerning "non-cultivable" mycoplasma
    contaminants in tissue cultures. Ann. N. Y. Acad. Sci.
    225: 265-276.
62. Chen, T. R. 1977. In situ detection of mycoplasma contamin-
    ation in cell cultures by fluorescent Hoechst 33258 stain.
    Exp. Cell Res. 104: 255-262.
63. Barile, M. F., and R. T. Schimke. 1963. A rapid chemical
    method for detecting PPLO contamination of tissue cell
    cultures. Proc. Soc. Exp. Biol. Med. 114: 676-679.
64. Levine, E. M. 1974. A simplified method for the detection
    of mycoplasmas. Methods Cell Biol. 8: 229-248.
65. Todaro, G. J., S. A. Aaronson, and E. Rands. 1971. Rapid
    detection of mycoplasma-infected cell cultures. Exp. Cell
    Res. 65: 256-257.
66. Russell, W. C., C. Newman, and D. H. Williamson. 1975. A
    simple cytochemical technique for demonstration of DNA in
    cells infected with mycoplasmas and viruses. Nature 253:
    461-462.
67. Stanbridge, E. 1971. Mycoplasmas and cell cultures. Bact.
    Reviews 35: 206-227.
68. Manischewitz, J. E., B. G. Young, and M. F. Barile. 1975.
    The effect of mycoplasmas on replication and plaquing ability
    of Herpes simplex virus. Proc. Soc. Exp. Biol. Med. 148:
    859-863.
69. Barile, M. F., and R. A. DelGiudice. 1972. Isolation of
    mycoplasmas and their rapid identification by plate epi-
    immunofluorescence. In: *A Ciba Foundation Symposium on
    Pathogenic Mycoplasma*. Elsevier, Amsterdam.
    pp. 165-186.
70. Kaklamanis, E., and M. Pavlatos. 1972. The immunosuppressive
    effect of mycoplasma infection. I. Effect on the humoral
    and cellular response. Immunology 22: 695-702.
71. Barile, M. F. 1967. Mycoplasma and leukemia. Ann. N. Y.
    Acad. Sci. 143: 557-572.

GENETIC EFFECTS OF MYCOPLASMA

Warren W. Nichols

Institute for Medical Research
Camden, N. J. 08103

In this paper I'll summarize the effects and the apparent effects of mycoplasma on chromosomes and genes. The best known genetic effects of mycoplasma are on chromosomes. This was first reported by Fogh and Fogh in 1965 (1). In this report chromosomes of the FL/amnion line had been followed for 9 years without appreciable change in number. When the cells were infected with mycoplasma there was a reduction in chromosome number and a rise in chromosome aberrations. The chromosome number gradually decreased from a range of 70-76 to 63-68. Chromosome aberrations included open breaks and stable and unstable rearrangements. These started during the first days after infection and developed slowly in mycoplasma-infected cultures. In subsequent work (2,3) it was demonstrated that after elimination of mycoplasma by aureomycin treatment the reduced chromosome number and stable rearrangements persisted, but unstable aberrations were reduced to pre-infection levels.

At approximately the same time Paton et al. (4) reported that *Mycoplasma orale* infection of human diploid fibroblasts increased the number of polyploid cells and the amount of chromosome breakage and rearrangement. These abnormalities were usually seen in 3 to 5 times the frequency of control cultures.

In our own laboratory, Dr. Aula (5) tested the effect of three mycoplasma strains: *M. salivarium, M. hominis type 2,* and *M. fermentans,* on human leukocyte cultures. When 10^6 CFU (colony forming units) were used mitotic inhibition was so severe that chromosomal analysis was impossible with the first two strains and somewhat less severe with *M. fermentans*. When 10^3 CFU were used no effect on the mitotic index was noticed and chromosome analysis

could be carried out. After three days of culture, the usual duration of lymphocyte culture for chromosome preparations, no abnormalities over control levels were noticed. However at five days
after initiation of culture the cells infected with *M. salivarium*
exhibited a 3-fold increase in chromosome abnormalities (5.6% to
18%). Since *M. salivarium* is a strain known to possess arginine
deaminase activity, the role of mycoplasma-induced arginine deficiency in the observed mitotic inhibition and chromosome breakage
was evaluated in cultures with 10^6 CFU *M. salivarium* and a
3-fold increase of arginine in the medium (up to 2 mM). Under these
conditions no mitotic inhibition was seen at 3 days, but by 5 days
of culture, although there was some increase in mitosis seen, the
number of mitotic figures was quite reduced when compared to
controls. The breakage frequency observed in cultures that had been
infected with 10^3 CFU in the presence of added arginine was the
same as control cultures in contrast to the 3-fold increase in
breakage observed in the absence of added arginine (Table 1).

The role of arginine depletion in the production of mitotic
inhibition and breakage was also studied by growing uninfected
leukocytes in an arginine-poor environment. Only arginine contained
in the serum was present and this amounted to between 0.4% and 1%
of the amount in control cultures. These cultures exhibited mitotic
inhibition and breakage equivalent to that seen with mycoplasma.
Shortly after that, Freed and Schatz (6) showed that cells deprived
of any essential amino acid exhibited mitotic inhibition and chromosome breakage. Some strains that don't produce an arginine decrease
and still break chromosomes may reduce another essential amino acid
(8). It is also known that deprivation of essential amino acids
leads to inhibition of DNA synthesis, and that although some strains
of mycoplasma do not deplete arginine, all strains do require
nucleic acid precursors for growth. There is morphologic similarity
between chromosome breakage produced by mycoplasma and by the
inhibitors of DNA synthesis. On the basis of this a common mechanism
or alternate mechanism may be the inhibition of DNA synthesis (4, 6,
13).

Several mycoplasma strains including the T strains now have
been reported to produce chromosome abnormalities (7,8,9,10),
although predominant types of abnormalities have varied somewhat.
Treatment of cultures with antibiotics that reduce the number of
mycoplasma reduces the chromosome damage (7), but dead mycoplasma
in large numbers exhibit at least mitotic inhibition (5, 9).

In one instance (11), the presence of mycoplasma was believed
to be the cause of a Robertsonian fusion of mouse chromosomes that
resulted in metacentric chromosome formation rather than the usual
mouse chromosome structure with a terminal centromere. Increased
chromosome abnormalities have also been found in amniotic fluid
cell cultures contaminated with mycoplasma (12) and the hazard of
incorrect prenatal diagnosis has been made.

Table 1

THE EFFECT OF ARGININE ON THE CHROMOSOME BREAKAGE CAUSED BY *M. SALIVARIUM* IN HUMAN LEUKOCYTES CULTURED FOR FIVE DAYS*

Inoculum		% of cells with breaks+		
		M.saliv. 10^3 CFU	*M.saliv.* 10^3 CFU + arginine 2 mM	Control
Exp.	I	17	ND	4
	II	22	6	4
	III	14	6	6
	IV	20	4	8
	V	17	8	6
Mean		18.0	6.0	5.6

+ Approximately 50 cells analyzed in each experiment

* From Aula, P. and Nichols, W.W., 1967 (5)

There is no direct evidence that mycoplasma can induce gene mutations in infected cells. However the high correlation observed between chromosome breakage and gene mutations would lead one to suspect that gene mutation induction by mycoplasma would be an excellent possibility. Whether or not mycoplasma produce gene mutations, it is clear that mycoplasma can interfere with the detection of gene mutations in somatic cell systems that depend on nucleoside pathways for selective methods. The presence of myco-plasma as a contaminant can prevent cells from utilizing a deoxy-riboside or its analogue by virtue of a nucleoside phosphorylase that breaks a deoxyriboside down to its free base which is taken up poorly by mammalian cells. That this interference occurred was first demonstrated by Nardone et al. (14) using autoradiography. The effects of this on a specific locus mutation system have been discussed by Clive et al. (15). These workers utilize mouse lymphoma cells that are heterozygous at the thymidine kinase locus (TK+/-). This system can be used to select for both forward and and reverse mutations. In the first case after treatment with a mutagen the cells are grown in the presence of BrdU. Mutated cells

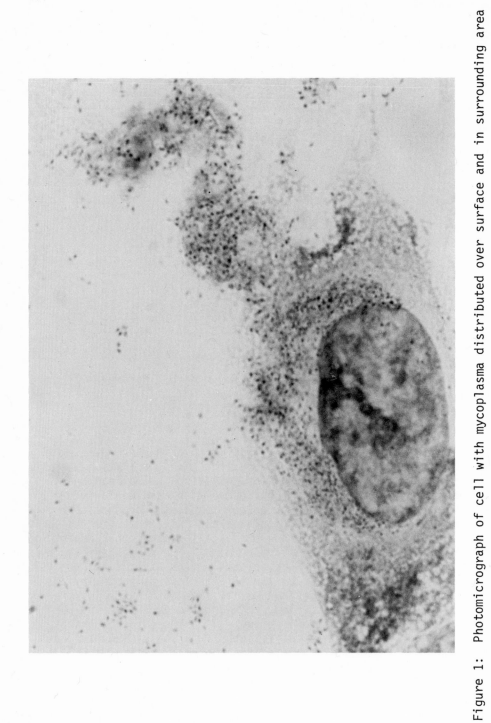

Figure 1: Photomicrograph of cell with mycoplasma distributed over surface and in surrounding area

that have lost the TK+ gene do not incorporate BrdU and are resistant, while the non-mutated cells take up BrdU and are killed
under the conditions of the experiment. In the presence of
mycoplasma the BrdU is not incorporated so all cells act like
mutants. Similarly, a population of TK -/- cells can be treated
with a mutagen and then selection made for back mutations to the
TK +/- state by growing the cells in selective medium containing
thymidine, hypoxanthine, and an antifolic acid compound (metho-
trexate) that prevents de novo cellular synthesis of pyrimidine and
purines. Only cells that can take up the exogenous pyrimidine can
survive. Mycoplasma prevents this and thus prevents this selection
too. Similarly, hypoxanthine phosphoribosyl transferase enzyme
(HGPRT) present in mycoplasma can be supplied to HGPRT-deficient
cells that are mycoplasma infected and interfere with selective
methods using this system.

In conclusion it should also be pointed out that cytogenetic
preparations can be used as one method of becoming suspicious that
a mycoplasma contamination has occurred. Fogh and Fogh (16) first
reported this in 1964. Cells stained for cytogenetic preparations
reveal heavy mycoplasma infections as small stained dots over the
cell surface (Fig. 1).

In summary, many strains of mycoplasma have been shown to be
capable of altering chromosome structure and number. The high
correlation between induced chromosome abnormalities and induced
gene mutations seen with chemical and physical agents make the
possibility of induced gene mutations by this biologic agent a
real one although no evidence for this currently exists. It has
been observed that tissue culture selective test systems for the
detection of gene mutations can be altered by the effects of
mycoplasma or cellular nucleoside chemistry.

References

1. Fogh, J. and Fogh, H. Chromosome changes in PPLO-infected FL human amnion cells. Proc. Soc. Exptl. Biol. Med. 119: 233-238, 1965.

2. Fogh, J. and Fogh, H. Karyotypic changes in mycoplasma-modified lines of FL human amnion cells. Proc. Soc. Exptl. Biol. Med. 129:944-950, 1968.

3. Fogh, J. and Fogh, H. Irreversibility of major chromosome changes in a mycoplasma-modified line of FL human amnion cells. Proc. Soc. Exptl. Biol. Med. 126:67-74, 1967.

4. Paton, G.R., Jacobs, J.P. and Perkins, F.T. Chromosome changes in human diploid cell cultures infected with mycoplasma. Nature 207:43-45, 1965.

5. Aula, P. and Nichols, W.W. The cytogenetic effects of mycoplasma in human leukocyte cultures. Jrl. Cell. Physiol. 70:281-290, 1967.

6. Freed, J.J. and Schatz, S.A. Chromosome aberrations in cultured cells deprived of single essential amino acids. Exptl. Cell Res. 55:393-409, 1969.

7. Stanbridge, E., Önen, M., Perkins, F.T. and Hayflick, L. Karyological and morphological characteristics of human diploid cell strain WI-38 infected with mycoplasma. Exptl. Cell Res. 57:397-410, 1969.

8. Kundsin, R.B., Ampola, M., Streeter, S. and Neurath, P. Chromosomal aberrations induced by T strain mycoplasmas. Jrl. Med. Genetics 8:181-187, 1971.

9. Copperman, R. and Morton, H.E. Reversible inhibition of mitosis in lymphocyte cultures by non-viable mycoplasma. Proc. Soc. Exptl. Biol. Med. 123:790-795, 1966.

10. Paton, G., Jacobs, J.P. and Perkins, F.T. The effect of mycoplasma on the karyology of normal cells. Ann. N.Y. Acad. Sci. 143:626-627, 1967.

11. Kuz'mina, S.V. Action of mycoplasmas on the chromosomal apparatus of mouse fibroblasts in tissue culture. Soviet Genetics 8:126-127, 1972.

12. Schneider, E.L., Stanbridge, E.J., Epstein, C.J., Golbus, M., Abbo-Halbasch, G. and Rodgers, G. Mycoplasma contamination of cultured amniotic fluid cells: potential hazard to prenatal chromosomal diagnosis. Science 184:477-480, 1974.

13. Stanbridge, E. Mycoplasmas and cell cultures. Bacteriological Rev. 35:206-227, 1971.

14. Nardone, R.M., Todd, J., Gonzalez, P. and Gaffney, E.V. Nucleoside incorporation into strain L cells: inhibition by pleuropneumonia-like organisms. Science 139:1100-1101, 1965.

15. Clive, D., Flamm, W.G. and Patterson, J.B. Specific-locus mutational assay systems for mouse lymphoma cells. In: CHEMICAL MUTAGENS, Vol. 3, edt. A. Hollaender, pp. 79-103, Plenum Press, 1973.

16. Fogh, J. and Fogh, H. A method for direct demonstration of pleuropneumonia-like organisms in cultured cells. Proc. Soc. Exptl. Biol. Med. 117:809-901, 1964.

MYCOPLASMAS IN RELATION TO AMNIOCENTESIS

DAVID TAYLOR-ROBINSON

Clinical Research Centre

Watford Road, Harrow, Middlesex HA1 3UJ, England

The purpose of this communication is to consider whether
mycoplasmas infect amniotic fluid, and, if so, the circumstances
under which infection occurs. Attention is drawn also to the
consequent effects of such infection both clinically and on cells
that are cultured from amniotic fluid that has been withdrawn by
amniocentesis.

Amniocentesis is a procedure in which a trochar and cannula
are inserted into the intrauterine amniotic sac and amniotic
fluid is withdrawn. It is carried out transabdominally or, rarely,
via the vaginal route and principally at (i) 14-20 weeks of
gestation for biochemical and particularly for cytogenetic studies,
and (ii) some time after 36 weeks when the main concern is the
maturity of the baby, which can be determined by assessing the
lecithin/sphingomyelin ratio, electrolytes and creatinine, and
the proportion of desquamated foetal cells which contain fat.
It is less usual for cytogenetic studies to be done at this late
time.

MYCOPLASMA FLORA OF THE HUMAN UROGENITAL TRACT

The mycoplasmas found in the human urogenital tract, of
both men and women, comprise M. fermentans, M. hominis and various
serotypes of Ureaplasma urealyticum (1). M. fermentans probably
constitutes about 1% only of all isolations. On the other hand,
M. hominis and U. urealyticum strains are often found, the latter
more frequently than the former. The occurrence of both microorganisms seems to be related, at least partially, to sexual

159

activity. Thus, as pointed out previously (2), isolations from
the female genital tract are made hardly ever in the case of nuns,
rarely before puberty, infrequently after the menopause, but very
frequently during the child-bearing years. In addition, greater
rates of isolation have been recorded in pregnant women than in
non-pregnant women (2,3), a point particularly relevant to the
present discussion.

PATHOGENICITY OF UROGENITAL MYCOPLASMAS

Some of the evidence which incriminates mycoplasmas found
in the urogenital tract as being actually or potentially
pathogenic is presented in Table 1. The undoubted pathogenicity
under certain circumstances of M. hominis and the ureaplasmas
clearly suggests that if they are present in amniotic fluid
then they have the capacity to damage the foetus or cause changes
in foetal cells. The question of whether mycoplasmas gain access
to amniotic fluid is obviously an important one.

Table 1.   Evidence that Urogenital Mycoplasmas are
Actually or Potentially Pathogenic

(a) M. hominis

(i) Sore throats in inoculated volunteers (4)

(ii) Puerperal fever (5,6)

(iii) Salpingitis ? (7)

(b) Ureaplasmas

Experimentally :

(i) Bovine strains produce pneumonia and mastitis
in cattle (8,9)

(ii) Human strains produce mastitis in goats (10)

(iii) Bovine and human strains produce mastitis in mice (11)

(iv) Human strains produce urethritis in men (12)

Table 2. Evidence that Mycoplasmas Infect Amniotic Fluid

Ref.	Gest-ation	Site tested	Membranes ruptured	No. cases	No. isol.	Mycoplasma
13	Term	Uterine cavity	YES	1	1	M. hominis
14	Term	Amniotic fluid	YES	1	1	M. hominis
15	Term	Amniocentesis	YES	6	1	M. hominis
	14-20 wks.	"	NO	44	3	M. hominis
16	Term	Amniotic side of placenta	YES	7	7	(M. hominis (2) (Ureaplasmas (5)
			?	113	0	
17	4 wks. prem.	Amniotic fluid	NO	1	1	Ureaplasma
18	Term	Placental membranes	YES	2	2	Ureaplasma
19	Term	Endometrium	YES	39	21 }	Mainly
		"	NO	40	8 }	ureaplasmas
20	14-20 wks.	Amniocentesis	NO	10	0	
21	Term	Placenta	YES	79	24 }	Mainly
		"	NO	44	4 }	ureaplasmas
22	Term	Amniocentesis	?	185	0	

MYCOPLASMA INFECTION OF AMNIOTIC FLUID

Evidence that mycoplasmas infect the amniotic cavity under certain conditions is presented in Table 2. Not all specimens were obtained by amniocentesis and where they were not, data on specimens obtained at Caesarian section only is recorded. Thus, mycoplasmal isolations which have been made from the products of conception are not due to their vaginal contamination. The main points which may be drawn from these data are (i) M. hominis strains and ureaplasmas have been found in amniotic fluid, the latter organisms more frequently than the former, (ii) both sorts of microorganism are most likely to be isolated after rupture of the membranes; the longer the interval since membrane rupture the more likely the chance of placental or amniotic fluid contamination (16). Furthermore, there is a greater chance of isolation being made following previous vaginal examination and prolonged labour (21), (iii) mycoplasmas are sometimes found in amniotic fluid even when the membranes are intact, and (iv) they are present probably less frequently in early than in late pregnancy, but there are insufficient data on this point. Finally, (v) culture of fluids obtained by the amniocentesis procedure has been carried out insufficiently to enable the precise frequency of mycoplasmal infection of amniotic fluid to be determined.

The fact that mycoplasmas, under certain conditions, may gain access to the amniotic cavity means that potentially they are able to cause certain pregnancy-related conditions, and contaminate amniocentesis cell cultures.

ASSOCIATION OF MYCOPLASMAS WITH PREGNANCY-RELATED CONDITIONS

Several clinical problems might arise as a result of mycoplasmal infection of amniotic fluid. For example, Shurin et al. (23) have isolated ureaplasmas, but not M. hominis, more frequently from cases of histologically severe chorioamnionitis than from those which were less severe or from those without disease and they and others (17) have suggested that chorio-amnionitis might be due to ureaplasmal infection. The evidence is indeed suggestive, but not conclusive. Ureaplasmas might also cause spontaneous abortion and there is a definite association between the occurrence of abortion and the presence of ureaplasmas in the cervix (24,25). However, the problem is whether the ureaplasmas invade the foetus and cause its death so that abortion ensues or whether the foetus dies for some other reason and is then invaded by the organisms. This is a difficult and contentious problem and not one that is particularly germane to the present discussion.

INFECTION OF AMNIOCENTESIS CELL CULTURES

From the preceding it is clear that there is far less chance of mycoplasmas gaining access to amniotic fluids at 14-20 weeks of gestation, and therefore being carried over into cell cultures derived from cells in the fluids, than there is of their gaining access closer to term. Since most cytogenetic studies are done on amnion cell cultures derived from early fluids this is an important consideration. If ureaplasmas do contaminate amniotic fluids it is possible that they might persist in cultures of cells derived from the fluids because Masover et al.(26) established a persistent infection of human fibroblast cell cultures by first treating the organisms with trypsin. However, such success in vitro is unusual and, indeed, Mazzali and Taylor-Robinson (27) found it impossible to set up a chronic infection of cell cultures simply because the growth cycle of the ureaplasmas was shorter than that of the cells so that when these were subcultured, viable ureaplasmas were not carried over.

On the other hand, although M. hominis is less likely than the ureaplasmas to contaminate amniotic fluid, theoretically it is more likely to persist in cell cultures. This is because the rate of decay of M. hominis organisms is slow so that viable organisms may be transferred when cells are subcultured. Because several subcultures may be necessary to establish sufficient cells for cytogenetic studies, the greatest danger must come from mycoplasmas which are given an opportunity to gain access during manipulation of the cells. In other words, not mycoplasmas in the genital tract of the mother, but those in the mouth of the operator, in other cell cultures and in the cell culture medium components. That such contamination of amnion cell cultures may occur has been clearly demonstrated (20) and since the organisms are capable of producing a variety of chromosomal abberations (Table 3), considerable confusion may arise in interpreting the results of chromosomal analyses.

Table 3. Mycoplasmal Contamination as a Cause of
Abnormal Chromosomes in Cultured Cells

Reference	Cell	Mycoplasma
28,29	FL human amnion	M. fermentans
30	WI-38 human lung	M. orale
31	WI-38 human lung	M. hominis
32	WI-38 human lung	M. fermentans
33	Human leucocytes	M. salivarium
34	WI-38 human lung	M. hyorhinis, M. orale M. pulmonis, A. laidlawii
35	Human lymphocytes	Ureaplasmas (human genital)

The foregoing leads to two conclusions. First, since most mycoplasmal contamination of amniocentesis cell cultures is likely to originate from sources other than the mother, it ought to be preventable. This means constant vigilance of the technique of handling cells, of the cell culture medium components, and of other factors that are needed to prevent infection (36). Second, preventive measures are apt to breakdown at some time and because mycoplasmas from the mother, M. hominis in particular, are occasionally going to persist in the cell cultures, the best mycoplasmal detection system is required : the best because a decision whether or not to perform an abortion may depend on the result. What is best is unknown at the present time, but in view of the existence of "non-cultivable" mycoplasmas (37) it would seem prudent to use one of the non-cultural methods along with the cultural techniques in the detection system.

REFERENCES

1. Taylor-Robinson, D. (1976). In: Scientific Foundations of Urology. Williams, D.I. and Chisholm, G.D. Eds. Vol. 1. Heinemann, London, pp. 223-227.
2. Taylor-Robinson, D. and Furr, P.M. (1973). Ann. N.Y. Acad. Sci. 225, 108-117.
3. Mårdh, P.-A. and Weström, L. (1970). Acta Path. Microbiol. Scand. 78, 367-374.
4. Mufson, M.A., Ludwig, W.M., Purcell, R.H., Cate, T.R., Taylor-Robinson, D. and Chanock, R.M. (1965). J. Amer. Med. Assoc. 192, 1146-1152.
5. Tully, J.G., Brown, M.S., Sheagren, J.N., Young, V.M. and Wolff, S.M. (1965). New Eng. J. Med. 273, 648-650.
6. Harwick, H.J., Purcell, R.H., Iuppa, J.B. and Fekety, F.R. (1971). Obstet. Gynecol. 37, 765-768.
7. Mårdh, P.-A. and Weström, L. (1970). Brit. J. Vener. Dis. 46, 179-186.
8. Howard, C.J., Gourlay, R.N. and Brownlie, J. (1973). J. Hyg., Camb. 71, 163-170.
9. Howard, C.J., Gourlay, R.N., Thomas, L.H. and Stott, E.J. (1976). Res. Vet. Sci. 21, 227-231.
10. Gourlay, R.N., Brownlie, J. and Howard, C.J. (1973). J. Gen. Microbiol. 76, 251-254.
11. Howard, C.J., Anderson, J.C., Gourlay, R.N. and Taylor-Robinson, D. (1975). J. Med. Microbiol. 8, 523-529.
12. Taylor-Robinson, D., Csonka, G.W. and Prentice, M.J. (1977). Quart. J. Med. In press.
13. Jones, D.M. (1967). J. Clin. Path. 20, 633-635.
14. Brunell, P.A., Dische, R.M. and Walker, M.B. (1969). J. Amer. Med. Assoc. 207, 2097-2099.

15. Harwick, H.J., Iuppa, J.B. and Fekety, F.R. (1969). Obstet. Gynecol. 33, 256-259.
16. Jones, D.M. and Tobin, B. (1969). J. Med. Microbiol. 2, 347-352.
17. Caspi, E., Herczeg, E., Solomon, F. and Sompolinsky, D. (1971). Amer. J. Obstet. Gynecol. 111, 1102-1106.
18. Solomon, F., Caspi, E., Bukovsky, I. and Sompolinsky, D. (1973). Amer. J. Obstet. Gynecol. 116, 785-792.
19. Lamey, J.R., Foy, H.M. and Kenny, G.E. (1974). Obstet. Gynecol. 44, 703-708.
20. Schneider, E.L., Stanbridge, E.J., Epstein, C.J., Golbus, M., Abbo-Halbasch, G. and Rodgers, G. (1974). Science 184, 477-480.
21. Caspi, E., Solomon, F., Langer, R. and Sompolinsky, D. (1976). Obstet. Gynecol. 48, 682-684.
22. Weissenbacher, E.-R., Bredt, W., Jonatha, W. and Zahn, V. (1976). Proc. Soc. Gen. Microbiol. iii (4), 145.
23. Shurin, P.A., Alpert, S., Rosner, B., Driscoll, S.G., Lee, Y.-H., McCormack, W., Santamarina, B.A.G. and Kass, E.H. (1975). New Eng. J. Med. 293, 5-8.
24. Kundsin, R.B. and Driscoll, S.G. (1970). Ann. N.Y. Acad. Sci. 174, 794-797.
25. Caspi, E., Solomon, F. and Sompolinsky, D. (1972). Israel J. Med. Sci. 8, 122-127.
26. Masover, G.K., Palant, M., Zerrudo, Z. and Hayflick, L. (1977). In: Nongonococcal Urethritis and Related Oculogenital. Infections. Holmes, K.K. and Hobson, D. Eds. Washington, D.C. In press.
27. Mazzali, R. and Taylor-Robinson, D. (1971). J. Med. Microbiol. 4, 125-138.
28. Fogh, J. and Fogh, H. (1965). Proc. Soc. Exp. Biol. Med. 119, 233-238.
29. Fogh, J. and Fogh, H. (1973). Ann. N.Y. Acad. Sci. 225, 311-329.
30. Paton, G.R., Jacobs, J.P. and Perkins, F.T. (1965). Nature 207, 43-45.
31. Allison, A.C. and Paton, G.R. (1966). Lancet ii, 1229-1230.
32. Paton, G.R., Jacobs, J.P. and Perkins, F.T. (1967). Ann. N.Y. Acad. Sci. 143, 626-627.
33. Aula, P. and Nichols, W.W. (1967). J. Cell Physiol. 70, 281-289.
34. Stanbridge, E., Önen, M., Perkins, F.T. and Hayflick, L. (1969). Exp. Cell Res. 57, 397-410.
35. Kundsin, R.B., Ampola, M., Streeter, S. and Neurath, P. (1971). J. Med. Genet. 8, 181-187.
36. McGarrity, G.J. (1976). In Vitro 12, 643-647.
37. Hopps, H.E., Meyer, B.C., Barile, M.F. and DelGiudice, R.A. (1973). Ann. N.Y. Acad. Sci. 225, 265-276.

EFFECTS OF MYCOPLASMAS ON LYMPHOCYTE CELL CULTURES

Gerard J. McGarrity

Department of Microbiology

Institute for Medical Research
Camden, New Jersey

I. Introduction

The use of human lymphocyte cultures for cytogenetic studies
was reported by Chrustschoff and Berlin in 1935 (1).
Because of difficulties in propagation and maintenance of lymphocyte cell cultures, work was limited. Normal leukocytes do
not ordinarily divide in peripheral blood although some do have
mitotic potential. Early studies were designed to determine what
factors could activate this latent potential. Plasma concentration,
oxygen tension and carbon dioxide had only minor effects. In 1955,
Rigas and Osgood reported the characteristics of phytohemagglutinin
(PHA), a mitogen present in the red kidney bean, Phaseolus vulgaris
(2). This plant extract was originally used to agglutinate erythrocytes in obtaining leukocytes from whole blood, and was shown to
induce mitosis in leukocytes.

Nowell reported that the mitogenic action of PHA did not involve
mitosis per se but the stage preceding mitosis involving the alteration of circulating monocytes and large lymphocytes to a state
where they are capable of mitosis (3,4). PHA stimulation resulted
in a loss of polymorphonuclear leukocytes within 36 hours with concomitant emergence of lymphocytes as the predominant cell type.
Large undifferentiated, mononuclear lymphoblasts are predominant
by 48 hours post-stimulation (5). PHA stimulation facilitated
examination of leukocyte chromosomes (6). However, PHA stimulated
cultures generally die after a few cell divisions.

Henle et al reported that irradiated cultured cells from
Burkitt's lymphoma that contained Epstein Barr virus (EBV) induced
normal peripheral leukocytes to grow (7). EBV transforms B lymphocytes. Lymphocytes from donors with previous EBV infections can
be established in long term culture. Lymphocytes from donors sero-
negative for EBV do not routinely achieve autonomous growth, but can
do so after EBV infection in vitro. The EBV genome is present in
cultured lymphocytes although no virus particle may be detectable (8).

Human lymphocyte cultures offer several advantages: 1)blood
as a source of cells; 2)the clonal nature of lymphocyte cell lines;
3)the relative ease of growing kilogram lots of cells; 4)survival
of the donor phenotype and genotype in vitro; 5) maintenance
of the chromosomal complement; 6)maintenance of specialized
immunologic functions; and 7)propagation of these lines without
apparent senescence. Lymphocyte cultures have been widely
used in studies on leukemia and other tumors, hematology,
cytology, immunology, cytogenetics, lymphocytotoxicity, differentiation and genetic diseases. Moore has reviewed these and
other uses (9).

Because of the increased use of lymphocyte cultures and the
numerous reported and potential effects of mycoplasmal infection,
regular mycoplasmal assays by proven technics should be used. The
purpose of this report is to list the potential sources of
infection and summarize the known and potential effects of mycoplasmal infection on this type of cell culture. Mycoplasmas can be
present in the original blood specimen, potentially influence
transformation, and exert various effects on long term lymphocyte
cultures. These points are summarized in Table 1.

TABLE 1.   Factors re Mycoplasmas and Lymphocyte Cell Cultures

        I.   Blood Carriage of Mycoplasma

       II.   Effects on Transformation

      III.   Effects on Cell Growth

             1. overall growth rate

             2. biochemical changes

             3. surface changes

             4. chromosome damage

             5. leukemoid potential

             6. interferon production

II. Source of Infection

The source of infection can be media, technicians, the original specimen itself or other infected cell cultures (10,11). Original tissues used to establish primary cell cultures were not found to be a major source of mycoplasmal infection. Barile has shown that only 0.5-1.0% of cell culture mycoplasmas over a 14 year period could be traced to original tissues. (11, these proceedings).

The incidence of mycoplasmas in peripheral blood used to establish lymphocyte cultures could be higher than 1% under certain conditions. Humans are colonized by mycoplasmas in the throat (10,12) and urogenital tract (13). It has been demonstrated that mycoplasmas can be present in the blood, especially during immunosuppression caused by disease or therapy. Murphy et al reported the isolation of 71 different strains of mycoplasmas from 1,950 patients. Specimens yielding mycoplasmas included bone marrow (0.7%), peripheral blood (15%), erythrocytes (3%), leukocytes (4.8%) and plasma (3.4%). These samples were obtained from both leukemic and apparently normal individuals (14). These findings indicated these organisms were isolated most frequently from leukemic children at diagnosis or when disease was in relapse. Other studies have reported the isolation of mycoplasmas from the blood of leukemic and normal patients (15,16).

The possibility that mycoplasmas might be present in peripheral blood specimens used to establish long term lymphocyte cultures must be recognized. Lymphocyte cultures must be tested for mycoplasma as soon as possible, and should be handled separately from clean cultures to prevent spread of infection. Introduction of a single infected culture into a laboratory can result in secondary infection of other cultures (10).

III. Effects of Mycoplasmal Infection

1. Mycoplasma in original tissue specimen

Since mycoplasmas can be present in peripheral blood, they can influence attempts to culture lymphocytes. Possible effects of mycoplasmas in whole blood specimens include 1)transformation, 2)alteration in growth rate and 3)CPE and eventual death of the culture. Like other mycoplasma-cell culture interactions, the precise effect will depend on the mycoplasmal strain, the cell culture and its micro-environment. The physiologic and genetic nature of the donor can also influence the host-parasite equilibrium. The published effects of mycoplasmas on lymphocytes are summarized in Table 2.

TABLE 2. Reported Effects of Mycoplasmas on Lymphocytes

MYCOPLASMA SPECIES	EFFECT	REFERENCE
M. PULMONIS	TRANSFORMATION	GINSBURG AND NICOLET (17)
M. PNEUMONIAE		FERNALD (18)
M. HOMINIS	TRANSFORMATION INHIBITION	BARILE AND LEVENTHAL (22)
M. ORALE		
M. ARTHRIDITIS		
M. ARTHRIDITIS	INTERFERON INDUCTION	RINALDO ET AL (23-25)
M. PULMONIS		COLE ET AL (32)
A. LAIDLAWII		
M. PNEUMONIAE		
M. SYNOVIAE		
M. FERMENTANS	LEUKEMOID INDUCTION	PLATA ET AL (33)
M. HOMINIS	MITOSIS INHIBITION	COPPERMAN AND MORTON (36)
M. SALIVARIUM	CHROMOSOME DAMAGE	AULA AND NICHOLS (37)
UREAPLASMA SP.		KUNDSIN ET AL (38)

2. Transformation

Ginsburg and Nicolet reported that M. pulmonis transformed rat lymphocytes at a high efficiency, 85% blast cells being detected within four days (17). These workers raised the possibility that lymphocyte donors might have been sensitized to M. pulmonis. Such transformation would be specific, similar to tuberculin sensitivity. However, specificity may not be essential since lymphocytes from specific pathogen free rats were also transformed by M. pulmonis (17).

Fernald showed that human lymphocytes from subjects with circulating antibodies to M. pneumoniae were transformed by this organism (18). Transformation was within the range of reactivity achieved by PHA. Statistical significance was found between responses in subjects with documented infection and sero negative individuals. This confirmed earlier findings volunteers infected by intranasal inoculation of M. pneumoniae (19). Lymphocytes from these volunteers were transformed by specific antigen.

While M. pulmonis and M .pneumoniae are not frequent cell culture isolates, results of the above studies indicate that mycoplasmas in blood samples from sensitized donors can influence transformation. This is relevant because M. salivarium and especially M. orale have been isolated from human blood specimens and have been isolated from cell cultures (14,20). In our laboratory, M. orale type 1 accounted for approximately 35% of 325 mycoplasmas isolated from 3,872 cell cultures over a five year period (unpublished results).

Data are not available to determine if there are differences in the transformation process mediated by mycoplasmas and other agents. Epstein-Barr virus is necessary for the transformation of human lymphocytes into continuous cells lines. Such lines exhibit primarily B cell properties and have been shown by immunofluorescence and molecular hybridization to contain EBV. Mycoplasma transformed lymphocytes may cause transformation directly or may activate EBV. M. arginini infection of human lymphocytes reduced the content of EBV capsid antigen in one study (21). The levels of interferon and macrophage inhibition factor were also reduced in this study.

Lymphocyte transformation by mycoplasmas were achieved by M. pneumoniae, and M. pulmonis, both fermentative organisms. Transformation was not achieved with M. hominis, M. orale, and M. arthriditis, species that derive energy not from glucose fermentation but arginine utilization (22). In this study, Barile and Leventhal showed that arginine utilizing species of mycoplasmas inhibited PHA action. The inhibition could be blocked with the addition of excess arginine.

Therefore, two effects on lymphocyte transformation can
be possible with mycoplasma: lymphocyte transformation with
fermentative non-arginine utilizers (M. pneumoniae, M. pulmonis,
A. laidlawii) or inhibition of PHA stimulation by non-fermentative arginine utilizers (M. hyorhinis, M. arginini, M. hominis,
M. salivarium, M. orale.

3. Interferon Induction

Rinaldo and co-workers induced inferon production in ovine
leukocytes with several mycoplamal species (23,24). Included were
human species and species commonly isolated from cell cultures.
A. laidlawii, M. pneumoniae, M. arthriditis and M. pulmonis
induced interferon in mice after intraperitoneal inoculation (25).
These initial studies did not induce interferon in vitro in murine
spleen cells, peritoneal exudate cells or peripheral blood leukocyte
cultures. This is similar to agents such as tilorone hydrochloride
which effectively induces interferon in mice, but not in murine
cells in vitro (26,27). Endotoxin can also induce interferon
in vivo (28), but only in low or undetectable levels in vitro
(29,30). The kinetics of the interferon response to mycoplasmal
infection are similar to that observed with non-replicating
viral inducers of interferon in mice, and suggests a similar
mechanism (31).

Rinaldo et al tried to enhance the in vitro interferon
inducing capacity of mycoplasma by treatment with specific antisera and trypsin (25). Preinfection of the mycoplasmas with the
mycoplasma virus (MVL51) did not induce interferon in murine
cells. MVL51 alone had no effect (25).

Results of more recent studies showed that M. pneumoniae
and M. synoviae induced interferon production in ovine and human
lymphocytes in vitro (32). These workers demonstrated that the
lymphocyte, and not the polymorphonuclear leukocyte was the
active interferon inducer and suggested that additional lymphocyte functions could be influenced by mycoplasmas.

As mentioned above, mycoplasmas can also reduce the levels
of interferon production in lymphocytes (21). Cole et al have
mentioned a number of variables that could qualitatively and
quantitatively influence interferon production by mycoplasmas (32).

4. Leukemoid Induction

Plata et al reported that certain strains of M. fermentans
freshly isolated from patients could induce both lethal toxicity
and leukemoid disease in certain strains of mice (33). The
leukemoid response followed 3-6 daily i.p. injections of 10^8 -
10^9 colony forming units (CFU), and was characterized by

enlarged lymph nodes, hepatosplenomegaly and a peripheral
leukocyte count two to fives times higher than normal, primarily
consisting of mature and immature granulocytes. These results
suggested that freshly isolated strains of mycoplasma can
differ significantly from laboratory strains in their pathogenicity
for animals.

Leukemoid reactions are difficult to distinguish from
leukemia. There are several criteria. Granulocytes in leukemoid
reaction are significantly higher in alkaline phosphatase
than chronic granulocytic leukemia. The leukemoid potential
and lethal toxicity of certain strains of M. fermentans
are independent (34). It is uncertain whether a loss in humoral
or cell mediated immunity could be initiated by mycoplasma to
establish the disease. Biberfeld and Sterner have reported that
M. pneumoniae infection can cause a transient depression of
cell mediated immunity (35).

5. Mitosis Inhibition and Chromosome Damage

Copperman and Morton demonstrated inhibition of mitosis in
human lymphocytes with nonviable M. hominis type 1 (33). This inhibition could be reversed by removal of the nonviable mycoplasmas.
Mitosis was initiated with PHA, stopped with nonviable mycoplasmas
and restarted without mycplasmas by changing the medium.

Aula and Nichols demonstrated mitotic inhibition of human
lymphocyte cultures with M. salivarium, M. hominis type 2 and
M. fermentans (37). In this study, an inoculum of 10^3 CFU of
M. salivarium signifcantly increased the incidence of chromosome
breaks. The effects of M. salivarium were shown to be mediated
by arginine depletion of the medium by the mycoplasma via the
arginine deiminase pathway. Arginine addition removed the mitotic
inhibition, and similar chromosomal changes could be induced by
arginine deficient medium without mycoplasmas.

Knudsin et al reported that two freshly isolated human
ureaplasmas induced chromosomal abnormalities in human
lymphocyte cultures obtained from normal subjects (38). These
workers noted that ureaplasmas do not possess arginine deiminase,
suggesting chromosomal damage in ureaplasma infected cells
by a mechanism other than arginine depletion.

Mycoplasma infected lymphocytes have not been subjected
to more thorough study by chromosome banding or sister chromatid exchange to determine the frequency of mutational events

mediated by mycoplasmas. Fogh and Fogh have examined infected
FL cells by trypsin banding (39). Results of these studies
indicated that chromosomes in cells infected with M. fermentans
exhibited banding patterns of normal chromosomes.

6. Mycoplasmas Recovered from Lymphocyte Cell Cultures

Mycoplasmas were isolated from 34 lymphocyte cell lines in
this laboratory. These cultures originated in one laboratory, and
all cultures yielded M. salivarium.   This species is rarely encountered in cell cultures and was not among the 1,374 isolates
reported by Barile et al (11). The nature of the donors of these
cell cultures is listed in Table 3. Mycoplasmas were detected
in these cultures by agar and broth inoculation. However, biochemical tests, including uracil conversion (Levine, these proceedings)
and the ratio of uptake of tritiated uridine to tritiated uracil
(Stanbridge, these proceedings) also detected mycoplasmal infection. Viability counts were performed on four cultures and showed
10^7-10^8 (CFU) of M. salivarium per ml suspension. The presence of
such concentrations of mycoplasmas will have profound biochemical
effects on the culture. Some of these cultures express a genetic
defect that allows a particular metabolic product to accumulate.
Depending on the nature of this product, it's release into
the medium, and the species of mycoplasma, the expression of
the genetic defect can be obliterated. This has been documented
separately by Stanbridge and Shinn and van Diggelen (these proceedings).

Lymphocyte cell cultures naturally infected with M. salivrium
died after 16 passages. This is illustrated in Figure 1. Mycoplasmas were detected when the culture from an apparently normal
patient, was first submitted to this laboratory at the third
passage. In controlled prospective studies, M. salivarium was
deliberately inoculated into normal lymphocyte cultures. The
cultures died 14-30 passages later. The lifespan was different
in different lines, but always significantly different from
uninoculated controls. Death is gradual with viability decreasing
from 90% to 30% over 4-8 passages. This delayed lethal effect
suggests that results of studies of mycoplasmal infection can
be influenced by the length of time the culture had been infected.
No difference in growth rates between infected and uninfected
controls was evident 2-3 passages after infection, even though
4.7x10^7 CFU M. salivarium per ml was present. However, large
differences in growth rates were evident after the infected

TABLE 3. M. Salivarium Infected Lymphocyte Cultures

Cell Culture Number	Donor Status
130, 131, 332, 351, 381 386, 388, 397, 398, 401, 462	Normal
387, 399, 400, 463, 464	Acute Lymphocytic Leukemia
395, 402, 460	Down's Syndrome
385	46 XX, −E
396, 461	Fanconi's Anemia
382, 383	Lesch-Nyhan
235, 384	Citrullinemia
389	Gaucher's Disease
353, 393	Mental Retardation
394	Maple Syrup Urine Disease
350	Pompe's Glycogen Storage II
352	Fructose 1-6 Diphosphate Deficiency
390	Hyper IgM

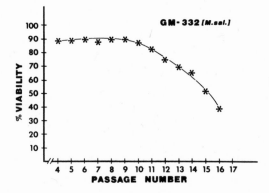

Figure 1. Viability of a human lymphocyte culture from an apparently normal subject. Culture contained Mycoplasma salivarium when first submitted to laboratory at Passage 3.

culture entered the death phase. Cytogenetic examination of
M. salivarium infected lymphocytes 3-4 passages after infection
showed no significant chromosomal damage compared to controls.

Studies are in progress to determine if M. salivarium infections
can influence lymphocyte membranes since mycoplasmas are associated
with cell membranes in infected cultures. Scanning electron
microscopy has confirmed this in M. salivarium infected
lymphocytes. Effects on membranes are particularly relevant in
lymphocyte cells since PHA attachment, histocompatibility antigen
and immunoglobulins among other reactions involve the cell membrane.
Expression of immunoglobulins, viral capsid antigen and nuclear
antigen of EBV was not affected by M. salivarium infection in
preliminary studies. These studies are continuing.

The original source of the M. salivarium infection is unknown.
Possible sources include: 1) whole blood specimen; 2)laboratory
personnel and 3)other cultures infected with the organism.
M. salivarium has been isolated from the blood of a leukemic child
(20), suggesting the blood as a possible source.   Twenty-five of
31 (80.1%) cell culture technicians carried M. salivarium in their
throats, and droplets carrying the organism were detected after
talking and sneezing (10). However, in spite of the prevelance of
the organism and its dissemination in the environment, it is a rare
cell culture isolate. Because of the high mycoplasmal concentrations
in infected cell cultures and the ease of generation of infective
droplets during routine cell culture procedures, we believe that
infected cell cultures are the most common source of further infection (10).

In other studies on M. salivarium, Parkinson and Carter reported the organism was phagocytosed by polymorphonuclear leukocytes
and monocytes (40). This mycoplasmacidal activity was exhibited
in the absence of detectable anti M. salivarium antiserum. Further
studies showed that mixtures of M. salivarium and non sensitized
mixed leukocytes released histamine. Histamine release occurred
independant of complement and specific antiserum (41).

    7. Conclusions

Accidental mycoplasmal infection can have profound effects on
lymphocyte cultures. The precise nature of these effects can not
be predicted, and will depend upon the specific properties of the
mycoplasma, the lymphocyte culture and other factors. Effective
quality control measures must be executed to prevent, detect and

control all forms of microbiological contamination, including mycoplasma. This includes periodic monitoring for mycoplasmal infection with technics of proven effectiveness, sterility testing of
serum and other media components, effective housekeeping and
disinfection procedures and quarantine facilities to handle cultures whose mycoplasmal status is unknown. These technics are
specified in a separate chapter and elsewhere (11,42-44).

Acknowledgement

These studies were supported in part by contracts #N01-GM-6-2119
and N01-AG-4-2865 from the National Institute for General Medical
Sciences and the National Institute on Aging. The technical
assistance of Victoria Ammen, Diane Meredith, Judi Sarama and
Veronica Vanaman is gratefully acknowledged.

References

1. Crustschoff, G.K. and E.A. Berlin. 1935. Cytological inves-
    tigations on cultures of normal human blood. J. Genet.
    31:243-251.

2. Rigas, D.A. and E.E. Osgood. 1955. Purification and proper-
    ties of the phytohemagglutinin of Phaseolus vulgaris.
    J. Biol. Chem. 212:607-609.

3. Nowell, P.C. 1960. Differentiation of human leukemic
    leukocytes in tissue culture. Exp. Cell Res. 19:267-277

4. Nowell, P.C. 1960. Phytohemagglutinin: an initiator of
    mitosis in cultures of normal human leukocytes. Cancer
    Res. 20:462-466.

5. Smith, G.F. 1973. The lymphocyte in culture: historic
    perspective. In: Birth Defects, Original Article Series,
    Long-term Lymphocyte Cultures in Human Genetics.
    The National Foundation -March of Dimes. Vol. IX (No. 1):
    5-8.

6. Moorhead, P.S., P.C. Nowell, W.J. Mellman, D.M. Battigs
    and D.A. Hungerford. 1960. Chromosome preparations of
    leukocytes cultured from human peripheral blood. Exp.
    Cell Res. 20:613-616.

7. Henle, W., V. Diehl, G. Kohn, H. zur Hausen, and G. Henle.
    1967. Herpes-type virus and chromosome marker in normal
    leukocytes after growth with irradiated Burkitt cells.
    Science 157:1064-1065.

8. Gerber, P. 1973. The role of Epstein-Barr virus in estab-
    lishing long term human lymphocyte cultures. In: Birth
    Defects Original Article Series. "Long-Term Lymphocyte
    Cultures in Human Genetics. Vol. IX (No. 1) The National
    Foundation-March of Dimes:20-30.

9. Moore, G.E. Jan. 1973. The future of cultured lymphocytes.
    In: "Birth Defects, Original Article Series," "Long-term
    Lymphocyte Cultures in Human Genetics." The National
    Foundation - March of Dimes. Vol IX (No. 1):13-19.

10. McGarrity, G.J. 1976. Spread and control of mycoplasmal
     infection of cell cultures. In Vitro 12:643-648.

11. Barile, M.F., H.E. Hopps, M.W. Grabowski and D.B. Riggs.
     1973. The identification and sources of mycoplasmas
     isolated from contaminated cell cultures. Ann. N.Y.
     Academy Sciences 225:251-264.

12. Crawford, Y.E. and W.H. Kraybill. 1967. The mixtures of
     mycoplasma species isolated from the human oropharynx.
     Ann. N.Y. Acad. Sciences 143:411-421.

13. Taylor-Robinson, D. and P.M.Furr. 1973. The distribution of
     T-mycoplasmas within and among various animal species.
     Ann. N.Y. Acad. Sciences. 225:108-117.

14. Murphy, W.H., C. Bullis, L. Cabick and R. Heyn. 1970.
     Isolation of mycoplasma from leukemic and nonleukemic
     patients. J. Nat. Cancer Inst. 45:243-251.

15. Murphy, W.H., C. Bullis, I.J. Ertel and C.J.D. Zarafonetis.
     1967. Mycoplasma studies of human leukemia. Ann. N.Y.
     Acad. Sci. 143:544-556.

16. Barile, M.F. 1967. Mycoplasma and leukemia. Ann. N.Y. Acad.
     Sci. 143:557-572.

17. Ginsburg, H. and J. Nicolet. 1973. Extensive transfor-
     mation of lymphocytes by a mycoplasma organism. Nature
     New Biol. 246:143-146.

18. Fernald, G.W. 1972. In vitro response of human lymphocytes
     to Mycoplasma pneumoniae. Infec. Immun. 5:552-558.

19. Levanthal, B.G., C.B. Smith, P.P. Carbone and E.M. Hersh.
     1967. Lymphocyte transformation in response to M. pneumoniae.
     In: Proceedings of the Third Annual Leucocyte Culture
     Conference (W.O. Rieke, ed.) Appleton-Century Crofts, N.Y.

20. Gregory, J.E. and J.L.Chisom. 1976. Mycoplasma salivarium
     in the blood of a child with leukemia. Abstract D70.
     Proceedings of the 76th Annual Meeting, American Society
     for Microbiology.

21. Archer, D.L. and B.G. Young. 1974. Control of interferon
     migration inhibition factor and expression of viral
     capsid antigens in Burkitt's lymphoma-derived cell
     lines: role of L-arginine. Infect. Immun. 9:684-689.

22. Barile, M.F. and B.G. Leventhal. 1968. Possible mechanism
     for mycoplasmal inhibition of lymphocyte transformation
     induced by phytohemagglutinin. Nature 219:751-752.

23. Rinaldo, C.R., Jr., B.C. Cole, J.C. Overall, Jr.,
     J. R. Ward and L.A. Glasgow. 1974. Induction of inter-
     feron in ovine leukocytes by species of Mycoplasma and
     Acholeplasma. Proc. Soc. Exp.Biol. Med. 146:613-618.

24. Rinaldo, C.R., Jr., J.C. Overall, Jr., B.C. Cole and
     L.A. Glasgow. 1973. Mycoplasma-associated induction of
     interferon in ovine leukocytes. Infect. Immunity 8:
     796-803.

25. Rinaldo, C.R, Jr., B.C. Cole, J.C. Overall, Jr. and L.A.
     Glasgow. 1974. Induction of interferon in mice by
     mycoplasmas. Infect. Immunity 10:1296-1301.

26. DeClerq, E. and T.C. Merigan. 1971. Bis-DEAE-fluorenone:
     mechanism of antiviral protection and stimulation of
     interferon production in the mouse. J. Infect. Dis.
     123:190-199.

27. Stringfellow, D.A. and L.A. Glasgow. 1972. Tilorone
     hydrochloride: an oral interferon-inducing agent.
     Antimicrob. Ag. Chemother. 2:73-78.

28. Stinebring, W.R. and J.S. Youngner. 1964. Patterns
     of interferon appearance in mice injected with
     bacteria or bacterial endotoxin. Nature 204:712.

29. Finkelstein, M.S., G.H. Bausch and T.C. Merigan. 1968.
     Interferon inducers in vivo: difference in sensitivity
     to inhibitors of RNA and protein synthesis. Science
     161:465-468.

30. Subrahmanyan, T.P., and C.A. Mims. 1970. Interferon pro-
     duction by mouse peritoneal cells. J. Reticuloendothel
     Soc. 7:32-42,

31. Stringfellow, D.A. and L. A. Glasgow. 1972. Hyporeactivity
     of infection: potential limitation to therapeutic use
     of interferon-inducing agents. Infect. Immunity 6:743-747.

32. Cole, B.C., J.C. Overall, Jr., P.S. Lombardi, and L.A.
     Glasgow. 1976. Induction of interferon in ovine and
     human lymphocyte cultures by mycoplasmas. Infec.
     Immun. 14:88-94.

33. Plata, E.J., M.R. Abell and W.H. Murphy. 1973. Induction of
     leukemoid disease in mice by Mycoplasma fermentans.
     Inf. Dis. 128:588-597.

34. Gabridge, M.G. and D.D. Gamble. 1974. Independance of
     leukemoid potential and toxigenicity of Mycoplasma
     fermentans. J. Inf. Dis. 130:664-668.

35. Biberfeld, G. and G. Sterner. 1976. Effect of Mycoplasma
     pneumoniae infection on cell mediated immunity.
     Infection (Suppl. 1) 17-20.

36. Coppermann, R. and H.E. Morton. 1966. Reversible inhibition
     of mitosis in lymphocyte cultures by non-viable myco-
     plasmas. Proc. Soc. Exp. Biol. Med. 123:790-795.

37. Aula, P. and W.W. Nichols. 1967. The cytogenetic effects
     of mycoplasma in human leukocyte cultures. J. Cell Physiol.
     70:281-290.

38. Kundsin, R.B., M. Ampola, S. Streeter and P. Neurath. 1971.
     Chromosomal aberrations induced by T strain mycoplasmas.
     J. Med. Gen. 8:181-187.

39. Fogh, J. and H. Fogh. 1973. Chromosome changes in cell
     culture induced by mycoplasma infection. Ann. N.Y.
     Acad. Sci. 225:311-329.

40. Parkinson, C.F. and P.B. Carter. 1975. Phagocytosis of
     Mycoplasma salivarium by human polymorphonuclear leuko-
     cytes and monocytes. Inf. Immun. 11:405-414.

41. Parkinson, C.F. 1975. Histamine release from human
     leukocytes when stimulated by Mycoplasma salivarium.
     Infec. Immunity 11:595-597.

42. McGarrity, G.J. 1975. Detection of mycoplasmas in cell
     culture. Tissue Culture Manual. 1:113-116.

43. McGarrity, G.J. 1975. Serum quality control. Tissue
     Culture Manual. 1:167-169.

44. McGarrity, G.J. 1975. Control of microbiological contamin-
     ation. Tissue Culture Manual 1:181-184.

CLINICAL IMPORTANCE OF DETECTING MYCOPLASMA CONTAMINATION OF

CELL CULTURES

Edward L. Schneider

Laboratory of Cellular and Comparative Physiology,
Gerontology Research Center, National Institute on Aging,
National Institutes of Health, PHS, U. S. Department of
Health, Education and Welfare, Baltimore, Maryland 21224

The preceding papers in this symposium have convincingly
detailed the wide range of cellular alterations induced by
mycoplasma infection. It is also apparent that considerable
advances have been achieved in the technology employed for
detecting mycoplasma contamination of cells in culture.
Therefore, it behooves the investigator working with cultured
cells to be certain that he is examining uncontaminated cell
cultures. It is also becoming increasingly clear that mycoplasma contamination may represent a hazard to successful
clinical use of cell cultures.

During the past 10 years, there has been explosive growth
in the field of human genetics. Genetic counseling centers
have been established at large numbers of hospitals and medical
centers. One important service of these centers is the pre-and
postnatal diagnosis of human biochemical and cytogenetic disorders
utilizing cultured human fibroblasts. While many of these laboratories have had considerable tissue culture experience, others
have only limited expertise in this area. Therefore, the risk
of mycoplasma contamination in this latter group is considerable.

Special Considerations in Culturing Amniotic Fluid Cells

The conditions for the culture of amniotic fluid cells has
been presented by Dr. Taylor-Robinson (1). However, I would
like to discuss a few important additional considerations in
dealing with these cell cultures. First, let us examine the
timing of the procedure and the length of the subsequent analytic

period. Amniocentesis is usually performed between the 14th
and 16th weeks of gestation. Chromosomal analysis of amniotic
fluid cells is usually possible three to four weeks after amniocentesis, while growing sufficient cells for biochemical analysis
can take as long as five to six weeks. Since abortion of affected fetuses is limited in some states after 20 gestational
weeks and in most states after 24 gestational weeks, there is
little time for repeat analysis. Certainly there is a great need
to produce uncontaminated cell cultures for chromosomal and
biochemical analysis on the first try.

Another important consideration is to avoid exposing the
pregnant mother to the risks of a second amniocentesis. Although
the risk may be quite low (2), the responsible investigator should
prevent this unnecessary situation. In practice, it is often the
case that a second amniocentesis is needed for the mother who was
hesitant to have the first procedure.

Lastly, since the results of biochemical and karyologic
determinations on these cells will influence the parents'
decision towards continuing or aborting the pregnancy, it is vital
that these determinations not be affected by laboratory artifacts.

Potential Hazards of Mycoplasma Infection of Cultured

Amniotic Fluid Cells

While maintaining a tissue culture facility which was
primarily utilized for culturing amniotic fluid cells, I decided
to examine the extent of mycoplasma contamination. Since our
previous studies had indicated that microbiologic testing alone
frequently failed to detect mycoplasma contamination (3, 4), it
was decided to use a battery of tests. These tests, run in parallel,
included Uridine/Uracil determinations, polyacrylamide gel electrophoresis of ^{3}H-uridine-labeled ribosomal RNA (PAGE), aceto-orcein
staining and microbiological culture of both cells and media
(Figure 1). The results of mycoplasma screening of replicate
amniotic fluid cell cultures are summarized in Table 1. Approximately half the cultures examined (11 of 20) revealed prominent
noneukaryotic ^{3}H-uridine-labeled ribosomal RNA peaks on gel
electrophoresis and reduced Uridine/Uracil ratios (5). Although
orcein staining was concordant with these results in 17 of 20
cultures, microbiological tests were consistently negative for
mycoplasma or other microorganisms. This disparity between microbiological, biochemical and morphological testing, which has been
reported by a number of laboratories, emphasizes the need for
multiple screening techniques.

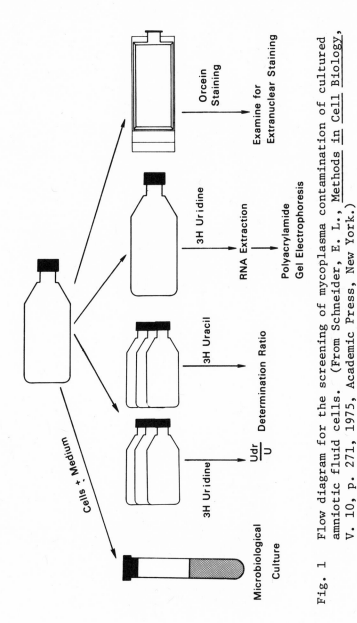

Fig. 1   Flow diagram for the screening of mycoplasma contamination of cultured amniotic fluid cells. (From Schneider, E. L., Methods in Cell Biology, V. 10, p. 271, 1975, Academic Press, New York.)

TABLE 1

Results of Biochemical, Histological, and Microbiological Screening
of Cultured Amniotic Fluid Cells

Cell Culture	Anti- biotic	$23S_E$ and $16S_E$ RNA's on PAGE	Udr/ U	Aceto-orcein staining	Microbio- logical culture
91	P*	−	840.0	+	−
96	P	−	699.0	−	−
98	P	−	408.0	+	−
98	A	−	374.6	−	−
99	P	−	492.5	−	−
99	A	−	681.0	−	−
107	P	−	482.4	−	−
107	A	−	778.5	−	−
115	P	−	850.0	−	−
90	P	+	176.5	+	−
90	G	+	1.4	+	−
91	G	+	4.3	+	−
95	P	+	4.6	+	−
95	G	+	10.4	+	−
96	G	+	8.7	+	−
97	P	+	215.0	+	−
97	G	+	178.0	+	−
110	P	+	62.7	−	−
110	A	+	82.7	+	−
115	A	+	57.9	+	−

*Amniotic fluid cell cultures were supplemented with antibacterial
drugs: penicillin (100 µg/ml) and streptomycin (100 µg/ml) (P),
gentamycin (Schering) (50 µg/ml) (G), or Aureomycin (Lederle)
(50 µg/ml) (A). From Schneider et al, Science 184:477-479, 1974.

Karyotypic analysis of these cultures revealed a significant increase in both chromosome breaks and gaps as well as increased aneuploidy in the mycoplasma contaminated cells when compared to controls (5). One mycoplasma-infected culture was of particular interest (115A) in that half the cells possessed a consistent pattern of multiple translocations. Although these chromosomal translocations were representative of mycoplasma contamination, they presented a difficult clinical decision. If these trans-locations were not mycoplasma induced, they might indicate an "unbalanced translocation" and lead to the birth of a child with multiple congenital abnormalities. Fortunately, all our amniotic fluid samples were divided into two equal aliquots and cultured under separate tissue culture conditions. Therefore, a parallel amniotic fluid cell culture was available for both mycoplasma testing and chromosomal analysis. This culture (115P) was negative on all screening tests and possessed normal karyology. We, thus, felt confident that the abnormal chromosomal findings in 115A were indeed due to mycoplasma contamination.

Another important potential hazard to successful prenatal diagnosis involves those human genetic disorders which feature chromosomal alterations and/or abnormalities in DNA repair. These syndromes can be diagnosed on the basis of their increased frequencies of chromosomal alterations. However, the known ability of mycoplasma to induce chromosomal alterations can lead to false positive results. The recent development of the BrdU-differential staining techniques (6, 7) now permits an additional means of diagnosing these disorders by measuring baseline and mutagen induced levels of sister chromatid exchanges (SCE). Although it is not yet known whether mycoplasma can induce SCE formation, it is known that viruses can induce SCE (8).

In addition to investigating potential problems with chromosomal diagnosis, we have explored the complications that could be created by mycoplasma contamination of amniotic fluid cell cultures used for prenatal biochemical diagnosis. Advances in human genetics now permit the biochemical prenatal diagnosis of over one-hundred inherited metabolic disorders (9). Among this group is the Lesch-Nyhan syndrome which features a markedly diminished level of the enzyme hypoxanthine-guanine phosphoribosyl-transferase (HGPRT) in cultured cells from these patients. To test for the potential effect of mycoplasma infection on these cells, we intentionally infected D98/AH-2, a permanent Hela-derived line with almost undetectable levels of HGPRT, with several mycoplasma strains (10). Mycoplasma infection resulted in the elevation of HGPRT levels to the normal range for Hela cells (Table 2). Gel electrophoresis of these infected cells revealed that the new HGPRT activities were of mycoplasma origin. These results indicate that mycoplasma contamination of cells from a

TABLE 2

HGPRT activities of A. laidlawii and M. hyorhinis in cell cultures

Sample	HGPRT activity (c.p.m. in inosinic acid/μg protein/min of assay)	Approximate no. of viable mycoplasmas/0.1 ml packed cell volume (± 0.5 $\log_{10}$)
A. laidlawii	27.46	3.0×10^9
M. hyorhinis	17.45	1.1×10^9
D98/AH-2 cells	No activity	Negative
D98/AH-2 cells infected with M. hyorhinis	18.27	1.9×10^8
D98/AH-2 cells infected with M. hyorhinis in the presence of 10^{-4} M hypoxanthine	5.58	8.0×10^7
D98/AH-2 cells infected with A. laidlawii	No activity	2.0×10^7
D98/AH-2 cells infected with A. laidlawii in the presence of 10^{-4} M hypoxanthine	2.87	2.0×10^7
HeLa	17.75	Negative

From Stanbridge, Tischfield & Schneider, Nature 256:329-331, 1975.

Lesch-Nyhan fetus might yield HGPRT levels in the normal enzyme range and thus yield a false negative diagnosis.

Suggested Approach for Mycoplasma Screening of Amniotic

Fluid Cells and for Prevention of Mycoplasma

Interference with Prenatal Diagnosis

Although antibiotics may obscure mycoplasma infection and, therefore, should probably not be used with permanent cell lines, their use is necessary in culturing amniotic fluid cell cultures since these cells cannot be easily replaced if lost. While no antibiotic can guarantee against mycoplasma infection, we have had particular success with chlorotetracycline.

Since quick diagnosis of contaminated cells is essential, rapid biochemical tests such as Uridine/Uracil or Uridine phosphorylase assays and morphological testing such as Hoechst 33258 staining are recommended, together with conventional microbiological tests.

It is also recommended that facilities for the culture of amniotic fluid cells be constructed to minimize contamination and that personnel be instructed in aseptic techniques. If possible, amniotic fluid obtained at amniocentesis should be divided into two equal aliquots and the cells cultured in separate tissue culture facilities by different technicians with different batches of media with diverse serum lots. In this way, a parallel, uncontaminated culture may be available for assessing results induced by mycoplasma contamination.

Finally, no cell cultures derived from other laboratories should be introduced into the amniotic fluid cell culture facility without prior mycoplasma screening.

Summary

Mycoplasma contamination appears to be as widespread in amniotic fluid cell cultures as in other cell types. It has been demonstrated that they represent a potential hazard to both biochemical and chromosomal prenatal diagnosis. Therefore, particular emphasis should be placed on preventing mycoplasma contamination as well as screening amniotic fluid cell cultures for these microorganisms. For screening, rapid testing (either biochemical or morphological) is recommended in addition to standard microbiological techniques.

References

1. Taylor-Robinson, D. Workshop on Mycoplasma Infection
    of Cell Cultures, Institute for Medical Research,
    Camden, New Jersey, March 22-23, 1977. In press.

2. Golbus, M. S. The prenatal diagnosis of genetic defects
    In Advances in Obstetrics and Gynecology, Williams and
    Wilkins, Baltimore, 1977.

3. Schneider, E. L., Epstein, C. J., Epstein, W. J.,
    Halbasch, G., and Betlach, M. Exp. Cell Res. 79:343-
    348, 1973.

4. Schneider, E. L., Stanbridge, E. J., and Epstein, C. J.
    Exp. Cell Res. 84:311-318, 1974.

5. Schneider, E. L., Stanbridge, C. J., Golbus, M., Halbasch,
    G. and Rodgers, G. Science 184:477-479, 1974.

6. Latt, S. A. Science 185:74-76, 1974.

7. Wolff, S. and Perry, P. Chromosoma (Berl) 48:341-353,
    1974.

8. Brown, R. L. and Crossen, P. E. Exp. Cell Res. 103:418-
    420, 1976.

9. Stanbury, J. B. Wyngaarden, J. B. and Fredrickson, D. S.
    The Metabolic Basis of Inherited Diseases, 3rd Edit.,
    McGraw-Hill, New York, 1972.

10. Stanbridge, E. J., Tischfield, J. A. and Schneider, E. L.
    Nature 256:329-331, 1975.

PHENOTYPIC ALTERATIONS IN MAMMALIAN CELL LINES AFTER MYCOPLASMA INFECTION

SEUNG-IL SHIN and OTTO P. VAN DIGGELEN[1]

Department of Genetics
Albert Einstein College of Medicine
Bronx, New York 10461

Contamination of cell cultures by mycoplasma can result in subtle or profound changes in cellular metabolism and function, and thereby produce serious experimental artifacts in studies of cellular biochemistry and physiology if the contamination remains undetected. Since many species of mycoplasmas do not cause overt cytopathic effects on the animal cells, and sometimes escape detection by the usual agar plate cultivation technique described by Hayflick (1), it is often difficult to state positively that a given cell culture is absolutely free of contaminating mycoplasmas. Particularly noteworthy in this regard are the "noncultivable" strains of Mycoplasma hyorhinis, which cannot be cultured in the absence of animal cells they parasitize. These host-dependent, cryptic strains of mycoplasma have recently emerged as frequent contaminants in cell cultures.{See, for example, the contributions by Barile, DelGuidice and McGarrity in this volume.}

Recently, we reported on the isolation and characterization of a cryptic variant of M. hyorhinis from a mouse cell clone that had been maintained for many cell generations in a medium containing 8-azaguanine (2). This strain of mycoplasma, which we shall designate M. hyorhinis (Einstein), appears to have an absolute requirement for an animal cell host for growth, and contains a very high level of endogenous hypoxanthine phosphoribosyltransferase (HPRT; E.C.2.4.2.8.) activity (2). Infection of animal cell lines by M. hyorhinis (Einstein) produces no apparent changes in gross

---

[1]Present address: Department of Cell Biology and Genetics, Faculty of Medicine, Erasmus University, Rotterdam, The Netherlands.

cell morphology and growth rate even when the titer of fully
infectious particles in the culture medium reaches 10^8 per ml.
However, the infection can cause profound alterations in several
important cellular phenotypes (2, 3).

In this paper, we will summarize our recent observations on
the phenotypic changes induced in mammalian cell cultures by
infection with several mycoplasma species, in order to illustrate
the potential problems that may be encountered by unrecognized
contamination with mycoplasma. We have employed the L-cell clone
L929 and its mutant derivative A9, which is deficient in HPRT
activity and reverts to the normal HPRT[+] phenotype with a very
low frequency (4). We take advantage of the fact that most, if
not all, mycoplasmas contain endogenous HPRT activity that can
easily be distinguished from the mammalian HPRT (5), which serves
as a convenient and quantitative measure of cell contamination.
Much of the experimental data have been described previously (2,
3, 5).

MATERIALS AND METHODS

Cell Culture Conditions Cells were maintained in the absence
of antibiotics in McCoy's 5a medium (GIBCO), supplemented with 10%
fetal bovine serum prescreened for the absence of mycoplasma. This
medium will be referred to as the control medium. The selective
media contained, in addition, 4×10^{-5} M 8-azaguanine (AG medium),
or 3×10^{-5} M 6-thioguanine (TG medium), or 10^{-4} M hypoxanthine
plus 4×10^{-7} M aminopterin plus 1.6×10^{-5} M thymidine (HAT medium)
(6).

Standard Strains of Mycoplasma The standard strains of
mycoplasma used in the study were kindly provided by Dr. Gerard J.
McGarrity, Institute for Medical Research, Camden, N.J. The cryptic
variant, M. hyorhinis (Einstein), was isolated in this laboratory
from a clone of A9 maintained in AG medium (2).

Assay of HPRT Activity in Cell Lysates Cell lysates were
prepared either by sonication of a suspension of trypsinized cells,
or by lysing a monolayer in situ for 20 min at 4°C with 1% Triton
X-100, in a buffer containing 5×10^{-3} M $MgCl_2$, 0.02 M potassium
phosphate buffer, pH 7.6, and 5×10^{-3} M 2-mercaptoethanol (7). The
assay of the cell-associated HPRT activity, which measures the
conversion of ^{14}C-hypoxanthine to ^{14}C-IMP with an excess of
5-phospho-ribosyl-1-pyrophosphate (PRPP), has been described (8).

Microassay of HPRT Activity in Intact Cells In each 6 mm well
of a microtest plate (MicroTest II, Falcon), 2×10^4 cells were
seeded and allowed to attach overnight. The medium was then replaced
with 0.1 ml fresh growth medium containing dialyzed serum, plus
0.1×10^{-3} M ^{14}C-hypoxanthine (30 mCi/mmole), and incubated for 6 hrs

at 37°C. To determine the "total cell uptake" of ^{14}C-hypoxanthine, cells were first washed twice with 0.2 ml phosphate-buffered saline and dissolved in 0.1 ml of 0.1 N NaOH. Each well was again washed with 0.1 ml of 0.1 N NaOH and the wash was combined with the cell lysate, suspended in 5 ml Aquasol (New England Nuclear Corp.), and counted in a liquid scintillation spectrophotometer.

Microassay of HPRT in Cell-Free Extracts Replicate cultures in microwells prepared as above were lysed in situ with 20 µl of 1% Triton buffer mentioned above, and incubated for 10 min at 37°C. The HPRT reaction was started by the addition of 20 µl of a reaction mixture to each well, so that the final 40 µl mixture would contain 60 x 10^{-3} M Tris-HCl buffer, pH 7.6, 5 x 10^{-3} M $MgSO_4$, 2 x 10^{-3} PRPP, and 1.0 x 10^{-4} M ^{14}C-hypoxanthine (30 mCi/mmole). After 60 min incubation at 37°C, the reaction was terminated by adding 10 µl of 0.1 M EDTA. Aliquots of the final mixture (20 µl) were spotted on DEAE paper (Whatman paper DE-81) and assayed for radio-activity in IMP as in the standard assay procedure.

Electrophoresis of HPRT Crude cell lysates, prepared by sonication, were subjected to electrophoresis on cellulose acetate gel (Cellogel, Reeve-Angel Co.) in phosphate buffer at pH 7.0, and the HPRT activity was identified by the fluorescence staining method we have described (9).

Autoradiography Cells grown on coverslips in control medium were labelled either with ^{3}H-thymidine (1 µCi/ml, 20 Ci/mmole) for 24 hr, or with ^{3}H-uridine (5 µCi/ml, 31 Ci/mmole) for 30 min. After labelling the cells were washed 3 times with phosphate-buffered saline, fixed in methanol-acetic acid (3 parts: 1 part) and dried in air. The coverslips were then dipped in Nuclear Track Emulsion (Kodak NTB2) and exposed for 6 days. After development, the cells were stained with Giemsa.

Electron Microscopy Electron microscopy of cells before and after infection with mycoplasma was carried out by Dr. David M. Phillips, The Population Council, New York, N. Y. For scanning electron microscopy, cells were grown on glass coverslips, fixed in 2.5% collidine-buffered glutaraldehyde, dehydrated in ethanol series and transferred to acetone. Coverslips were critical point dried with liquid CO_2 in a Sorvall Critical Point Drying System, coated with gold using an Edwards 306 coater and viewed in an ETEC autoscan. For transmission electron microscopy, cells were grown on Falcon plastic petri dishes. Cells were fixed in 2.5% collidine-buffered glutaraldehyde, postfixed in 1% OsO_4, dehydrated through alcohol and embedded in Epon. {See the contribution by Phillips, this volume.}

The Nude Mouse Colony   The nude mouse colony was established
from a stock backcrossed to BALB/c and maintained in sterile-air
laminar flow cage racks (Lab Products, Inc., Garfield, N.J.), as
described previously (10).

Transplantation and Re-initiation of Cell Lines after Passage
in Nude Mice   These procedures have been described earlier (11).
Briefly, cells were trypsinized, counted and resuspended in
phosphate-buffered saline, and 0.2 ml aliquots were injected
subcutaneously at a single site.   Trypsinization reduced the cell-
associated mycoplasma titers considerably in the infected cultures,
but did not eliminate the mycoplasma completely from the cells.
The original maximal titers were regained within a few days after
trypsinization if the cells were kept in culture.   When progressively
growing tumors developed in injected mice, they were removed
aseptically from the animals, washed in phosphate-buffered saline,
minced and sieved through a stainless steel mesh to produce single
cell preparations.   The cells were then plated in the culture
medium.   Unattached cells were washed away after overnight
incubation.   Vigorous monolayer cultures were obtained in all cases.

Staining of Cells with Bisbenzimid (Hoechst 33258) for
Mycoplasma   Cells were seeded on glass coverslips and allowed to
incubate for at least 4 days before examination to maximize the
mycoplasma titer.   The procedures for fixing and staining with the
bisbenzimid dye (Hoeschst 33258) as described by Chen (12) were
followed.   The stained cells were screened and photographed under
a Zeiss fluorescence microscope.

RESULTS AND DISCUSSION

Apparent Transfer of Mycoplasma-Specific HPRT Activity to
HPRT-Deficient Cells   The mouse cell mutant A9 was originally
isolated by Littlefield by growing the mouse L929 cells in a medium
containing 8-azaguanine (13).   A9 cells are highly resistant to
both 8-azaguanine and 6-thioguanine, and almost completely deficient
in HPRT activity; as a result, they are unable to grow in HAT medium
(14).   Because of the high endogenous HPRT activity of M. hyorhinis
(Einstein), the infection of HPRT-deficient cells such as A9 by this
mycoplasma results in the rapid appearance of a cell-associated
HPRT activity that reaches a saturating level within 4 days after
infection (2).

That this "acquisition" of new HPRT activity by the animal
cells is due to the mycoplasma HPRT, and not due to the reexpression
of the mouse isozyme in the mutant cell, can be shown by the fact
that the A9-associated HPRT is still characteristic of the mycoplasma-specific enzyme.   The mycoplasma-coded HPRT activity can be

distinguished from the mouse isozyme on the basis of differences in electrophoretic mobility, antigenic crossreactivity and inhibition by cytotoxic guanine analogues (2). These differences are summarized in Table 1. In addition, the transfer of HPRT activity to A9 cells by M. hyorhinis is abolished completely by a pretreatment of the mycoplasma stock with a monospecific antiserum prepared against a standard strain of M. hyorhinis (ATCC) (2). (See Table 2.)

Table 1. Comparison of HPRT Activities from
Mouse Cells and M. hyorhinis (Einstein)

Enzyme Parameter	Source of HPRT	
	Mouse L929	M. hyorhinis
Km for hypoxanthine (M)	1.7×10^{-5}	5.0×10^{-5}
Km for PRPP (M)	5.0×10^{-5}	5.7×10^{-4}
Inhibited by:		
8-azaguanine	+	+
6-thioguanine	+	+++
Inactivated by 70°C, 2 min (%)	9	98
Crossreactivity to antiserum against mouse HPRT (%)	100	<10
Electrophoretic mobility	Fast	Slow

(Data from Van Diggelen, Phillips and Shin, ref. 2)

However, due to the unique catalytic properties of the HPRT coded by M. hyorhinis (Einstein), A9 cells infected by this mycoplasma acquire the high level of cell-associated HPRT activity without at the same time becoming resistant to HAT medium or becoming sensitive to 8-azaguanine or 6-thioguanine. We have shown earlier(2) that this paradoxical phenotype may be due to the elevated substrate binding constants of the HPRT activity produced by the mycoplasma, especially for PRPP (see Table 1). In intact cells, where the intracellular concentration of PRPP is suboptimal for the mycoplasma HPRT, exogenous hypoxanthine cannot be utilized. However, in the usual cell-free assays of HPRT activity with cell extracts, a saturating level of PRPP is added in the reaction mixture so that the mycoplasma enzyme becomes fully functional. This interpretation is consistent with the data summarized in Table 3.

Therefore, HPRT-deficient mutant cells contaminated with M. hyorhinis (Einstein) can, even if maintained continuously in AG- or TG-medium, acquire an apparently wild-type level of HPRT activity when assayed in cell-free extracts.

Table 2. Transfer of Mycoplasma-Specific HPRT to A9 Cells
          after Infection by M. hyorhinis (Einstein)

Cells and Additions	HPRT Activity Associated with A9 Cells (CPM)	Origin of HPRT [a]
A9 + None	475	-
A9 + M. hyorhinis	42,560	Mycoplasma
A9 + M. hyorhinis, pretreated with antiserum b	488	-

Uninfected control medium or Millipore-filtered mycoplasma
stock cultures containing 10^3 infectious particles were added
to 15,000 A9 cells, and assayed for cell-associated HPRT
activity 4 days later as described in Materials and Methods.

a Determined by electrophoretic mobility.

b Preincubated with monospecific antiserum against M.
  hyorhinis (ATCC) for 1 hr at 1/100 dilution.

(Data from Van Diggelen, Phillips and Shin, ref. 2)

Table 3. Failure to Utilize Exogenous Hypoxanthine by A9
          Cells Deliberately Infected with M. hyorhinis

Cells	Conversion of Hypoxanthine to IMP by Cell Extract [a] (CPM)	Uptake of Hypoxanthine by Intact Cells [b] (CPM)
A9	11	305
A9, infected with M. hyorhinis (Einstein)	4,360	197
L929	9,740	21,986

a Total conversion of ^{14}C-hypoxanthine by lysates of 2×10^4
  cells at PRPP concentration of 2×10^{-3} M.

b Total cellular uptake by 2×10^4 cells of ^{14}C-hypoxanthine
  in 6 hr, in the absence of added PRPP in culture medium.

(Data from Van Diggelen, Phillips and Shin, ref. 2)

Phenotypic Alterations in Cellular Resistance to HAT Medium

A more striking phenotypic alteration with respect to cellular resistance to selective media is the finding that normal wild-type (HPRT⁺) cells such as L929 become extremely sensitive to HAT medium after infection with M. hyorhinis (Einstein). Data presented in Table 4 show that L929 cells deliberately infected with M. hyorhinis (Einstein) fail to grow in HAT medium, despite the fact that the cells are still producing normal levels of endogenous HPRT and unable to grow in AG-medium. Similar phenomenon has been reported by Holland and coworkers (15), and has been explained in terms of depletion of thymidine in the culture medium by the nucleoside phosphorylase produced in the mycoplasma.

Table 4. Resistance to Selective Media of HPRT⁺ and
HPRT⁻ Cells before and after Deliberate
Infection with M. hyorhinis (Einstein)

	Efficiency of Plating (%) by:			
Growth Medium	A9	A9+Mh[a]	L929	L929+Mh[a]
Control medium (CM)	61	43	57	43
CM + 8-azaguanine	45	39	0	0
CM + 6-thioguanine	54	49	0	0
CM + HAT	0	0	41	0

  a A9 and L929 cells deliberately infected.

(Data from Van Diggelen, Phillips and Shin, ref. 2)

The most significant conclusion from this observation is that HPRT-deficient cells preselected for 8-azaguanine resistance will not yield viable HAT-resistant cell hybrids after artificial cell fusion with HPRT⁺ cells if either of the cell populations used is contaminated with a mycoplasma such as M. hyorhinis (Einstein).

Failure to Incorporate Exogenous Thymidine by Contaminated Cells

One of the tests used commonly for mycoplasma infection in cell cultures utilizes the fact that all mycoplasma species have an absolute requirement for exogenous purines and pyrimidines for growth (16). Growth of test cultures with ³H-thymidine followed by autoradiography of fixed cells can thus be used to reveal the presence of cell-associated mycoplasmas as silver grains over the cytoplasmic and intercellular areas (17). In uncontaminated cultures, silver grains should be localized only over the cell nuclei.

Contrary to this expectation, however, A9 cells deliberately infected with M. hyorhinis (Einstein) do   not incorporate exogenous ^{3}H-thymidine from the culture medium at all, even though uninfected control A9 cells are clearly labelled in the nuclei under identical conditions (see Fig. 1, a and b). When these cultures are pulse-labelled for 30 min with ^{3}H-uridine, on the other hand, uninfected control A9 cells are labelled only over the nuclei but A9 cells deliberately infected with the mycoplasma are labelled mostly over the cytoplasm (Fig. 1, c and d).

The surprising failure to incorporate exogenous thymidine in the culture medium by the mycoplasma-infected A9 cells may be due also to the very high level of nucleoside phosphorylase activity of the mycoplasma. In any case, this observation suggests that the screening of cell cultures for mycoplasma contamination by autoradiography of fixed cells (17) or by sucrose gradient sedimentation of supernatant fluids from cultures after incubation of cells with ^{3}H-thymidine (18) may produce misleading results.

Reduction in Cellular Tumorigenicity The hairless mouse mutant called nude is genetically athymic and deficient in cell-mediated immunity (19, 20). These mice therefore provide an ideal means of determining the neoplastic growth potential in vivo of a variety of transformed cell lines regardless of the species or tissue of origin (10, 21).

Uninfected A9 cells are highly tumorigenic in nude mice, and produce rapidly growing lethal tumors in 100% of animals injected with at least 10^4 cells. At lower cell doses, the frequency of tumor formation decreases, but even as few as 100 cells per mouse can still produce tumors in about half of the mice (11). The lag time between the injection of cells and the first appearance of a detectable tumor nodule is also a function of the cell dose (3). Data given in Table 5 show, for instance, that when 10^6 cells are injected, detectable nodules appear at the site of injection within 7 to 13 days, but when 10^3 cells are injected, this lag time is increased to over 21 days. Since the cell doubling time for A9, at least in vitro, is about 16 hrs, this increase in lag time is unlikely to be due solely to the time it takes for the 10^3 injected cells to expand to 10^6 cells.

In contrast, A9 cells deliberately infected with M. hyorhinis (ATCC) and A. laidlawii have slightly longer lag time for tumor initiation and significantly slower tumor growth rate compared to the uninfected controls (see Table 5). In fact, tumors developed from A9 cells infected with M. hyorhinis (A9Mh) are all growth-arrested and never reach the usual large sizes regularly observed with the uninfected A9 cells. Many of the mice injected with mycoplasma-infected cells develop cachexia and a severe liver disease characteristic of the wasting syndrome described by others (19, 22).

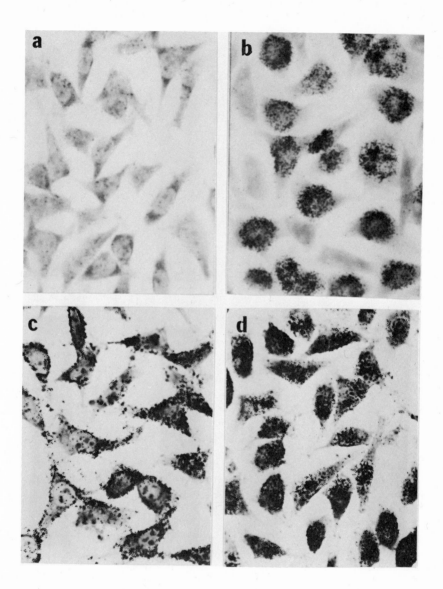

Figure 1. Autoradiographs of infected and uninfected control
A9 cells, after labelling with ^{3}H-thymidine for 24 hr during the
logarithmic growth phase, or with ^{3}H-uridine for 30 min.
  <u>a</u> Infected A9 cells, labelled with thymidine for 24 hr
  <u>b</u> Uninfected A9 cells, labelled with thymidine for 24 hr
  <u>c</u> Infected A9 cells, labelled with uridine for 30 min
  <u>d</u> Uninfected A9 cells, labelled with uridine for 30 min

(From Van Diggelen, Phillips and Shin, ref. 2)

Table 5. Tumor Initiation and Growth Rate of Uninfected Control and Mycoplasma-Infected A9 Cells in Nude Mice

Cell Line	Origin of Cell Line	No. Cells Injected	Days before Tumor first Detected (days)	Final Weight of Tumor [a] (g)	Duration [b] of Experiment (days)	No. Mice with Tumor/ No. Injected
A9	Uninfected control	10^3	21-28	3	50	3/5
		10^4	15-19	3	45	10/10
		10^5	10-20	5	40	10/10
		10^6	7-13	7-11	35	15/15
A9Mh	A9, infected with M. hyorhinis (ATCC)	2×10^6	14-22	0.04-0.2	38-52	4/6
A9Al	A9, infected with A. laidlawii	10^6	10-16	0.2-1.5	33	5/5
		2×10^6	10,16	1.6,2.0	35	2/3
		4×10^6	12,14	0.3,2.5	36	2/2

A9 cells were infected deliberately with standard ATCC strains of M. hyorhinis or A. laidlawii and maintained in regular growth medium until the mycoplasma titer reached the maximal level according to the HPRT assay. Cells were then harvested by trypsinization and injected into nude mice subcutaneously as described in Materials and Methods. a Final weight of tumors when each series was terminated. Single values represent the average of the group; otherwise the range of weights is given. b Days post-injection, when the tumors were recovered or the experiment terminated. (From Van Diggelen, Shin and Phillips, ref. 3)

Above data indicate that extreme care should be taken in studies of cellular tumorigenicity in nude mice in order to avoid the complications that can arise through unrecognized contamination of the test cells by mycoplasma.

Surface Morphological Changes in A9 After Infection with M. hyorhinis and A. laidlawii Both M. hyorhinis (ATCC) and A. laidlawii can establish a persistent covert infection in A9 cells without causing detectable alterations in cell doubling time, plating efficiency or gross morphology when examined under phase optics at low magnification (Van Diggelen and Shin, unpublished observations). However, when glutaraldehyde-fixed cells are examined by electron microscopy, striking changes in the cell surface morphology are evident (3).

The scanning electron micrographs in Fig. 2 show A9Mh cells, which have been infected with M. hyorhinis 4 days previously and have reached the maximal titer of the mycoplasma as determined by the assay of mycoplasma-specific HPRT activity. The most striking feature of A9Mh cells is that the exposed surface of all interphase cells are literally saturated with the pleiomorphic, roughly spherical particles (Fig. 2). In an earlier study, we have shown that these more or less uniform spherical particles are present only on the external side of the cell membrane and have the diffuse, non-electron dense cores characteristic of mycoplasmas (2). Furthermore, these particles can be released from the cells by a gentle trypsinization, and the culture medium of A9 cells containing a maximal titer of M. hyorhinis may contain up to 10^8 infectious particles per ml (2).

Elimination of Mycoplasmas from Infected Cells after Passage in Nude Mice Both M. hyorhinis and A. laidlawii possess high levels of endogenous HPRT activity (23), which can be distinguished from the mouse HPRT by a number of criteria discussed earlier (see Table 1) (5). The mycoplasma-specific HPRT activity can thus be used as a quantitative measure of the infection of A9 cells by the two mycoplasma strains. As shown in Table 6, uninfected A9 cells have negligible HPRT activity, but acquire the mycoplasma-derived HPRT activity following a deliberate infection with M. hyorhinis or A. laidlawii. The increase in the HPRT activity is correlated with the increase in the number of mycoplasma particles in the culture as determined by the HPRT transfer assay (Table 2) as well as by scanning electron microscopy and the DNA-staining method (12).

Contamination of A9 cells by either M. hyorhinis or A. laidlawii results in a significant reduction in cellular tumorigenicity as determined in the nude mouse (Table 5). However, when the tumors which eventually develop from the infected A9 cells are removed from the nude mice and new cultures are established from them, these cultures are found to be free of the mycoplasmas (3).

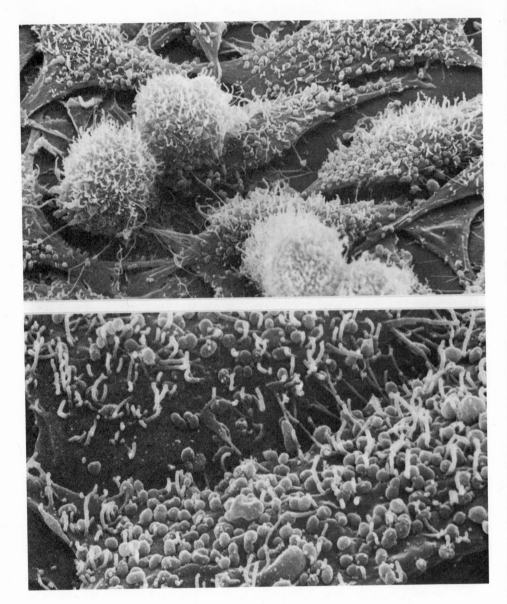

Figure 2. Scanning electron micrographs of A9Mh, mouse A9 cells deliberately infected with M. hyorhinis (ATCC) and allowed to reach the saturating level of mycoplasma titer. Cells were grown on glass coverslips, fixed and photographed as described in Materials and Methods. In a, a pair of recently divided cells can be seen at the left. In b, numerous mycoplasma particles and microvilli can be seen at a higher magnification on parts of two interphase cells.

Table 6.   Elimination of Mycoplasmas from Infected
A9 Cells by Transplantation in Nude Mice

| Cell Line | Cell-Associated HPRT Activity [a] (CPM) | Presence of Mycoplasma Particles Detected by: | | |
		DNA Staining [b]	Scanning EM [c]
Uninfected controls			
L929	82,600	—	—
A9	247	—	—
A9 cells deliberately infected			
A9Mh [d]	78,400	+++	+++
A9A1 [e]	14,200	+++	++
Infected A9 cells, passaged once through nude mice			
A9Mh-nu1	120	—	—
A9Mh-nu2	189	—	—
A9Mh-nu3	151	ND [f]	ND
A9Mh-nu4	266	ND	ND
A9A1-nu1	176	—	—
A9A1-nu2	216	—	ND
A9A1-nu3	230	—	ND
A9A1-nu4	145	ND	ND
A9A1-nu5	84	ND	ND

A9 cells were infected deliberately with M. hyorhinis and A.
laidlawii, and after the maximal titers were reached, harvested
and injected into nude mice. Tumors which developed were removed
aseptically and used to re-establish cultures as described in
Materials and Methods. The 9 tumor-derived lines listed here are
from the same experimental series summarized in Table 5.

    a Total HPRT activity in cell extract prepared in situ with
       Triton X-100 from confluent monolayers in 60 mm petri dish.
    b According to the Hochst 33258 method of Chen (12).
    c See Fig. 2 and 3.
    d Infected with M. hyorhinis (ATCC).
    e Infected with A. laidlawii.
    f ND: Not done.

(Data from Van Diggelen, Shin and Phillips, ref. 3)

This surprising result has been confirmed in 9 independent trials, 4 from A9 cells infected with M. hyorhinis (A9Mh) and 5 from A9 cells infected with A. laidlawii (A9Al) (see lower half of Table 6).

The absence of mycoplasmas from the "cured" A9 cells recovered from the nude mice was first demonstrated by the absence of the mycoplasma-derived HPRT activities in cell extracts (Table 6), and later by microscopic examination of fixed cells that have been grown for over 4 weeks in the control medium.   The scanning electron micrographs of A9Mh-nul cells, which are the cells that have been re-introduced into culture after one passage of A9Mh cells in nude mice, are presented in Fig. 3.   A comparison with the scanning elctron micrographs of A9Mh cells before the passage in nude mice (Fig. 2) demonstrates cearly that a single passage of mycoplasma-infected A9 cells in the immune-deficient mice has resulted in the complete elimination of the mycoplasma from the culture.   This conclusion is confirmed also by the results of screening the A9Mh and A9Mh-nul cells with the fluorescent dye Hoechst 33258, shown in Fig. 4.

Essentially identical results were obtained also with A9 cells infected with A. laidlawii (Table 6).   However, whether these observations are applicable generally to cell lines and mycoplasma strains other than A9 and M. hyorhinis and A. laidlawii remains to be seen.

When the "cured" A9 cells recovered from the tumors grown in nude mice, A9Mh-nu and A9Al-nu, were once again injected into nude mice, the lag time for tumor initiation and subsequent tumor growth rate were now comparable to those of the uninfected control A9 cells.   Therefore, the failure or delay in tumor growth following the first injection of A9Mh and A9Al cells observed in Table 5 was due to the presence of mycoplasmas in the cultures, and not caused by an irreversible change in cellular tumorigenicity (3).

Generality of the Phenotypic Alterations by Mycoplasma Contamination   The major phenotypic alterations caused in the mouse L cells by infection with M. hyorhinis described so far are summarized in Table 7.   These results are based mostly on our studies with the cryptic strain of mycoplasma, M. hyorhinis (Einstein).

Are these phenotypic alterations general phenomena applicable to other mycoplasma strains as well, or are they due to properties unique to certain select strains of M. hyorhinis?   In order to answer this question, we have screened five representative species of mycoplasma that are commonly encountered as contaminants of animal cell cultures (5).   These species are listed in Table 8. It was found that all of these mycoplasma species contain variable but significant levels of endogenous HPRT activity.   In terms of greater heat sensitivity, exaggerated inhibition by 6-thioguanine,

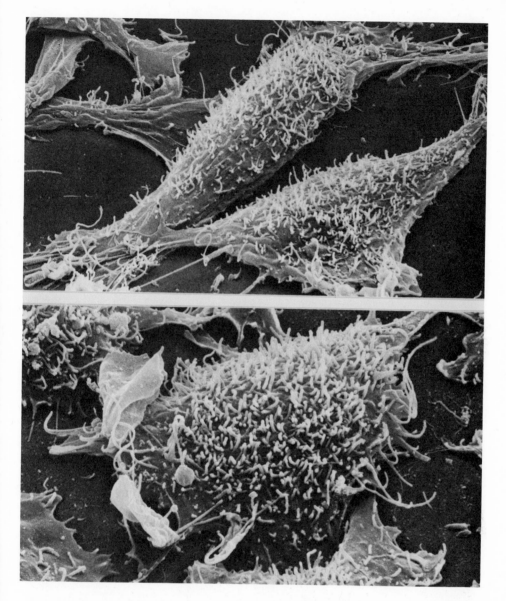

Figure 3. Scanning electron micrographs of A9Mh-nul, cells
derived from A9Mh cells after a single passage in nude mice. Note
the striking absence of the mycoplasma particles originally seen
on these cells before injection into the mice (Fig. 2). External
"blebs" sometimes appear on uninfected cells, as in b, but these
structures can be distinguished easily from the spherical mycoplasma
particles that are smaller and more uniform in size and shape.

Table 7. Phenotypic Alterations in Mouse Cells after
          Deliberate Infection with M. hyorhinis (Einstein)

	Cell Lines			
Apparent Phenotype	Control L929	Infected L929	Control A9	Infected A9
HPRT activity[a]	+++	+++	−	+++
Resistance to HAT medium	+	−	−	−
Resistance to 8-azaguanine	−	−	+	+
Uptake of ^{3}H-thymidine	+	−	+	−
Tumorigenicity in nude mice	+++	±	+++	±

a HPRT activity found in lysates prepared from trypsin-
   disaggregated, washed cells.

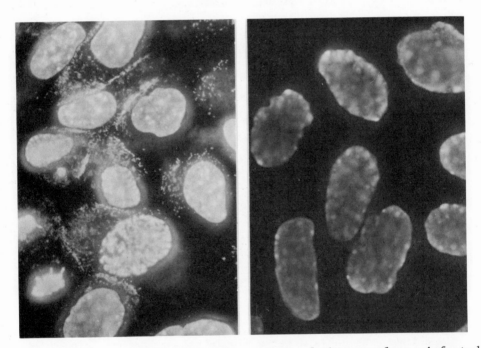

Figure 4. Fluorescence micrographs of the mycoplasma-infected
A9Mh cells (left), and the "cured" A9Mh-nul cells recovered from a
nude mouse tumor (right). Cells were grown for 4 days on glass
coverslips, fixed and stained with Hoechst 33258 according to Chen
(12). In A9Mh cells, numerous bright particles are visible in
extranuclear areas, but the A9Mh-nul cells show only nuclear
fluorescence indicating the absence of mycoplasma. (From 400 X)

Table 8. Endogenous HPRT Activity in Mycoplasmas:
Specific Activity, Heat Sensitivity and
Inhibition by 6-Thioguanine

Species	Specific Activity [a]	Heat Sensitivity [b]	Inhibition by 6-Thioguanine [c]
A. laidlawii	176	19.0	92.7
M. arginini	86	0.7	99.6
M. hyorhinis (ATCC)	27	3.1	97.5
M. hyorhinis (Einstein)	362	5.6	98.2
M. orale	75	0.4	99.6
M. salivarium	68	0.3	99.4
Mouse L929 cells	187	91.0	56.0

a nmoles of IMP formed/hr/mg protein at 37°C.
b % of original HPRT activity remaining after 2 min at 70°C.
c % of HPRT activity inhibited by equimolar concentration of
   6-thioguanine in the standard reaction mixture.
   (Data from Van Diggelen, McGarrity and Shin, ref. 5)

and slower electrophoretic mobility, the HPRT activity specified by
each of these mycoplasmas was similar to the HPRT activity of M.
hyorhinis (Einstein) and clearly different from the mammalian
enzymes(5) (Table 8). In electrophoresis on the cellulose acetate
gel in neutral pH (9), the fastest-migrating HPRT of mycoplasma
(A. laidlawii) is slightly slower than the Syrian hamster HPRT,
which is itself the slowest-migrating mammalian HPRT known so far
(9) (see Fig. 5).

In addition, each of the five mycoplasma species that we have
screened can transfer its HPRT activity to A9 cells, and render the
normally HAT-resistant L929 cells sensitive to HAT medium. These
data are summarized in Table 9.

These results therefore suggest that the alterations in
cellular phenotypes observed in the mouse A9 and L929 cells after
infection by M. hyorhinis or A. laidlawii probably do occur in
other cell lines infected with other species of mycoplasmas.
From this perspective, it would seem that many experimental data
that describe unusual or unexpected cellular behavior may in fact
have been generated by unrecognized contamination of the cell
cultures by mycoplasmas. As we have shown, certain strains of
mycoplasma can easily escape conventional detection methods.

Table 9. Transfer of Mycoplasma-Specific HPRT to
          A9 Cells after Deliberate Infection, and
          Loss of HAT-Resistance in Infected L929 Cells

| Infecting Mycoplasma | A9 | | L929 |
	Cell-Associated HPRT Activity (CPM) a	Growth in HAT Medium	Growth in HAT Medium
None	31	−	+++
A. laidlawii	17,430	−	−
M. arginini	824	−	−
M. hyorhinis (ATCC)	6,254	−	−
M. hyorhinis (Einstein)	54,180	−	−
M. orale	365	−	−
M. salivarium	733	−	−

Uninfected control A9 and L929 cells were first screened for
the absence of mycoplasma contamination by the DNA-staining method,
and 15,000 cells were seeded in each Linbro well. Standard stock
solutions containing the mycoplasma species in excess of 10^3
particles were added to each well, and after 4 days of incubation
in the control medium, cell-associated HPRT activity was assayed
by the micro assay technique described in Materials and Methods, or
cellular resistance to HAT medium was determined by plating 10^5
cells in each 60 mm Falcon petri dish in control medium plus HAT.
The uninfected L929 cells had a plating efficiency of at least
40% in the control medium; none of the mycoplasma-infected cultures
produced a single viable clone in HAT medium.

(Data from Van Diggelen, McGarrity and Shin, ref. 5)

SUMMARY

The results presented in this paper demonstrate that unrecognized contamination of cell cultures by mycoplasmas can significantly
alter the apparent physical, biochemical and genetic properties
of the cells. In particular, the following specific phenotypic
alterations have been documented:

(a) Due to the high endogenous HPRT activity in all common
     mycoplasma species, mutant cells deficient in this enzyme
     may appear to have "reverted" to the normal HPRT-positive
     phenotype after contamination by a mycoplasma.

(b)   Both HPRT-positive and HPRT-negative cells may become
      extremely sensitive to HAT medium when infected with
      mycoplasma. As a result, cell lines contaminated with
      mycoplasmas may fail to yield viable cell hybrids if
      the HAT selection method is used for their isolation.

(c)   Cells infected with certain strains of mycoplasma do not
      incorporate exogenous nucleosides from the culture
      medium. Mycoplasma-contaminated cells can therefore
      produce misleading results in studies of cellular
      incorporation of ^{3}H-thymidine or ^{3}H-uridine.

(d)   Mycoplasma infection of normally tumorigenic cells may
      result in a significant reduction in, or a complete
      failure to express, the tumorigenic potential when the
      cells are assayed by injection into nude mice.

(e)   At least with the mouse A9 cells deliberately infected
      with M. hyorhinis and A. laidlawii, a single trans-
      plantation in the nude mouse and subsequent recovery of

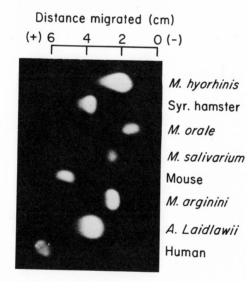

Distance migrated (cm)

(+) 6   4   2   0 (-)

M. hyorhinis

Syr. hamster

M. orale

M. salivarium

Mouse

M. arginini

A. Laidlawii

Human

Figure 5.   Electrophoresis of HPRT activities of five common
strains of mycoplasma and three mammalian species. See the text.
Syr. hamster: BHK-21; Mouse: L929; Human: HeLa.
(From Van Diggelen, McGarrity and Shin, ref. 5)

the cells from the tumor can result in the complete
elimination of the mycoplasma from the cell cultures.

(f) Our data indicate that at least some of the above
     observations on phenotypic alterations induced by M.
     hyorhinis (Einstein) are applicable also to other
     mycoplasma species that commonly contaminate cell
     cultures. These species include A. laidlawii, M. argi-
     nini, M. hyorhinis (ATCC), M. orale and M. salivarium.

ACKNOWLEDGMENTS

    We are greatly indebted to Dr. David M. Phillips for the
electron micrographs, and to Dr. Gerard J. McGarrity for supplying
us with the standard strains of mycoplasma as well as for helpful
suggestions and discussions. This work was supported by PHS
research grants 5 RO1 GM21015 and 1 PO3 GM19100 (Genetics Center
Grant to Albert Einstein College of Medicine), and a research grant
from the National Science Foundation (PCM-76-07573). S.S. is a
recipient of a Faculty Research Award from the American Cancer
Society.

REFERENCES

1. Hopps, H.E., B.C. Meyer, M.F. Barile and R.A. DelGiudice. 1973.
    Problems concerning "non'cultivable" mycoplasma contaminants
    in tissue culture. Ann. N.Y. Acad. Sci. 225:265.

2. Van Diggelen, O.P., D.M. Phillips and S. Shin. 1977. Endoge-
    nous HPRT activity in a cryptic strain of mycoplasma and its
    effect on cellular resistance to selective media in infected
    cell lines. Exp. Cell Res. 106:191.

3. Van Diggelen, O.P., S. Shin and D.M. Phillips. 1977. Reduct-
    ion in cellular tumorigenicity after mycoplasma infection
    and elimination of mycoplasma from infected cultures by
    passage in nude mice. Cancer Res. 37:2680.

4. Shin, S., R. Caneva, C.L. Schildkraut, H.P. Klinger and M.
    Siniscalco. 1973. Cells with phosphoribosyl transferase
    activity recovered from mouse cells resistant to 8-azaguanine.
    Nature 241:194.

5. Van Diggelen, O.P., G.J. McGarrity and S. Shin. 1978. Endo-
    genous HPRT activity in mycoplasmas isolated from cell
    cultures. (Submitted for publication)

6. Szybalski, W., E.H. Szybalska and G. Ragni. 1962. Genetic studies with human cell lines. Nat. Cancer Inst. Monogr. 7:77.

7. Sharp, J.D., N.E. Capechi and M.R. Capecchi. 1973. Altered enzymes in drug-resistant variants of mammalian tissue culture cells. Proc. Nat. Acad. Sci. 70:3145.

8. Shin, S., P. Meera Khan and P.R. Cook. 1971. Characterization of hypoxanthine-guanine phosphoribosyl transferase in man-mouse somatic cell hybrids by an improved electrophoretic method. Biochem. Genet. 5:91.

9. Van Diggelen, O.P. and S. Shin. 1974. A rapid fluorescence technique for electrophoretic identification of hypoxanthine phosphoribosyltransferase allozymes. Biochem. Genet. 12:375.

10. Freedman, V.H. and S. Shin. 1974. Cellular tumorigenicity in nude mice: Correlation with cell growth in semi-solid medium. Cell 3:355.

11. Freedman, V.H., A.L. Brown, H.P. Klinger and S. Shin. 1976. Mass production of animal cells in nude mice with retention of cell specific markers. Exp. Cell Res. 98:143.

12. Chen, T.R. 1977. In situ detection of mycoplasma contamination in cell cultures by fluorescent Hoechst 33258 stain. Exp. Cell Res. 104:255.

13. Littlefield, J.W. 1964. Three degrees of guanylic acid-inosinic acid pyrophosphorylase deficiency in mouse fibroblasts. Nature 203:1142.

14. Littlefield, J.W. 1964. Selection of hybrids from fibroblasts in vitro and their presumed recombinants. Science 145:709.

15. Holland, J.F., R. Korn, J. O'Malley, H.J. Minnemeyer, and H. Tieckelmann. 1967. 5-Allyl-2'-deoxyuridine inhibition of nucleoside phosphorylase in HeLa cells containing mycoplasma. Cancer Res. 27:1867.

16. Stanbridge, E. 1971. Mycoplasmas and cell cultures. Bacteriol. Rev. 35:206.

17. Nardone, R.M., J. Todd, P. Gonzalez, and E.V. Gaffney. 1965. Nucleoside incorporation into strain L cells: Inhibition by pleuropneumonia-like organisms. Science 149:1100.

18. Todaro, G.J., S.A. Aaronson and E. Rands. 1971. Rapid detection of mycoplasma-infected cell cultures. Exp. Cell Res. 65:256.

19. Flanagan, S.P.   1966.   "Nude", a new hairless gene with
        pleiotropic effects in the mouse.   Genet. Res. 8:295.

20. Pantelouris, E.M.   1968.   Absence of thymus in a mouse mutant.
        Nature 217:370.

21. Shin, S., V.H. Freedman, R. Risser and R. Pollack.   1975.
        Tumorigenicity of virus-transformed cells in nude mice is
        correlated specifically with anchorage independent growth
        in vitro.   Proc. Nat. Acad. Sci. 72:4435.

22. Scheid, M.P., G. Goldstein and E.A. Boyse.   1975.   Different-
        iation of T cells in nude mice. Science 190:1210.

23. Stanbridge, E.J., J.A. Tischfield and E.L. Schneider.   1975.
        Appearance of hypoxanthine guanine phosphoribosyltransferase
        activity as a consequence of mycoplasma contamination.
        Nature 256:329.

METHODS OF PREVENTION, CONTROL AND ELIMINATION

OF MYCOPLASMA INFECTION

Gerard J. McGarrity, Veronica Vanaman and Judith Sarama

Department of Microbiology

Institute for Medical Research, Camden, New Jersey

INTRODUCTION

Mycoplasma infected cell cultures should not be used for experimental or diagnostic work. Many reports have been published in
this text and elsewhere on the effects of mycoplasma infection on
cultured cells. These reports represent only a small portion of
the total effects of infection. In a particular infected culture,
the possible simultaneous effects are numerous, including: alterations in nucleic and amino acid metabolism, depletion of nutrients
from the medium, chromosomal damage, phenotypic alteration, enzyme
induction, induction of interferon, and membrane changes. An alteration in one characteristic can induce additional changes in other
characteristics. Aula and Nichols demonstrated that chromosome damage
by mycoplasmas was caused by depletion of arginine from the medium
(1). Therefore, the overall effect of infection can be the additive
or synergistic total of all mycoplasmal effects. Some effects may
not become immediately produced and may become apparent only after
10, 20 or more population doublings following infection. For these
reasons, studies showing no apparent difference between infected and
non-infected cultures as a rationale to use infected cultures should
be viewed skeptically.

The best safeguard is prevention. This is preferable and much
easier than rectifying the damage caused by widespread infection
in the laboratory. All cell cultures should be viewed as potentially
infected and handled accordingly. Preventive and control measures
must consider the major modes of transmission of mycoplasma
infection in the laboratory, i.e., how infection is introduced
into the laboratory and how it spreads from culture to culture.

The rate of mycoplasma infection of cell cultures is influenced primarily by the population sampled. Infection rates in long term cell cultures, cell cultures with antibiotic containing media, and cell cultures handled in laboratories having chronic mycoplasma problems tend to be higher than primary cultures, cultures in low passage number, cultures without antibiotics, and in cultures handled in laboratories with effective quality control programs. Barile et al have reported infection rates of approximately 15% over a 16 year period (2). We have examined more than 5,200 cell cultures over a 6 year period and found an infection rate of 7.4% (3). In our studies, the annual rate of infection has ranged from 3.4% to 14.9%, dependant primarily on the nature of the cultures tested. Most of our studies were on cell cultures in relatively early passage, 5th or less, and were performed primarily on cultures submitted for cell banking. The rate of infection was lower in these cultures.

The major mycoplasma species isolated by Barile et al and ourselves have been human, bovine and porcine (2,3). This tends to incriminate laboratory technicians, bovine serum and trypsin (derived from porcine stomach) as the primary sources of mycoplasma infection. We have noted that when a cell culture from a particular laboratory contained mycoplasma, most, perhaps all, cell cultures in that laboratory were likewise infected with the same mycoplasma species (4).

EPIDEMIOLOGY OF MYCOPLASMAL INFECTION OF CELL CULTURES

To be effective, a quality control program must be based on a clear understanding of the epidemiology of mycoplasma infection. This consideration must include the sources of mycoplasmas and the mode of transmission to explain: a)the predominance of human, bovine and porcine mycoplasma species; and b)the all or none pattern of infection of all cultures in a particular laboratory.

Figure 1 illustrates the primary and secondary sources of mycoplasma infection of cell culture. The terms primary and secondary are used epidemiologically, referring to chronological sequence. They do not refer to frequency or relative importance of these sources. The primary sources include bovine serum, trypsin, the tissue specimen used to initiate the cell culture and laboratory personnel. The secondary source of infection is other infected cell cultures. These sources will be analyzed from the standpoint of frequency of contamination, mycoplasmal concentration in these sources and ease of dissemination into the environment.

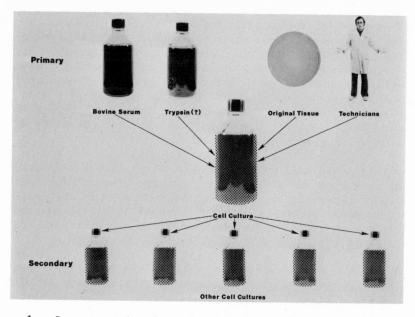

Figure 1. Sources and modes of transmission of mycoplasmal infection of cell cultures.

Bovine Serum

    Bovine serum is a requirement to grow virtually all types of animal cells. McKeehan et al have shown that the requirements of fetal bovine serum protein can be less than 25 g/ml (0.05%) serum in defined media for WI-38 cell cultures. Such defined media (MCDB 104) can be used only for prescribed cell types (5).

    Wide variation can occur in different lots of bovine serum from different suppliers and from individual suppliers. Because of the potential effects of chemical and microbiological con- tamination total quality control of bovine serum will be covered, not only problems associated with mycoplasma. In an extensive quality control survey on fetal bovine serum Boone et al found significant variations in inter and intra suppliers in certain parameters (6). Significant differences were detected in total growth-supporting capacity under certain conditions, total protein, hemoglobin, lactic dehydrogenase and free fatty acids. No significant differences were found in specific gravity and a lipid panel consisting of total lipids, neutral fats, and choles- terol. Sera were not examined for steroids other than cholesterol. The only parameter that correlated with growth-promoting capacity

in this study was the concentration of free fatty acids: the higher
the free fatty acid concentration the poorer the growth promotion.
Human fetal lung cells were used as indicators of growth in this
study. Other more fastidious cells could possibly be influenced
by variations other than free fatty acids. For example, lactic
dehydrogenase can be a measure of leukocytolysis as well as
hemolysis. Leukocytolysis can contaminate serum with activated
lysosomal hydrolases that can degrade serum components to form
products toxic for some cultures.

While certain cell cultures can be maintained in low serum
media or in serum-free media for 1-2 passages, serum free media
for routine culture is not likely to be available in the near
future. To minimize the effects of biochemical variations and to
prevent introduction of adventitious agents, suppliers and users
must institute stringent quality control measures.

Unprocessed bovine serum collected in the abattoir is grossly
contaminated. Abattoir collected serum is centrifugated and filtered
to reduce the incidence of contamination. Many microorganisms have
been isolated from bovine serum used in cell culture media. These
organisms are listed in Table 1 and include various types of bacteria, several viral agents, mycoplasmas, yeast, fungi and bacteriophage. Processed sera are generally free of gross microbiological
contamination and subjected to sterility testing by suppliers.
An incidence of contamination of approximately 10% was detected
in commercial fetal bovine serum in one study (6). The incidence
of contamination among four suppliers ranged from 5 to 29%. Sterility tests vary, but generally include multiple microbiological
media and incubation temperatures and should include specific
assays for mycoplasma. Mycoplasma testing should utilize the
large volume test method of Barile and Kern (7). This technique
involves the inoculation of a minimum of 25 ml of the test serum
into mycoplasma media. Only those serum lots that pass such tests
are sold commercially.

Table 1   ORGANISMS ISOLATED FROM BOVINE SERUM

            Acholeplasma laidlawii
            Mycoplasma arginini
            Mycoplasma hyorhinis
            Infectious bovine rhinotracheitis
            Bovine virus diarrhea
            Parainfluenza 3
            Bovine enterovirus
            Bovine syncytial virus
            Bacteriophage
            Bacteria (many)
            Yeast
            Fungi

Any contamination (especially mycoplasmal) that is undetected by these test procedures will generally be difficult to detect and of a low order of magnitude. This low incidence of contamination will be in the range of Poisson distribution (8). Poisson is a discrete distribution which can be applied to a sequence if a random variable, x, is distributed among a parameter X according to the equation:

$$P\ (X{=}x)\ =\ e^{-\ \lambda}\ \lambda^{\ x} \over X\ !$$

where x = a count, 1,2...; e = 2.7181 (natural logarithm base); and λ is the mean and the variance (square of the standard deviation) of the distribution, i.e., $\lambda = \mu = \sigma^2$

Poisson distribution can be used to explain mycoplasmal con-tamination of bovine serum. The event p(contamination) is very rare but n (no. of bottles) is so large that the mean number of contam-inated bottles (p x n) is a finite constant equal to X. Assume the usual mycoplasmal containination rate of bovine serum bottles under present conditions is small (p = .01), i.e., 1% and in sterility tests of 1,000 bottles, 6 are found to be contaminated. The probability of 6 or more contaminations occurring can be determined by Poisson distribution where X = n x p = 1,000 x 0.001 = 1.0. From tables of Poisson probability functions, the probability of having 6 bottles contaminated is very rare = 0.0006. This low order of probability will influence the chances of detecting low levels of contamination and indirectly the sampling size required.

Gerwe has calculated that sterility testing of a small number of samples, ten or twenty, out of a large lot can only detect gross contamination, and may not detect levels of contamination of 1% or less (9). Kundsen, using binomal expansion and theoretical values demonstrated that probability of acceptance of lots of vary-ing assumed degrees of contamination were little affected by differ-ences in lot size, but greatly affected by differences in sample size, particularly for lots of higher defectiveness (10).

Brewer devised probability tables that list the 95% confi-dence level for acceptance of lots as sterile (11). The data are presented in Table 2. The probability that a 1% contaminated lot will be accepted as sterile is 82% when 20 samples are assayed. At this contamination level, contamination will usually be missed even when 50 samples are assayed. With a contamination rate of 0.1%, assay of 100 consecutive samples would yield a probability of 91% of missing the contamination. Therefore, the sterility test procedure must be designed with media, incubation conditions and controls to detect low levels of contamination and fastidious contaminants as efficiently as possible. Quality control procedures for bovine serum are outlined later in this chapter.

Table 2   RELATIONSHIP OF PROBABILITIES OF ACCEPTANCE OF LOTS OF
             VARYING ASSUMED DEGREES OF CONTAMINATION OF SAMPLE SIZE

% Contamination

N*	0.1	0.3	0.5	1
10	.99	.98	.96	.91
20	.98	.94	.90	.82
50	.95	.86	.78	.61
100	.91	.74	.61	.37
200	.82	.55	.36	.13
300	.74	.41	.22	.05
400	.67	.30	.13	.02
500	.61	.22	.08	.01

N* - Number of samples tested.   From Brewer, 1957 (11).

Two problems are inherent in all sterility test procedures:
sample size and appropriate growth media. Generally, the entire
volume of the test material cannot be sampled. The sterility of
the whole is presumed on the basis of testing a relatively small
sample. This assumption can be erroneous; low levels of contamination can be undetected by random sampling. Further, the media used
in sterility tests will not support growth of all microorganisms.
Therefore, even elaborate test procedures are selective. The U.S.P.
states, "Interpretation of the results of sterility tests must allow
for the possibility that the degree of contamination is of a low
order of magnitude" (12).

Routine testing of serum does not always include screens for
viruses, although this can be a serious problem. Technics are
available for detection of bovine viruses in serum (13,14).
Molander et al in one series reported in 1968 demonstrated
that approximately 10% of serum lots contained bovine viruses,
particularly bovine virus diarrhea virus, infectious bovine
rhinotracheitis virus and parainfluenza virus (15). Bovine
herpes virus has also been isolated from serum (13).

From the above consideration it is clear that negative
sterility tests do not guarantee sterility of the specimen (12).
If mycoplasmas are present in bovine serum that has been tested
by large volume technics, they will be present in low concentrations
and in a small number of bottles per lot. If bovine serum is the
only source of bovine mycoplasmas isolated from cell cultures, one

would expect that infection by these species (primarily A. laidlawii
and M. arginini) would follow the same Poisson distribution of
bovine serum contamination. This would mean that virtually all
laboratories would be subject to such random mycoplasma infection
regardless of preventive measures, and that infection within a
laboratory would be sporadic, one or two cultures being contaminated.
This is not the case. We conclude that while bovine serum is
chronologically a primary source of infection and necessary to
initiate infection in a laboratory, other factors are needed to
explain the observed pattern of infection.

Trypsin

Trypsin is a suggested source of infection. This is based
on the isolation of the porcine species Mycoplasma hyorhinis
from cell cultures. Barile et al have shown that M. hyorhinis
accounts for approximately 21% of all mycoplasma isolates
from cell cultures (16). The incidence in our survey is far less -
on the order of 2-3%. This difference may be due to populations
sampled, and to the periods of sampling, our surveys started in
1971 while Barile et al were initiated years before. The heretofore
unrecognized fastiduous strains of this organism may alter these
statistics. All cell cultures should be tested for this specific
fastidious strain.

Trypsin routinely used to disaggregate cell culture monolayers
is derived from porcine stomach. It has been postulated that
the organism is introduced into cell cultures in this manner.
However, M. hyorhinis has never been isolated from trypsin.
Our studies show that trypsin treatment will kill mycoplasmas
with death curves being influenced by the number of mycoplasmal
organisms and the presence of mycoplasma clumps (3). MacMorine
has reported that overnight exposure of mycoplasmas to trypsin
results in complete killing of the organism (personal communicaton).
Therefore, the relative importance of trypsin as a source of
mycoplasma is unclear.

An alternate transmission route of M. hyorhinis is bovine
serum. Swine and cattle are occasionally processed through the
same slaughterhouse, bovine serum may become contaminated with
swine mycoplasma during collection and processing. The organism
has been isolated from serum (16,17).

Of particular interest is the finding by Gois et al (18).
In this study, 7 of 51 strains of M. hyorhinis could be detected
in the lungs of pigs by immunofluorescent, but not culture
techniques. This indicates the possibility that the fastidious
strains of M. hyorhinis may not necessarily be cell culture adapted
strains of the organism, but can exist in vivo as well. These
may represent true obligate parasites in pig lungs. Conversely,
the inability of these strains to grow could be due to the mycoplasmacidal activity of some lung suspensions (19).

Whether these fastidious strains of M. hyorhinis cell culture
adapted strains or fastidious wild types should be determined.
If the latter is true, fastidious strains of other species, unable
to propagate on cell free media, should be considered. Gois et al
demonstrated that certain strains of M. arginini, M. hypopneumoniae
and M. hyosynoviae could be detected in lungs of pigs by immunofluorescence but not by culture (18).

Regardless of whether M. hyorhinis is introduced via serum
or trypsin it can be concluded that trypsin itself is not the major
source of all M. hyorhinis isolated from cell cultures for the same
reasons listed for bovine serum.

Original Tissue Specimen

The original tissue specimen used to initiate cell cultures
can theoretically be a source of microbiological, including
mycoplasmal, contamination, dependent particularly upon the
anatomical site of the tissue. Tissue specimens, even from skin
and colon, can be adequately sterilized by antibiotic treatment
for the first passage. Mycoplasmas have been isolated from the
mouth, throat, lower respiratory tract, blood, hands and urogenital
tracts. Barile has shown that the tissue specimen itself was not
a major source of mycoplasma infection (2,9,16). In these studies,
between 0.5 and 1.0% of original tissue specimens contained
mycoplasmas. Although precise quantitative data are not available
from our laboratory our observations are similar. Of more than
1,000 human skin fibroblast cultures tested, less than five were
infected with human mycoplasmas in the second passage or less
(unpublished results).

Other supportive evidence comes from the fact that the
major mycoplasma species isolated are human, bovine and porcine
despite the fact that many cell cultures of other animal species
are handled in the laboratory. We have assayed hundreds of mouse
cell cultures without isolating murine mycoplasmas. On the other

hand we have isolated bovine mycoplasmas from mouse, human, cat, dog and monkey cell cultures. Further, Barile has reported an infection rate of approximately 1% in primary cultures with increasing frequency as passage levels increase (20). Based on these observations one can conclude that the original tissue specimen is not a major source of mycoplasma infection.

Special consideration is required for lymphocyte cultures. Murphy et al and Barile et al have isolated mycoplasmas from peripheral blood (21,22). Murphy et al have shown that mycoplasmas could be isolated from apparently normal individuals, although the frequency of isolation increases significantly during immuno-suppression caused by underlying disease or therapy. Mycoplasma infection should be considered in the initiation of lymphocyte cultures and mycoplasma testing should be performed as soon as possible after establishment of continuous lymphocyte cell lines (23).

Personnel

Since a significant percentage of mycoplasma isolates from cell cultures are human species, laboratory personnel must be considered as potential sources. Numerous reports have been published on human carriage of mycoplasma in the throat and oral cavity (24-27). A significant percentage of normal healthy humans harbor mycoplasma in these sites based on isolations by culture or serology.

Purcell et al demonstrated distinct antibody patterns for human mycoplasmas in different age groups (24). Antibody to M. orale type 1 was observed in 50-90% of all age groups. Antibody to M. salivarium was detected in more than 90% of individuals older than 10 years of age. This was the most frequently encountered mycoplasma in this study, which we confirmed by isolating the organism from 24 of 31 (80.4%) cell culture personnel (4). Kundsin and Praznik demonstrated that 84% of their study group yielded M. orale type 1 or M. salivarium in pharyngeal cultures (25).

In a Japanese study, only 5 of 66 throat swabs (7.6%) and 18 of 117 sputa samples (15.4%) yielded mycoplasmas (26). However, in this study, 8 of 23 strains (34.8%) isolated from sputa and throat swabs were M. orale and 15 as M. salivarium. Further, the highest incidences of mycoplasmal species were the dental calculus (88%), the inflammed or degenerative crevice (56.8%) and the healthy gingival crevice (52.6%). All isolates from gingival crevices and dental calculi were identified as M. salivarium.

The role of M. salivarium and M. orale in the mouth is unclear. The results of Kumagai et al suggested that M. salivarium
is an inhabitant of the gingival sulci, although the conclusion
might be based on an analysis of the predominant population of
oral mycoplasmas (26). Razin et al has also isolated this organism from gingival crevices (27). M. salivarium could originate
in gingival areas and be transported to other exudates e.g.,
throat and saliva.

M. orale type 1 might originate from tissues away from the
gingival areas, especially tonsils, and deeper oropharyngeal areas.
Crawford and Kraybill isolated M. orale with increasing frequency
from patients with acute respiratory disease (28). The incidence
of the organism was higher in the sputa from patients with chronic
respiratory disease (26).

The significance of the oral cavity as a source of cell cultures is not clearly understood. We have been unable to detect
M. orale in throats of personnel from laboratories having chronic
infection of cell cultures due to this organism. Conversely, although M. salivarium is the predominant oral mycoplasma, it is only
rarely isolated from cell cultures. It was not among the 1,376 cell
culture isolates reported by Barile et al (2). We have isolated the
organism from lymphocyte cultures from two laboratories.

Oral microorganisms can be disseminated into the environment
via droplets generated by talking, sneezing and other activities.
M. salivarium was recovered from droplets after talking and
sneezing by human volunteers. M. orale was not detected in the
same studies (4).

What mycoplasmal infection that is transmitted via oral droplets
should be eliminated by antibiotic free media and use of hand or pro
pipettes. Oral droplets contain a variety of microorganisms, including staphylocci, streptococci, diplococci, neisseria, and perhaps
yeast and mycoplasma. Introduction of these droplets into cell
cultures with antibiotic free media would result in rapid microbial
growth, gross turbidity and destruction of the cell cultures within
one-two days. With antibiotics, however, most of these microorganisms
are killed. Yeast and mycoplasmas would be the most resistant.
Antibiotics would select mycoplasmas and other fastidious organisms
as contaminants that could reproduce under these conditions. Typicall
such contaminants would be slow growing, be difficult to detect
and not produce gross turbidity or other apparent changes in the
culture. They could remain undetected for years. Mouth pipetting
can generate these droplets under certain conditions. Use of hand
pipettes and a practice of no talking when handling cell cultures
should eliminate this possible mode of transmission. Various hand
pipettes are available (29).

Conclusions from Consideration of Primary Sources

Consideration of serum, trypsin, original tissue specimens and personnel as primary sources indicates that mycoplasmas are either present in low numbers in these sources or, in the case of personnel, the microorganisms are not generated and disseminated in large numbers into the environment. Mycoplasmas would be present in these sources according to Poisson distribution. If these were the only factors of mycoplasma infection, infection rates would also follow Poisson distribution. One would expect a sporadic incidence of infection on a random basis in all laboratories, perhaps one every 2-3 years, infecting only a small portion of the cell cultures. This can happen, but it is not the normal observation. Preventive measures, especially sterility testing, would not significantly alter the incidence.

Infected Cell Cultures

Other mechanisms are needed to explain the observed pattern of widespread infection of all cultures in a laboratory. Infected cultures themselves offer such an explanation. In infected cultures, concentrations of mycoplasmas are typically 10^6-10^8 CFU/ml. Additional organisms are associated with the plasma membrane of the cultured cells. Infected cultures contain 2-3 more logs of mycoplasmas than cells. These cultures could alternately be viewed as mycoplasmal cultures contaminated with cells. A comparison of mycoplasmal concentrations between the primary and secondary sources of infection shows approximately six logs greater concentration in the secondary source. Mycoplasmal infected cell cultures can serve as a secondary source of infection.

We and others have noted the existence of so-called low levels of infection, on the order of 10^1-10^3 CFU/ml. We now believe that low level infections are artifacts, caused by improper sampling, presence of antibiotics, poor quality of media, or other variables. Improper sampling includes assays performed on old or post confluent cultures, assay of media but not cells, presence of additives such as trypsin, dimethyl sulfoxide, or certain antibiotics. Handling of the cell culture can affect the number of mycoplasmas present (3). We have performed mycoplasmal viable counts on more than 100 infected cell cultures when the cells were in late log-early stationary phase of growth. We have never detected less than 10^5 CFU/ml. In these proceedings, DelGiudice and Hopps have reported sparse levels of growth with some strains of Serogroup 38, although these were not quantitated.

Cell culture mycoplasmas can be readily disseminated into the environment. All routine laboratory procedures with liquid media can generate droplets (30,31). Pipetting, decanting, centrifuging, sonicating and other routine procedures generate relatively large droplets. Such droplets will not remain airborne, but will sediment within seconds into the immediate environment, onto hands, work surfaces, supplies, equipment, etc. A droplet of 0.05 ml from an infected culture will contain, on the average, 5×10^5 (10^7 CFU/ml x .05 ml) mycoplasma organisms. These sedimented droplets can serve as a source of further infection. We have detected mycoplasmas on equipment, hands, supplies and the work surfaces during and after trypsin-ization and passage of 3T6 cell cultures infected with Acholeplasma laidlawii (4). Even gentle removal of a T-50 flask of an A. laidlawii infected 3T6 culture from the incubator resulted in heavy contamination of the lip of the flask. Pipettes, hands, propipettes, outside of flasks, work surfaces and the outside of disinfectant pans all yielded mycoplasmas (4).

Additional supplies used with infected cell cultures will also become contaminated. Contaminated coverslips, hemocytometers, trypan blue, centrifuge tubes, needles, syringes, animals receiving injections of infected cell cultures, can disseminate the organism in the environment.

Mycoplasmas are remarkably resistant to dehydration and can survive drying for days. Separate cell culture supernatants con-taining M. orale or A. laidlawii were detected 4-7 days after inoculation onto a work surface (4). Kundsin demonstrated that aerosols of M. pneumoniae, M. orale type 1 and M. hominis could survive in aerosol, even when the count mean diameter of the aerosol was 2.1 μm (32). Wright et al showed the survival of air-borne mycoplasmas was influenced by relative humidity (33).

These characteristics of cell culture mycoplasmas: 1)concentrations of 10^6-10^8; 2)easy generation of droplets; and 3)prolonged survival of dried mycoplasmas lead us to conclude that mycoplasmal infected cell cultures are themselves the biggest single source of infection. These characteristics would also explain how, after initial introduction into a laboratory, mycoplasmas eventually infect all other cell cultures in the laboratory. If the initial introduction into cell cultures is from serum, personnel, tissue specimens, the inoculated mycoplasma undergo logarithmic growth in the first 4-7 days. The mycoplasma concentration increases from the 10^0-10^1 levels in the primary sources to the 10^6-10^8 ml typically seen in infected cultures.

Mycoplasmas could also be brought into the laboratory in infected cultures. Several situations have been encountered in which laboratories have had their initial infection after receiving cultures from laboratories that had chronic mycoplasma problems. Regardless of the source of the infection, it is clear that once in the laboratory, it is only a matter of time before the infection spreads, unless stringent measures are taken. Under controlled conditions, we trypsinized and passed a culture free of mycoplasma immediately after work with an infected culture was completed. No disinfectant or safeguards were practiced for the purposes of this experiment. Within three weeks the originally clean culture was infected with the same mycoplasma species as was present in the first cell culture. This demonstrates the ease of spread and the need for adequate control measures, especially chemical disinfection of the immediate environment following work with each individual cell line.

These data also demonstrate the breakdown in the integrity of aseptic barriers around individual cultures. These results on mycoplasma spread could also relate to other types of contamination-infection. Mycoplasmas can serve as an indicator of how other microorganisms, particularly viruses, could be similarly spread to infect other cell cultures and serve as a biohazardous risk to personnel. The same mechanism could also explain the widespread contamination of animal cell cultures by HeLa and other cell cultures reported independently by Gartler and Nelson-Rees (34,35). The same preventive measures, careful aseptic technic and thorough chemical disinfection of work surfaces, should control spread of all (36,37).

These breaks in aseptic barriers can also result in contamination of cell cultures by microorganisms in the environment. The hair, clothing and hands of personnel, air, and organisms growing in moist areas are particularly significant sources. It is not generally possible to determine the source of environmental contamination. We have, on occasion, been able to document the source of bacterial and fungal contamination. These are listed in Table 3. The first six of these have been reported previously (38); the final four are described here.

Table 3   SOURCES OF CELL CULTURE CONTAMINATION

Cell Culture	Contaminant	Source
Aedes aegypti	Torula sp.	Serum
Glial cells	Torula sp.	Serum
Henle's intestine	Staphylococcus albus	Hand lotion dispenser
Fathead minnow	Pseudomonas sp.	Floor mat
Chinese hamster	Pseudomonas sp.	Trypsin
F 483	Flavobacterium sp.	Faucet
3T3 4 C	Pasteurella sp.	Rat
RIII - MT	Pseudomonas sp.	Water bath
HEL	Mycobacterium	Technician (?)
Nine cultures	Bacillus sp.	Media during sterility test

The pasteurella organism evidently was transferred from rats by an investigator who handled the cell culture only once, 20-30 minutes after handling rats in the animal colony. The organism had a bi-polar staining characteristic, and was also isolated from the rats that were handled.

A water bath, constantly filled and maintained at 37°C was the source of pseudomonas contamination in RIII-MT and several other cell lines. Only cultures that were trypsinized in this laboratory became contaminated. Pseudomonas sp. was isolated from all contaminated cultures. Analysis showed that the trypsin was removed from the refrigerator and warmed in the water bath before use. The water contained more than 10^5 CFU of pseudomonas organisms per ml. The isolates from the cell culture and the water bath were of the same pyocin type (39).

A technician was believed to be the source of Mycobacterium smegmatis contamination. Only cultures handled by this technician contained the organism although cultures, media and facilities were shared with other personnel. Ten to fifteen cultures yielded the organism over a several month period. M. smegmatis has been isolated from skin and genitals; sampling of the technician's hands failed to recover the organism.

A Gram positive rod was introduced into McCoy's medium
during sterility testing. Four different microbiological
media inoculated with the McCoy's were sterile. The last procedure
in the sterility protocol was to add 5 ml of the McCoy's test
specimen to a sterile tube. The organism, a Bacillus sp. and
ubiquitous in the environment was isolated from the last tube
containing only McCoy's. Subsequent tests showed the contaminant
could readily grow in all four media, and the organism was not
isolated from other bottles of McCoy's, even with membrane filtration of 450 ml. It was concluded that the organism contaminated
the media during the final step of the sterility test. The contamination was originally interpreted as a false positive,
and the media was used in several cell cultures, all of which
were destroyed in 24 hours by the Bacillus sp.

PREVENTIVE MEASURES

An effective preventive and control program must consider both
the primary and secondary sources of infection. Quality control
measures must be practiced on all aspects of the culture facility,
including media components, personnel, environment, tissue specimens and other specifics that could influence the sterility of
cultures or culture components. The recommendations listed in this
section are specific for mycoplasma. However, many can also be
appplied to a broader control program for bacterial and fungal
contaminants. Other reviews for detection and control of non
mycoplasmal microorganisms are available (4,36,37,38,40,41).

Although sterility testing of bovine serum is performed by
commercial suppliers, this institute also conducts sterility tests
on lots of serum before purchase. When the in-house supply of
serum drops below a defined level the supplier is contacted and an
entire lot is reserved. Three bottles from that lot are sent for
sterility and growth promotion testing. Growth promotion comparisons are made with a previously accepted lot. The type of indicator cell culture used should be representative of the types
used in each facility. Two human skin fibroblast lines are used
in this institution.

Sterility testing is performed using two different growth temperatures (30°C and 37°C) and five different microbiological media.
Media include fluid thioglycolate, brain-heart infusion, Sabaroud
dextrose, trypticase soy broth and mycoplasma broth and agar media.
Mycoplasma testing is by large volume mycoplasma procedure of

Barile and Kern (7). If sterility and growth test results are acceptable, the entire lot of bovine serum is purchased. Smaller laboratories can request a 100 ml serum from a lot before purhase. This quality control procedure has resulted in the rejecting of two sera lots for microbiological contamination and three lots for poor growth promotion over the past 10 years. Microbiological contamination was caused by torula yeasts and diphtheroids. Additional sterility testing is performed on each individual bottle of serum by laboratory technicians. Other media components are tested by incubating dispensed aliquots of media at 37°C for 14 days.

Even so, problems can occur. Figure 2 is a bottle of unopened bovine serum from a lot that was tested by the supplier and our laboratory and found free of detectable contamination. Mold was observed in this unopened refrigerated bottle, demonstrating that no sterility test protocol can guarantee the complete absence of microbiological contamination in a lot. Frequent examination of cell cultures can minimize the potential risks of low level contamination.

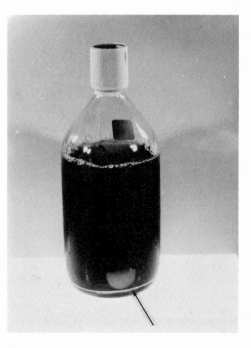

Figure 2. Fungal contamination in an unopened bottle of fetal bovine serum from a serum lot that was accepted as sterile.

Mycoplasmas could be introduced in the same fashion. Spontaneous mycoplasmal infection was encountered in this laboratory within the past 6 months. Two cell cultures previously shown to be mycoplasma free by exhaustive tests developed mycoplasma infection within a three week period following thawing and expansion of frozen stock. Extensive repeat testing of frozen and expanded cultures confirmed these results. Both infected cultures yielded Acholeplasma laidlawii. The two cell cultures were handled in separate laboratories, and used different bottles from the same lot of serum. Extensive sampling of the frozen cell stocks, the lot of bovine serum and the environment in each laboratory followed. All failed to detect A. laidlawii. No other cultures were infected. It is assumed although not proven, that this infection was introduced via the bovine serum. This is based on the isolation of a bovine mycoplasma. Calculations have shown that if this lot of serum contained mycoplasma it would be on the average 1 infectious unit per 10.5 liters of serum.

This was an unusual situation and was the only time during the past ten years that such mycoplasma infection arose spontaneously. The fact that no additional cultures in either of the two laboratories became infected attests to the efficiency of the control measures in effect.

Original tissue specimens, explants and biopsies should be assayed for mycoplasma and other microbiological contaminants as soon as possible. Antibiotics are routinely used for biopsy material only. This generally includes penicillin, 1,000 units per ml and streptomycin, 100 mcg per ml. Gentamycin at a concentration of 100 mcg per ml or a combination of oxacillin 20 mcg/ml and gentamycin, 50 mcg/ml (40). Penicillin-streptomycin treatment has been acceptable for human skin fibroblasts, and has resulted in a very low level of contamination - on the order of 1% (A.E. Greene, personal communication). Continued antibiotic treatment beyond the first passage does not generally eliminate microorganisms and is usually futile.

Infected Cultures

Since infected cultures constitute the major source of infection, special care must be undertaken to prevent culture to culture spread. One should assume that all cultures in the laboratory are infected and proceed accordingly.

New cell cultures should be acquired only from reliable sources and should be accompanied by a statement listing the last

date of mycoplasma testing, methods used and test results. Several
situations have been encountered in which the initial mycoplasmal
infection in a laboratory occurred shortly after introduction of
cultures from laboratories with known mycoplasmal problems.
By the time cultures were assayed and mycoplasmas were detected,
the infection spread to other cultures. The practice of
acquiring cultures from collaborators and colleagues without mycoplasma assay is a potentially disasterous one and should be
avoided. If possible, cultures should be acquired from reliable
cell repositories who have performed standardized tests on all
cell cultures. The possibility exists that even cultures from such
repositories may contain mcyoplasma, especially since many cells
were deposited before the existence of fastidious strains of
Mycoplasma hyorhinis was recognized (42,43). The standard
tests performed by most repositories, agar and broth inoculation,
would not have detected these strains. We have isolated
M. orale from several cultures from a cell repository (44).

     Cultures should be retested after they are introduced into
the laboratory and periodically thereafter. The type of test
procedure employed will depend upon the capabilities of the individual laboratory. Different technics are described elsewhere
in this text. Until test results are available, cultures should
be handled in a quarantine facility. This should consist of
a separate laboratory used to handle only those cultures whose
mycoplasma status is unknown. It should include separate media,
supplies, equipment and handling. If this is not feasible, quarantine cultures can be handled at the end of the workday after work
with clean cultures has been completed.

     The frequency of mycoplasma testing thereafter will be influ-
enced by several factors, including the past history of the laboratory with regard to mycoplasma infection. Laboratories having a
chronic mycoplasma problem require more frequent testing. Frequency of testing would also depend on the number of cell cultures
used, those handling more cultures should institute frequent test
programs. The number of cultures introduced into the laboratory
from other sources is another consideration. Those laboratories
handling small numbers of cell cultures, approximately 5, and
having no past history of mycoplasma infection based on standardized
effective test procedures, should test their cell cultures every
3-6 months. Laboratories handling an increased number of cell
cultures; receiving numerous cultures from outside laboratories;
or having mycoplasma problems in the past should institute
more frequent testing. Laboratories using indirect methods should
have their results confirmed periodically by a combination of agar
and broth inoculation and immunofluorescence for M. hyorhinis.

The sensitivity and limitations of the mycoplasma screening
method should be known. For example, microbiological culture
alone will not detect all strains of M. hyorhinis and ratio of
uptake of uridine to uracil can yield false results in cell
cultures showing poor growth. The limitations on all procedures
are described in detail elsewhere in this text. Distinctions
should be made between presumptive and diagnostic tests.

Positive and negative controls must be included. Use of mycoplasma
infected cultures to serve as positive controls may be unacceptable
to some laboratories. One alternative is to send cultures to outside laboratories for mycoplasma testing. For epidemiological
purposes and to determine possible sources of infection, all mycoplasma isolates should be identified.

Because of the large concentrations of mycoplasmas in infected
cultures and the ease of droplet formation, thorough and efficient
chemical disinfection of work surfaces after work with individual
cultures is crucial. Aside from the need to monitor for mycoplasmas, this control measure is the most important in preventing
spread of infection through the laboratory. Many efficient disinfectants are available. Chloro-phen (Rochester Germicide,
Rochester, N.Y.) has been routinely used in this laboratory at a
concentration of 2 ounces per gallon. Just as important as the
selection of the disinfectant is its proper use. Concentration,
length of exposure, and presence of extraneous protein are factors
that will influence the efficiency of disinfection. The disinfectant solution should be generously applied to the work surface
when work with a particular cell culture has been completed, and
allowed to remain on the surface for approximately 5 minutes.
Rubber gloves should be worn to avoid skin irritation.

Some laboratories place cotton gauze or other materials
soaked with disinfectant on the work surface during cell culture
manipulations. These can dry out in mass air flow rooms or laminar
air flow cabinets. Glass or plastic wares placed on the soaked
pad can become slippery because of the presence of detergents
in disinfectant solutions.

Personnel Practices

The major preventives against personnel contamination include
the use of antibiotic free media for all stock cultures and the
prohibition of mouth pipetting. For certain experiments having an
increased risk of contamination due to extraordinary manipulations

or large numbers of specimens, e.g. virus titrations, antibiotics can be incorporated into the test cultures for the duration of the experiment. This should only be in the experimental vessels, not stock cultures.

Laboratory personnel should wear protective clothing when performing aseptic operations. This can be either a clean laboratory coat worn over street clothing or, preferably, special laboratory clothing worn in place of street clothes. Cell culture personnel should don special laboratory coats for travel to more contaminated zones, such as administrative areas and animal laboratories. Since hands can become contaminated with mycoplasmas, effective hand washing should be performed after work with a particular cell culture has been completed.

Aseptic technics should be regularly reviewed and updated with laboratory personnel. Most of the published laboratory work is performed not by the principle investigator, but by the laboratory technologist. The decisive battle against contamination will be fought at the laboratory bench by the technologist. Investigators should regularly discuss potential problems of contamination with the technologist. We reported an overall contamination rate of 1% when a number of technicians made repeated serial dilutions in sterile broth tubes (28). Most technicians performed the entire procedure perfectly, but sporadic contamination did occur. Even a low level of contamination of 1% during procedures could result in significant problems over 12 months based on the assumption that cell cultures are either passed and/or refed twice weekly. A culture handled 104 times per year with a contamination potential at each handling of 1%, would be contaminated within the year. New equipment and supplies introduced into the laboratory should be analyzed for the potential as a source or reservoir of contamination. Especially troublesome are items that either store liquids (CO_2 incubators and water baths) or are difficult to clean.

Ventilated Safety Cabinets

The microbial content of laboratory air is the sum of the the number of organisms present in incoming air and by the number generated by personnel and procedures in the laboratory. We have demonstrated that airborne bacteria increased inside a conventially ventilated transfer room during routine procedures (38). Efficient filtration and ventilation can reduce the threat of airborne contamination. Airborne transmission is probably a minor route of transfer for mycoplasma infection of cell cultures. However, many other environmental microorganisms can contaminate cultures via the airborne route.

The airborne route of contamination can be effectively eliminated by mass airflow (MAF) or laminar airflow (LAF) units. The filters in these units, high efficiency particulate air, or HEPA filters, are 99.7% efficient in removal of particles having an effective diameter of 0.3 m (45). The efficiency of filtration actually <u>increases</u> for particles smaller than 0.3 microns because of a <u>longer</u> path of particles through the filter due to Brownian movement (46).

Mean diameter of viral elementary bodies is less than 0.3 m. However, airborne microorganisms generally do not exist as naked particles but ride on larger particles of hair, skin, dust, dried sputum, etc. HEPA filtration will effectively remove all viable airborne microorganisms by direct filtration or dehydration of organisms on the filters. If required, used HEPA filters can be gas sterilized prior to removal in some units (47).

In LAF ventilation, HEPA filtered air is uniformly introduced into an enclosure throughout an entire ceiling (or wall) and moves vertically (or horizontally) at a relatively high velocity, 100 ft/ min. Contamination generated in the enclosure is removed by the rapidly moving airstream within seconds for recirculation and fil- tration.

Work with potentially biohazardous material should be per- formed in LAF biological safety cabinets (47). Different designs are available. The basic design and performance of these units is currently regulated by standards promulgated by the National Sanitation Foundation (NSF) (48). To meet NSF standards, LAF biological safety cabinets must pass engineering, physical and biological criteria, including in-use test procedures. Biological testing includes challenge of the unit with spore suspensions of <u>Bacillus</u> <u>subtilis</u> var niger to determine dissemination of contamination inside the cabinet, protection of the product inside and protection of the personnel outside the cabinet. The biological safety cabinet should be located away from doors, air vents, traffic and other areas of activity. Generation of air turbulence by walking and other activities can compromise the protective air curtain at the front of the unit. Placement of materials inside the working cabinet can also affect efficiency. Overloading the cabinet can negate the advantages of the uniform air distribution and the air curtain. Purchase of LAF biological safety cabinets should only be from manufacturers who have met NSF specifications. The basic design of the LAF safety cabinet can be modified to increase the volume of exhaust air and charcoal filtration for work with potentially mutagenic and carcinogenic materials (Labconco Corp., Kansas City, Mo.)

For procedures where there is no, or minimal biohazard, the work can be performed in MAF units. These utilize a remotely located HEPA filter and a ceiling distribution system with velocities considerably less than LAF, typically on the order of 25 fpm. These units have been shown effective in various biomedical environments (38,49-51). Advantages of mass air flow include reduced purchase, maintenance and air conditioning costs, and reduced noise levels. The operator can sit in the MAF enclosures without the physical separation of LAF safety cabinets.

Efficient use of LAF and MAF systems will essentially eliminate the airborne route as a major source of contamination. However, quality control measures are needed to guarantee the effectiveness of filtration and ventilation. A significant number of laminar airflow safety cabinets had detectable leaks in the filter and improper air distribution in one study (52). These can negate the advantages of air flow systems. Quality control measures should include checking the integrity of the filter media, the filter gasket and the filter seal. Airflow, and where appropriate, air curtains should be checked. Test procedures are available. Names of firms who perform commercial testing of LAF and MAF units are available from NSF and manufacturers.

Waste Disposal

Spent media and discard cultures should also be viewed as potentially infected. Spent media should be carefully decanted into a pan of disinfectant. The same criteria of factors influencing disinfection apply here. Disinfectant solutions of 3X strength should be used in discard pans. The concentration of disinfectant will be decreased by addition of liquids and inactivation by the addition of protein solutions from cell cultures, serum, etc. Spent media should not be discarded into sinks. Vacuum lines should contain in-line HEPA filters to eliminate infectious aerosols.

Phenolic disinfectants leave residues on glassware and autoclaves. This can corrode autoclave parts, although we have not experienced any significant problem in more than 10 years of autoclaving disinfectant solutions. Disinfectant residues on glassware can be eliminated by thorough rinsing of glassware in high purity water. Autoclaving of disinfectant solutions will not be a serious problem if two autoclaves are available in the kitchen, one for sterilization of discarded wares and the second for sterilization of clean, wrapped glassware for laboratory use. If two autoclaves are not available, non-corrosive disinfectants can be used.

Glassware should be completely immersed in the disinfectant
solution to insure proper killing action and to prevent clogging
of small orifices with dried proteinaceous material. Disinfection in the pan also reduces the potential microbial hazard of
transporting glass and plastic wares to the kitchen for autoclaving. Transporting wares in pans with lids or covers is another
alternative.

ELIMINATION OF MYCOPLASMA INFECTION

Many reports have been published on elimination of mycoplasmas from infected cultures (53-57). These reports have utilized
various procedures including antibiotics, antisera, injection into
nude mice and hypotonic solutions. This laboratory has investi-
gated several published procedures with uniformly poor results.
Mycoplasma sampling conducted immediately after treatment have
usually been negative, but repeat testing performed 2-3 weeks
later have generally resulted in detection of the same species
of mycoplasma as originally isolated. Possible explanations for
this include a small residuum of mycoplasma remaining after treatment or reinfection of the 'cured' cell cultures by other infected
cultures in the laboratory. Either is possible. Controlled prospective studies using genetically marked organisms could determine
which of these two factors are more important.

Regardless of the efficacy of these treatments, the initial
question regarding elimination is why should attempts be made
to cure the infection? Mycoplasma infection indicates that a minimum
of 10^8 organisms of mycoplasma have been present in the culture
during the period of infection, which may be weeks, months,
even years. The infection will exert tremendous effects on the
cell culture. These can range from transient to permanent
and include parameters such as population growth, cytopathology,
alterations in nucleic acid and amino acid metabolism and chromosome
abberations. These effects hae been reviewed in this text and
elsewhere (58). In addition to the gross biochemical effects,
the effects of selective pressure must also be considered. The
cell population resultant from mycoplasmal infection may be
significantly different from the original population. Additionally,
the elimination procedure will also select sub-populations from the
culture.

We recommend prompt elimination of infected cultures from the
laboratory by autoclaving. This avoids such cultures serving as a
source of further infection. The infected culture is essentially
an unknown culture that cannot be compared to noninfected cultures

of the same type. Reports have stated that mycoplasma infection
does not influence the specific parameter of interest in a cell
culture study. This is generally based on short-term controlled
studies with and without mycoplasma infection measuring a single
cell parameter. The effect of mycoplasma infection changes
with time. No difference may be detectable shortly after infection.
In one study, we first noted discernible changes in a culture 14
passages after mycoplasmal infection (23).

The key to minimizing effects of mycoplasma is prevention
and control of infection. Cultures that are of interest should
be frozen in early passage to serve as a reserve in case of mutation
or mycoplasma infection. The preventive and control measures
outlined here are prudent steps to minimize possibility of erroneous
results and should be viewed as part of an overall effective and
practical quality control program. These measures have proven
effective. A large number of infected and non-infected cultures
are continuously being submitted to the cell repositories housed
at this institute. No documented case of accidental cross infection
has ever occurred when cultures were in quarantine. Even when
mycoplasmal infection developed in the two non-quarantine laboratories
described above, no further infection developed.

Effective cell culture quality control measures serve as a
life insurance program to the cell culture laboratory contributing
to the continued productivity of the laboratory even when challen-
ged with disaster.

References

1. Aula, P. and W.W. Nichols. 1967. The cytogenetic effects of
     mycoplasma in human leucocyte cultures. J. Cell Physiol.
     70:281-289.

2. Barile, M.F., H,E. Hopps, M.W. Grabowski, D.B. Riggs and R.
     delGiudice. 1973. The identification and sources of mycoplas-
     mas isolated from contaminated cell cultures. Ann. N.Y. Acad.
     Sci. 225:251-54.

3. McGarrity, G.J. 1977. Factors influencing microbiological
     detection of mycoplasmas in cell cultures. Submitted for pub-
     lication.

4. McGarrity, G.J. 1976. Spread and control of mycoplasmal infection
     of cell cultures. In Vitro 12:643-648.

5. McKeehan, W.L., K.A. McKeehan, S.L. Hamilton and R.G. Ham.
   1977. Improved medium for clonal growth of human diploid
   fibroblasts at low concentrations of serum protein. In
   Vitro 13:399-416.

6. Boone, C.W., N. Mantel, T.D. Caruso, Jr., E. Kazam and R.E.
   Stevenson. 1972. Quality control studies on fetal bovine
   serum used in tissue culture. In Vitro 7:174-189.

7. Barile, M.F. and J. Kern. 1971. Isolation of Mycoplasma arginini
   from commercial bovine sera and its implication in contaminated
   cell cultures. Proc. Soc. Exp. Biol. Med. 138:432-437.

8. Bahn, A.K. 1972. Basic Medical Statistics pp. 182-183, Grune and
   Stratton, New York.

9. Gerwe, E.G. 1956. Safety testing of poliomyelitis vaccine by
   tissue culture technic. Dagli Atti del 2 Congresso Internaz-
   ionale de Standardizazione Immunomicrobiologica. Rome.

10. Knudsen, L.F. 1949. Sample size of parenteral solutions for
    sterility testing. J. Amer. Pharm. Assoc. 38:332-337.

11. Brewer, J.H. 1957. In: Antiseptics, Disinfectants, Fungicides and
    Sterilization. Second edition (G.L. Reddish, ed.) Lea and
    Febiger. Philadelphia, Pa. pp. 160-161.

12. The United States Pharmocopeia, Nineteenth edition. 1975 Mack
    Printing Co., Easton, Pa.

13. Molander, C.W., A.J. Kniazeff, C.W. Boone, A. Paley and
    D.T. Imagawa. 1972. Isolation and characterization of
    viruses from fetal calf serum. In Vitro 7:168-173.

14. Federoff, S., V.J. Evans, H.E. Hopps, K.K. Sanford and C.W.
    Boone. 1972. Summary of proceedings of a workshop on serum
    for tissue culture purposes. In Vitro 7:161-165.

15. Molander, C.W., A. Paley, C.W. Boone, A.J. Kniazeff and D.T.
    Imagawa. 1968. Studies on virus isolation from fetal calf
    serum. In Vitro 4:148.

16. Barile, M.F., H.E. Hopps and M.W. Grabowski. 1977. Incidence
    and sources of mycoplasma contamination: a brief review.
    These proceedings.

17. Barile, M.F. 1973. Mycoplasma contamination of cell cultures:
    mycoplasma-virus-cell culture interactions. In: Contamination
    of Tissue Cultures (J. Fogh, ed.) Academic Press, N.Y. pp.
    517-520.

18. Gois, M., F. Sisak, F. Kuksa and M. Sovadina. 1975. Incidence
    and evaluation of the microbial flora in the lungs of pigs
    with enzootic pneumonia. Zbl. Ved. Med. B. 22:205-219.

19. Kaklamanis, E., L. Thomas, K. Stavropoulos, I. Borman and
    C. Boshwitz. 1969. Mycoplasmacidal action of normal tissue
    extracts. Nature 221:860-862.

20. Barile, M.F. 1967. Mycoplasma and cell cultures. NCI Monograph 29:
    201-204.

21. Murphy, W.H., C. Bullis, L. Dabick, R. Heyn and C.J. Zarafonetis.
    1970. Isolation of mycoplasma from leukemic and nonleukemic
    patients. J. Nat. Cancer Inst. 45:243-251.

22. Barile, M.F., G.P. Bodey, J. Synder, D.B. Riggs and M.W.
    Grabowski. 1966. Isolation of Mycoplasma orale from leukemic
    bone marrow and blood by direct culture. J. Nat. Cancer Inst.
    36:155-159.

23. McGarrity, G.J. 1977. Effects of mycoplasmas on lymphocyte
    cell cultures. These proceedings.

24. Purcell, R.H., R.M. Chanock and D. Taylor-Robinson. 1969. Serol-
    ogy of the mycoplasmas of man. In: The Mycoplasmatales and
    the L-Phase of Bacteria (L. Hayflick, ed.) Appleton-Century
    Crofts, New York pp. 221-264.

25. Kundsin, R.B. and J. Praznik. 1967. Pharyngeal carriage of
    mycoplasma species in healthy young adults. Amer. J. Epidem-
    iol. 86:579-593.

26. Kumagai, K., T. Iwabuch, Y. Hinuma, K. Yuri and N. Ishida.
    1971. Incidence, species and significance of mycoplasma species
    in the mouth. J. Infect. Dis. 123:16-21.

27. Razin, S., J. Michmann and Z. Shimshoni. 1964. The occurrence of
    mycoplasmas (pleuropneumonia-like organisms) (PPLO) in the oral
    cavity of dentulous and edentulous subjects. J. Dent. Res. 43:
    402-405.

28. Crawford, Y.E. and W.H. Kraybill. 1967. The mixture of myco-
    plasmas of man. Ann. N.Y. Acad. Sci. 143:411-421.

29. Halbert, M.M., J. Krober, D. Vesley and N. Vick. 1975. Catalog
    of pipetting aids and other safety devices for the biomed-
    ical laboratory. University of Minnesota School of Public
    Health, Minneapolis.

30. Dimmick, R.L., W.F. Vogl and M.A. Chatigny. 1973. Potential for
    accidental aerosol transmission in the biological laboratory.
    In: Biohazards in Biological Research (A. Hellman, M.N.
    Oxman and R. Pollack, eds.). Cold Spring Harbor Laboratory,
    Cold Spring Harbor, N.Y., pp. 246-266.

31. Kenny, M.T. and F.L. Sabel. 1968. Particle size distribution
    of Serratia marcescans aerosols created during common labor-
    atory accidents. Appl. Microbiol. 10:1146-1150.

32. Kundsin, R.B. 1968. Aerosols of mycoplasmas, L forms and bac-
    teria: comparison of particle size, viability, and lethality
    of ultraviolet radiation. Appl. Microbiol. 16:143-146.

33. Wright, D.N., G.D. Bailey and M.T. Hatch. 1968. Survival of
    airborne mycoplasma as affected by relative humidity. J.
    Bacteriol. 95:251-252.

34. Gartler, S.N. 1967. Genetic markers as tracers in cell culture.
    NCI Monograph 26:167-194.

35. Nelson-Rees, W.A. and R.R. Flandermeyer. 1977. Inter and intra
    species contamination of human breast tumor cell lines HBC
    and BrCa5 and other cell cultures. Science 195:1343-1344.

36. McGarrity, G.J. 1975. Serum quality control. TCA Manual 1:
    167-169.

37. McGarrity, G.J. 1975. Control of microbiological contamination.
    TCA Manual 1:181-184.

38. McGarrity, G.J. and L.L. Coriell. 1971. Procedures to reduce con-
    tamination of cell cultures. In Vitro 6:257-265.

39. Bruun, J., G.J. McGarrity, W.S. Blakemore and L.L. Coriell
    1976. Epidemiology of Pseudomonas aeruginosa infection by
    pyocin typing. J. Clin. Microbiol. 3:264-271.

40. Armstrong, D. 1973. Contamination of tissue culture by
    bacteia and fungi. In: Contamination in Tissue Culture.
    (J. Fogh, ed.). Academic Press, N.Y.

41. McGarrity, G.J. 1977. Cell culture facilities. TCA Manual.
    In press.

42. Hopps, H.E., B C. Meyer, M.F. Barile and R.A. DelGiudice.
    1973. Problems concerning "non-cultivable" mycoplasma
    contaminants in tissue cultures. Ann. N.Y. Acad. Sci.
    225:265-276.

43. DelGiudice, R.A. and H.E. Hopps. 1977. Microbiological
    methods and fluorescent microscopy for the direct demon-
    stration of mycoplasmal infection of cell cultures.
    These proceedings.

44. McGarrity, G.J. and L.L. Coriell. 1973. Detection of
    anaerobic mycoplasmas in cell cultures. In Vitro 9:17-18.

45. Anonymous. 1972. Federal Standard No. 209 b, U.S. Govt.
    Printing Office, Washington, D.C.

46. Whitby, K.T. and D.A. Lundgren. 1965. Mechanics of air
    cleaning. Trans. A.S.A.E. 8:342-352.

47. Coriell, L.L. and G.J. McGarrity. 1968. Biohazard hood to
    prevent infection during microbiological procedures.
    Appl. Microbiol. 16:1895-1900.

48. National Sanitation Foundation Advisory Committee for bio-
    hazard Cabinetry. 1976. National Sanitation Foundation
    Standard No. 49 for Class II (Laminar Flow) Biohzard
    Cabinetry. NSF, Ann Arbor, Michigan.

49. Coriell, L.L., G.J. McGarrity and J. Horneff. 1967. Medical
    applications of dust-free rooms I: elimination of airborne
    bacteria in a research laboratory. J. Amer. J. Public
    Health Nat. Health 57:1824-1836.

50. Coriell, L.L., W.S. Blakemore and G.J. McGarrity. 1968.
    Medical applications of dust-free rooms: II. elimination
    of airborne bacteria from an operating theatre. J. Amer.
    Med. Ass. 203:1038-1046.

51. McGarrity, G.J., L.L. Coriell, A.E. Greene, R.W. Schaedler,
    and R.J. Mandle. 1969. Medical applications of dust-free
    rooms: use in an animal care laboratory. Appl. Microbiol.
    18:142-146.

52. Wedum, A.G., W.E. Barkley and A. Hellman. 1972. Handling of infectious agents. J.Amer. Vet. Med. Ass. 16:1557-1567.

53. Pollock, M.F. and G.E. Kenny. 1963. Mammalian cell cultures contaminated with pleuro-pneumonia-like organisms. III. elimination of pleuro-pneumonia like organisms with specific antiserum. Proc. Soc. Exp. Biol. Med. 112:176-181.

54. Perlman, D., S.B. Rahman and J.B. Seman. 1967. Antibiotic control of mycoplasma in cell culture. Appl. Microbiol. 15:82-85.

55. Gori, G.B. and D.Y. Lee. 1964. A method for eradication of mycoplasma infections in cell cultures. Proc. Soc. Exp. Biol. Med. 117:918-921.

56. Mardh, P.H. 1975. Elimination of mycoplasmas from cell cultures with sodium polyanethol sulphonate. Nature 254:515-516.

57. VanDiggelen, O., S. Shin and D. Phillips. 1977. Reduction in cellular tumorigenicity after mycoplasma infection and elimination of mycoplasma from infected cultures by passage in nude mice. Cancer Res. 37:2680-2687.

58. Stanbridge, E. 1971. Mycoplasmas and cell cultures. Bacteriol. Rev. 35:206-227.

CELL CULTURE MYCOPLASMAS: A BIBLIOGRAPHY

Compiled by Gerard J. McGarrity, Diane Meredith,
Dorothy Gruber, and Marcella McCall

Institute for Medical Research
Camden, New Jersey

INTRODUCTION

The purpose of this bibliography is to list all available
references on the various aspects of mycoplasma infection of
animal cell cultures. Topics covered include: general reviews
and textbooks; basic properties of mycoplasmas; incidence,
detection and identification of cell culture mycoplasmas; effects
of mycoplasmas on various cell culture parameters; effects of
mycoplasmas on organ cultures; antibiotic sensitivities and
potential methods of elimination; and preventive measures. Many
sources were utilized in this literature search. Major sources
were Volumes I, II and III of the mycoplasma bibliographies
published by Domermuth and Rittenhouse, a Medlars II search conducted by the National Library of Medicine's National Interactive
Retrieval Service for this Institute, and our own personal files.

This bibliography has been assembled without selection and
prejudice. Cross referencing has been used. A paper reporting
the effects of mycoplasma infection on chromosomes in cells infected with influenza virus would be listed under both cytogenetics
and viruses. The references under each heading are in alphabetical
order of the first author. The authors would be happy to be informed of any omissions which can be incorporated into a future
publication.

INDEX

REFERENCES

1. GENERAL REVIEWS AND TEXTBOOKS

Anonymous. 1971. Summary of proceedings of a workshop on serum
for tissue culture purposes. In Vitro 8(3):161-7.

Anonymous. 1972. Pathogenic mycoplasmas. A Ciba Foundation Symposium. Elsevier Excerpta Medica. North Holland.

Brown, A. and J.E. Officer. 1968. Contamination of cell cultures
by mycoplasma (PPLO). In: Methods in Virology. K. Maramorosch
and H. Koprowski, ed. 4:531-564. New York, Academic Press

Domermuth, C.H. and J.G. Rittenhouse. 1971. Mycoplasmataceae: A
Bibliography and Index 1852-1970. Virginia Polytechnic Institute and State University. Blacksburg, Va.

Domermuth, C.H. and J.G. Rittenhouse. 1973. Mycoplasmatales: A
Bibliography and Index 1970-1972. Virginia Polytechnic Institute and State University. Blacksburg, Va.

Domermuth, C.H. and J.G. Rittenhouse. 1976. The Mycoplasmas:
A Bibliography and Index 1973-1975. Virginia Polytechnic Institute and State University. Blacksburg, Va.

Fogh, J. (ed.) 1973. Contamination of Tissue Cultures. Academic
Press, N.Y.

Fogh, J., N.B. Holmgren, P.P. Ludovici. 1971. A review of cell
culture contaminations. In Vitro 7(1):26-41.

Hayflick, L. (ed.) 1969. The Mycoplasmatales and the L Phase
of Bacteria. Appleton-Century-Crofts, N.Y.

Hayflick, L. (consult. ed.) 1967. Biology of the Mycoplasma.
Ann. N.Y. Acad. Sci. vol. 143.

Hayflick, L. 1965. Tissue cultures and mycoplasmas. 1965. Tex.
Rep. Biol. Med. 23: Suppl. 1:285-302.

Kagan, G.Y. 1966 and 1967. Mycoplasma: infections of man,
animals, and tissue cultures. Genetics of Microorganisms
53-67, No. 10B774.

Krudy, E.S. and D. Shiers. 1977. Mycoplasma: A Bibliography. Information Retrieval. Washington, D.C. and London.

Ludovici, P.P., N.B. Holmgren. 1973. Cell culture contaminants. Methods Cell Biol. 6:143-208.

Maniloff, J. and H. J. Morowitz.1972. Cell biology of the myco-plasmas. Bact. Rev. 36(3):263-90.

Maniloff, J. and A. Liss. 1973. The molecular biology of myco-plasma viruses. Ann. N.Y. Acad. Sci. 225:149-58.

Maramorosch, K. (ed.) 1973. Mycoplasma and Mycoplasma-like Agents of Human, Animal, and Plant Diseases. Ann. N.Y. Acad. Sci. vol. 225.

Mattman, L. 1974. Cell wall deficient forms. 411p. Illus. CRC Press, Cleveland, Ohio.

Razin, S. 1969. Structure and function in mycoplasma. Ann. Rev. Microbiol. 23:317-56.

Sharp, J.T. (ed.) 1970. The Role of Mycoplasmas and L Forms of Bacteria in Disease. Charles C. Thomas, Springfield, Ill.

Smith, P.F. 1971. The Biology of Mycoplasmas. Academic Press, N.Y.

Stanbridge, E. 1971. Mycoplasmas and cell cultures. Bacteriol. Rev. 35(2):206-27.

Taylor-Robinson, D. and P.M. Furr. 1973. The distribution of T-mycoplasmas within and among various animal species. Ann. N.Y. Acad. Sci. 225:108-17.

Thomas, L. 1969. Mechanisms of pathogenesis in mycoplasma infec-tion. Harvey Lect. 63:73-98.

Tully, J.G. and S. Razin. 1977. The Mollicutes. In: Handbook of Microbiology, vol. 1, 2nd edition. A.I. Laskin and H. Lechevalier (eds.) Chemical Rubber Co., Cleveland, Ohio (in press).

2. BASIC PROPERTIES OF MYCOPLASMAS

Addey, J.P., et al.1970. Viability of mycoplasmas after storage in frozen or lyophilised states. J. Med. Microbiol. 3:137-45.

Al-Aubaidi, J.M. and J. Fabricant. 1971. Methods for purification
of mixed cultures of mycoplasma. Cornell Vet. 61(4):559-72

Altucci, P., G.L. Varone and G. Catalano. 1969. On a mycoplasma
inhibitor obtained from disrupted mycoplasma cells: isolation
and some biological properties. Chemotherapy 14(4):258-63.

Altucci, P., G.L. Varone, G. Catalano and L. Manguso. 1971.
Mycoplasmas in human genito-urinary pathology. Pathol. Microbiol. 37(2):89-98.

Anderson, D.R., Manaker, R.A. 1966. Electron microscopic studies of
mycoplasma (PPLO strain 880) in artificial medium and in tissue
culture. J. Natl. Cancer Inst. 36(1):139-54.

Anderson, D.L., M.E. Pollock and L. F. Brower. 1965. Morphology
of Mycoplasma laidlawii type A. I. comparison of electronmicro-
scopic counts with colony-forming units. J. Bact. 90(6):1764-7.

Bailey, G.D., D.N. Wright and M.T. Hatch. 1967. Survival of mcyoplasma in the aerosol state. Bact. Proc. 1967-71.

Bailey, J.S., H.W. Clark, W.R. Felts, R.C. Fowler and T. McP.
Brown. 1961. Antigenic properties of pleuropneumonia-like
organisms from tissue cell cultures and the human genital area.
J. Bact. 82(4):542-7.

Bailey, J.S., H.W. Clark, W.R. Felts and T. McP. Brown 1963.
Growth inhibitory properties of mycoplasma antibody. J.
Bact. 86(1):147-50.

Balashova, V.V. 1972. Morphological properties of M. laidlawii.
Mikrobiologya 41(1):173-5.

Balducci, L, M. Midulla, L. Bertolini. 1968. Peculiarities
of a strain of Mycoplasma hominis, type I isolated by tissue
culture. Boll. Soc. Ital. Biol. Sper. 44(9):856-8.

Barile, M.F. 1965. Mycoplasma (PPLO), leukemia and autoimmune
disease. Wistar Inst. Symp. Monogr. 4:171-85.

Barile, M.F., R.T. Schimke and D. B. Riggs. 1966. Presence of the
arginine dihydrolase pathway in mycoplasma. J. Bact. 51(1):
189-92.

Bashmakova, M.A. and V.M. Soldatova. 1972. The survival of Mycoplasma hominis under various conditions of culture conservation.
Lab. Delo. 4:243-5.

Bennett, A.H., R.B. Kundsin and S.S. Shapiro. 1973. T-strain mycoplasmas, the etiologic agent of non-specific urethritis: a
venereal disease. J. Urol. 109:427-9.

Berg, R.B. and T.E. Frothingham. 1961. Hemadsorption in monkey
kidney cell cultures of mycoplasma (PPLO) recovered from rats.
Proc. Soc. Exp. Biol. Med. 108(3)616-18.

Bergold, G.H., R. Mazzali. 1970. Problems using density gradients. Brief report. Arch. Gesamte Virusforsch 31(1):168-74.

Black, F.T. and A. Krogsgaard-Jensen. 1974. Application of
indirect immunofluoresence, indirect hemagglutination and
polyacrylamide-gel electrophoresis to human T-mycoplasmas.
Acta Pathol. Microbiol. Scand. 82(3):345-353-B.

Brostoff, J., A. Freedman, I.M. Roitt. 1973. Leucocyte migration
inhibition of Mycoplasma fermentans in patients with rheumatoid
arthritis. Int. Arch. Allergy Appl. Immunol. 45(5):690-6.

Butler, M. and B.C.J.G. Knight. 1960. The survival of washed
suspensions of mycoplasma. J. Gen. Microbiol. 22:470.

Caspi, E., E. Herczeg, F. Soloman and D. Sompolinsky. 1971.
Amnionitis and T strain mycoplasmemia. Am. J. Obstet. Gynecol.
111(8):1102-6.

Caspi, E., F. Solomon and D. Sompolinsky. 1972. Early abortion
and mycoplasma infection. Isr. J. Med. Sci. 8(2):122-7.

Cole, R.M., J.G. Tully, T.J. Popkin et al. 1973. Morphology,
ultrastructure and bacteriophage infection of the helical
mycoplasma-like organism (Spiroplasma citri gen. nov. sp. nov.)
cultured from "Stubborn disease" of citrus. J. Bacteriol. 115:
367-84.

Cozine, W.S. 1968. Some factors influencing the survival of
Mycoplasma pneumonia in aerosols. Diss. Abstr. 29(10-12):3845-B

Cuccurullo, L. and A. Violante. 1969. Electron microscope
observations of a mycoplasma cultured in acellular medium
and fibroblast culture: a review. Boll. 1st Sieroter,
Milan 48(6):561-71.

Czekalowski, J.W., D.A. Hall and P.R. Woolcock. 1973. Studies
on proteolytic activity of mycoplasmas: gelatinolytic
property. J. Gen. Microbiol. 75(1):125-33.

Das, J. and J. Maniloff. 1975. Replication of mycoplasmavirus
   MVL51. J. Replicative intermediates. Biochem. Biophys. Res.
   Commun. 66(2):599-605.

DeLouvois, J., M. Blades, R.F. Harrison, R. Hurley and V.C.
   Stanley. 1974. Proceedings: Mycoplasmas and human infertile
   couples. Lancet 1:1073-5.

DeLouvis, J., M. Blades, R.F. Harrison, R. Hurley and V.C.
   Stanley. 1974. Proceedings: Mycoplasmas and human infertility.
   J. Clin. Path. 27(6):514.

Dmochowski, L., H.G. Taylor, C.E. Grey, D.A. Dreyer, J.A. Sykes,
   P.L. Langford, T. Rogers, C.C. Shullenberger and C.D. Howe.
   1965. Viruss and mycoplasma (PPLO) in human leukemia. Cancer
   18(10):1345-68.

Domermuth, D.H. 1960. Antibiotic resistance and mutation rates
   of mycoplasma. Avian Dis. 4:456-66.

Dajani, A.S. and E.M. Ayoub. 1969. Mycoplasmacidal effect of
   polymorphonuclear leucocyte extract. J. Immunol. 102(3):
   698-702.

Edward, D.G. ff. 1971. Determination of sterol requirement for
   mycoplasmatales. J. Gen. Microbiol. 69:205-210

Edward, D.G. ff., E.A. Freundt, R. M. Chanock, J. Fabricant,
   L. Hayflick, R.M. Lemcke, S. Rasin, N.L. Somerson, J.G.
   Tully and R.G. Wittler. 1972. Proposal for minimal standards
   for descriptions of new species of the order Mycoplasmatales.
   Int. J. Syst. Bact. 22(3):184-8.

Edwards, G.A. and J. Fogh. 1960. Fine structure of pleuropneumonia-like organisms in pure culture and in infected
   tissue culture cells. J. Bact. 79(2):267-76.

Eveland, W.C. 1970. Fluorescent staining with labeled mycoplasma antigen: direct reaction with antibody-producing cells.
   Arch. Environ. Health 21(3):397-401.

Fallon, R.J. 1966. Leukemia and lymphosarcoma in animals and man.
   2. The relationship between mycoplasmas and human leukemia.
   Vet. Rec. 79:700-2.

Fallon, R.J. and D.K. Jackson. 1967. The relationship between
   a rodent mycoplasma, Mycoplasma pulmonis, and certain mycoplasmas isolated from tissue cultures inoculated with material
   from patients with leukaemia. Lab. Anim. 1(1):55-64.

Fallon, R.J., et al. 1968. Relation between mycoplasmas and leukaemia and related diseases. Brit. Med. J. 4:225-8.

Fox, H., R.H. Purcell and R.M. Chanock. 1969. Characterization of a newly identified mycoplasma (Mycoplasma orale type 3) from the human orapharynx. J. Bact. 98(1):36-43.

Fraser, K.B., P.V. Shirodaria, M. Haire, D. Middleton. 1971. Mycoplasmas in cell cultures from rheumatoid synovial membranes. J. Hyg. (Camb.) 69(1):17-25.

Furness, G., F.J. Pipes and M.J. McMurtrey. 1968. Susceptibility of human mycoplasmata to ultraviolet and X irradiations. J. Infect. Dis. 118(1):1-6.

Furness, G. 1969. Differential responses of single cells and aggregates of mycoplasma to ultraviolet irradiation. Appl. Micro-biol. 18(3):360-4.

Girardi, A.J., L. Hayflick, A.M. Lewis and N.L. Somerson. 1965. Recovery of mycoplasmas in the study of human leukaemia and other malignancies. Nature. 205(4967):188-9.

Glan, P.V. and V.V. Neustroeva. 1968. Incorporation of H³-tagged thymidine into cells of mycoplasma-contaminated cultures. Zh. Microbiol. Epidemiol. Immunobiol. 45(12):21-3.

Gourlay, R.N., J. Bruce and D.J. Garwes. 1971. Characterization of mycoplasmatales virus laidlawii 1. Nature New Biol. 229:118-9.

Gourlay, R.N. 1971. Mycoplasmatales virus-laidlawii 2, a new virus isolated from Acholeplasma laidlawii. J. Gen. Virol.12: 65-7.

Gourlay, R.N. and S.G. Wyld. 1971. Some biological characteris-tics of Mycoplasmatales virus-laidlawii 1. J. Gen. Virol. 14 (1):15-23.

Gourlay, R.N. and S.G. Wyld. 1973. Isolation of Mycoplasmatales virus-laidlawii 3, a new virus infecting Acholeplasma laid-lawii. J. Gen. Virol. 19(2):279-83.

Hall, R.H. and A. Mittleman. 1964. Characterization of the nucleic acids of a mycoplasma (PPLO-880) isolated from ex-tracts of human tissue. Int. Congr. Biochem. 6(1):58.

Hatanaka, M., R. DelGiudice, C. Long. 1975. Adenine formation from adenosine by mycoplasmas: adenosine phosphorylase activity. Proc. Natl. Acad. Sci. USA 72(4):1401-5.

Hayflick, L. and W.R. Stinebring. 1955. Intracellular growth of
pleuropneumonia-like organisms. Anat. Rec. 121:477-78.

Hellung-Larsen, P., Frederiksen, S. 1976. Influence of mycoplasma
infection on the incorporation of different precursors into
RNA components of tissue culture cells. Exp. Cell Res. 99(2):
295-300.

Hirth, R.S., W.N. Plastridge and M.E Tourtellotte. 1967. Survival
of mycoplasma in frozen bovine semen. Amer. J. Vet. Res. 28
(122):97-9.

Holland, J.F., H. Minnemeyer, J. T. Grace, Jr., R. Block,
J. O'Malley and H. Tieckelmann. 1963. 5-Allyl-2'deoxyuridine
(AVdR) (anti-tumor agent) activity on metabolism of pyrimidine
deoxynucleosides by HeLa cells infected with mycoplasma.
Proc. Amer. Assoc. Cancer Res. 4(1):29.

Holland, J.F., R. Korn, J. O'Malley, H.J. Minnemeyer and H.
Tieckelmann. 1967. 5-Allyl-2'deoxyuridine inhibitin of nucleo-
side phosphorylase in HeLa cells containing mycoplasma (human).
Cancer Res. 27(10 part 1):1867-73.

Hopps, H.E., B.C. Meyer, M.F. Barile and R. A. DelGiudice. 1973.
Problems concerning "noncultivable" mycoplasma contaminants
in tissue cultures. Ann. N.Y. Acad. Sci. 225:265-76.

Hummeler, K., N. Tomassini and L. Hayflick. 1965. Ultrastructure
of a mycoplasma (negroni) isolated from human leukemia. J.
Bact. 90(2):517-23.

Hung, M.H. 1971. Studies on PPLO (mycoplasma). III. Mycoplasmas
in human saliva and their relation to dentition. J. Formosan
Med. Assoc. 70:242-50.

Jagielski, M., Kaluzewski, S. 1972. Contamination of cell cultures
with mycoplasma. II. Properties of isolated mycoplasma. Med. Dosw.
Mikrobiol. 24(4):323-31.

Jansson, E., U. Vainio, O. Snellman, S. Tuuri. 1971. Search for
mycoplasma in rheumatoid arthritis. Ann. Rheum. Dis. 30(4):
413-8.

Jansson, E., et al. 1974. Letter:Mycoplasma antibodies in
sarcoidosis. J. Clin. Pathol. 27(6):510-11.

Jasper, D.E. and N.C. Jain. 1966. Histochemical observations on mycoplasma after staining with acridine orange. Appl. Microbiol. 14(5):720-3.

Jezequel, A.M., M.M. Shreeve and J.W. Steiner. 1967. Segregation of nucleolar components in mycoplasma-infected cells. Lab. Invest. 16(2):287-304.

Johnson, L., H. Hayashi and D. Soll. 1970. Isolation and properties of a transfer ribonucleic acid deficient in ribothymidine. Biochem. 9(14):2823-2831.

Joncas, J., A. Chagnon, G. Lussier and V. Pavilanis. 1969. Charactreristics of a Mycoplasma hyorhinis strain contaminating a human fetal diploid cell line. Can. J. Microbiol. 15(5):451-4.

Jurmanova, K., P. Veber, J. Lesko and L. Hana. 1975. Drying and irradiation of calf and horse serum: II. Influence on mycoplasma content of the calf sera. Zbl. Bakt. Hyg. I. Abt. Orig. A. 231(4):514-18.

Kaklamanis, E, L. Thomas, K. Stavropoulos, I. Borman, C. Boshwitz. 1969. Mycoplasmacidal action of normal tissue extracts. Nature 221(183):860-2.

Kato, H. T. Murakami, K. Aita, K. Ono and K. Aoyama. 1972. Effects of suspension media on the survival of mycoplasma during storage at -20 C. J. Fac. Agricult. Iwate Universtity 10(3):125-31.

Knudson, D.L. and R. MacLeod. 1970. Mycoplasma pneumoniae and Mycoplasma salivarium: Electron microscopy of colony growth in agar. J. Bact. 101(2):609-17.

Koshimizu, K., K. Yamamoto and M. Ogata. 1973. Mycoplasmas isolated from dogs with malignant lymphoma. Jap. J. Vet. Sci. 35(2):123-32.

Koski, T.A., G.G. Christianson, F.L. Cole. 1976. Inactivation of mycoplasmas by use of phenol, formalin and beta-propiolactone. J. Biol. Stand. 4(2):151-4.

Kundsin, R.B. 1966. Characterization of mycoplasma aerosols as to viability, particle size, and lethality of UV irradiation. J. Bact. 91(3):942-4.

Kundsin, R.B. 1968. Aerosols of mycoplasmas, L-forms and bacteria: Comparison of particle size, viability, and lethality of ultraviolet radiation. Appl. Microbiol. 16(1):143-6.

Kundsin, R.B. 1970. The role of mycoplasmas in human reproductive failure. Ann. N.Y. Acad. Sci. 174(2):794-7.

Kurzepa, H., et al. 1969. Growth of parasitic mycoplasma without serum or serum fraction. J. Bact. 99:908-9.

Levashov, V.S., T.N. Klushina. 1969. Biological properties of reversed cultures of various mycoplasmas isolated from tissue cultures and normal bovine serum. Zh Mikrobiol. Epidemiol. Immunobiol. 46(6):107-10.

Liebisch, A. 1963. Phase-contrast and light microscopy of pleuro-pneumonia-like organisms on solid media. Beitr. Trop. Subtrop. Landw. Tropen. Vet. Med. 2:120-30.

Liska, B., P.F. Smith. 1974. Requirements of Acholeplasma laidlawii A, strain LA1, for nucleic acid precursors. Folia Microbiol. (Praha) 19(2):107-17.

Liska, B. and L. Tkadlecek. 1975. Electron-microscopic study of a Mycoplasmatales virus, strain MV-Lg-pS2-L 172. Folia Microbiol. 20(1):1-7.

Liss, A. and J. Maniloff. 1971. Isolation of Mycoplasmatales viruses and characterization of MVL1, MVL 52 and MVG51. Science 173(3998):725-7.

Liss, A. and J. Maniloff. 1972. Transfection mediated by Mycoplasmatales viral DNA. Proc. Natl. Acad. Sci. USA 69(11): 3423-7.

Liss, A. and J. Maniloff. 1973. Characterization of Mycoplasmatales virus DNA. Biochem. Biophys. Res. Commun. 51(1): 214-8.

Liss, A. and J. Maniloff. 1973. Infection of Acholeplasma laidlawii by MVL51 virus. Virology 55(1):118-26.

Liss, A. and J. Maniloff. 1974. Effect of EDTA and competitive DNA on mycoplasmavirus transfection of Acholeplasma laidlawii. Microbios 11A(46):107-14.

Liss, A. and J. Maniloff. 1974. Intracellular replication of mycoplasma-virus MVL51. J. Virol. 13(4):769-74.

Liss, A. 1975. Mycoplasmatales virus group L1: Isolation, characterization, growth and transfection studies. Diss. Abstr.
35(8):4055-B.

Lloyd, L.C. and J. R. Etheridge. 1974. Survival of mycoplasmas
in aerosol particles. Victorian Vet. Proc. 32:9.

Loveday, R.K. 1964. Lactational failure in the sow. J.S. Afr.
Vet. Med. Ass. 35:229-33.

Low, I.E., A.A. Jacobs, A.J. Sbarra. 1973. Mycoplasmacidal
activity of a leukocytic myeloperoxida peroxide-halide system.
J. Infect. Dis. 127:Suppl:S72-6.

Lynn, R.J. and H.E. Morton. 1956. The inhibitory action of agar
on certain strains of pleuropneumonia-like organisms. Appl.
Microbiol. 4(6):399-341

Manchee, R.J., D. Taylor-Robinson. 1968. Haemadsorption and
haemagglutination by mycoplasmas. J. Gen. Microbiol. 50(3):
465-78.

Manchee, R.J., D. Taylor-Robinson. 1969. Utilization of neuraminic acid receptors by mycoplasmas. J. Bacteriol. 98(3):
914-9.

Maniloff, J. and A. Liss. 1973. The molecular biology of mycoplasma viruses. Ann. N.Y. Acad. Sci. 225:149-58.

Mannheim, W. and G. Wolf. 1972. The temperature requirements of
growth of some mycoplasmas. Zentralbl. Bakt. Parasitenk.
Infektions-krankh Hyg. 221A(2):232-49.

Mardh, P.A., D. Taylor-Robinson. 1973. The differential effect of
lysolecithin on mycoplasmas and acholeplasmas. Med. Microbiol.
Immunol (Berl) 158(3):219-26.

Mazzali, R. and D. Taylor-Robinson. 1971. The behaviour of T-
mycoplasmas in tissue culture. J. Med. Microbiol. 4(1):125-38.

Meloni, G.A. 1968. On some aspects of the development of Mycoplasma
hominis type I in acellular and cellular media. G. Mal Infett.
Parassit 20(6):498-510.

Metz, J. and W. Bredt. 1971. Electron microscopy studies of Mycoplasma hominis (strain W 463-69). Z. Med. Mikrobiol. Immunol.
156(4):368-78.

Meyer, D.M. and D.J. Blazevic. 1971. Differentiation of human mycoplasma using gas chromatography. Can. J. Microbiol. 17(2)297-300.

Milne, R.G., G.W. Thompson and D. Taylor-Robinson. 1972.
Electron microscope observations on Acholeplasma laidlawii
viruses. Arch. Gesamte Virusforsch 37(4):378-85.

Mishima, K. 1973. Hemolysis of oral mycoplasmas. J. Jap.
Stomatol. Soc. 40:389-403.

Naeye, R.L. 1975. Editorial: Causes and consequences of chorio-
amnionitis. New Engl. J. Med. 293(1):40-1.

Nakamura, M. and H. Sakamoto. 1967. Stability of human strains of
mycoplasma to heat, pH and shaking. Jap. J. Bact. 22(10):595-9.

Nakamura, M. and M. Kawaguchi. 1972. Ultrastructure of M. orale
Serotype 1 in agar growth. J. Gen. Microbiol. 70(2):305-14.

Nakamura, M., T. Ito and N. Hirata. 1974. Mycoplasmasin, a new
bacteriolysin of mycoplasmas. Igaku No Ayumi 91(5):201-2

Neimark, H.C. 1964. DNA activity from "lactic PPLO." Nature 203
(4944)549-50.

Okano, H., et al. 1970. Effect of trypsin and nagarse on various
mycoplasma organisms. Jap. J. Bact. 25:321-8.

Okano, H., H. Chosa and J.Y. Homma. 1970. Effect of proteolytic
enzymes on several kinds of mycoplasma organisms. Jap. J. Exp.
Med. 40(3):213-20.

Oswald, E.J., et al. 1968. Survival of mycoplasma in dry-state,
semisynthetic antibiotics. Antimicrob. Agents Chemother. 8:
471-3.

Pachas, W.N. 1970. The role of mycoplasma in some unusual conditions of the kidney and the urinary tract. Ann. N.Y. Acad.
Sci. 174:786-93.

Parkinson, C.E. 1975. Histamine release from human leukocytes
when stimulated by Mycoplasma salivarium. Infect. Immun. 11
(3):595-7.

Parkinson, C.F. 1975. Reactivity of mast cells to Mycoplasma
salivarium. Infect. Immun. 11(3):598-600.

Parkinson, C.F. and P.B. Carter. 1975. Phagocytosis of _Mycoplasma salivarium_ by human polymorphonuclear leukocytes and monocytes. Infect. Immun. 11(2):405-14.

Patriarca, P., S. Beckerdite, P. Pettis, P. Elsbach. 1972. Phospholipid metabolism by phagocytic cells. VII. The degradation and utilization of phospholipids of various microbial species by rabbit granulocytes. Biochim. Biophys. Acta 280(1):45-56.

Perez, A.G., J.H. Kim, A.S. Gelbard, B. Djordjevic. 1972. Altered incorporation of nucleic acid precursors by mycoplasma-infected mammalian cells in culture. Exp. Cell Res. 70(2): 301-10.

Peterson, A.M. and M. Pollock. 1969. DNA homology and relative genome size in mycoplasma. J. Bact. 99(3):639-44.

Pratt, W.B., S.R. Gross, L. Aronow. 1968. Endosymbionts as a source of cytoplasmic satellite deoxyribonucleic acid. J. Mol. Biol. 33(2):521-5.

Provost, A. 1969. Cytotoxic effect of anti-mycoplasma mycoides serum on bovine lung cells in vitro. Rev. Immunol. (Paris) 33(1): 1-6.

Prozorovckii, S.V., G.M. Bochko, I.V. Rakovskaia, T.I. Mit'kina. 1967. Features specific to the cultivation and antigenic properties of mycoplasma isolated from the oral cavity. Stomatologiia (Mosk.) 46(4):34-8.

Purcell, R.H., J.R. Valdesuso, W. L. Cline, W.D. James and R.M. Chanock. 1971. Cultivation of mycoplasmas on glass. Appl. Microbiol. 21(2):288-94.

Raccach, M., S. Rottem, S. Razin. 1975. Survival of frozen mycoplasmas. Appl. Microbiol. 30(2):167-71.

Rakovskaya, I.V., Z.A. Postnikova, T.D. Morgunova and G. Y. Kagan. 1972. Study of immunodepressive effect of Mycoplasma laidlawii on the formation of humoral antibodies in mice. Bull, Eksp. Biol. Med. 74(10):60-62.

Randall, C.C., L.G. Gafford, G.A. Gentry, L.A. Lawson. 1965. Lability of host-cell DNA in growing cell cultures due to mycoplasma. Science 149(688):1098-9.

Razin, S. and B.C.J.G. Knight. 1960. The effects of ribonucleic acid and deoxyribonucleic acid on the growth of mycoplasma. J. Gen. Microbiol. 22:504.

Razin, S. 1961. Nucleic acid precursor requirements of saprophytic mycoplasma (PPLO). Bull. Res. Counc. Israel Sect. E. Exp.
   Med. 9(2):56.

Razin, S. and M. Argaman. 1961. Properties of the Mycoplasma
   (PPLO) cell envelope. In: II. General Microbiology. Bull.
   Res. Counc. Israel Sect. E. Exp. Med. 129E(3/4):121-2.

Razin, S., A. Knyszynsky and Y. Lifshitz. 1964. Nucleases of
   mycoplasma. J. Gen. Microbiol. 36(2):323-31.

Razin, S. 1968. Mycoplasma toxonomy studied by electrophroesis
   of cell proteins. J. Bact. 96(3):687-94.

Razin, S. 1969. Organization of protein and lipid in the mycoplasma
   membrane. J. Gen. Microbiol. 57:8-9.

Razin, S. and J.G. Tully. 1970. Cholesterol requirements of
   mycoplasmas. J. Bacteriol. 102:306-10.

Razin, S. 1973. In: Advances in Microbial Physiology 10:1-80.
   A.H. Rose and D.W. Tempest (eds.). Academic Press, N.Y.

Razin, S. 1975. In: Progress in Surface and Membrane Science.
   9:257-312. D.A. Cudenhead, J.F. Danielli and M.D. Rosenberg
   (eds.). Academic Press, N.Y.

Razin, S. and S. Rottem. 1976. In: Biochemical Analysis of Membranes. p.3-26. A.H. Mady (ed.). Chapman Hall Ltd., London.

Robertson, J., et al. 1972. Virus-like particles in Mycoplasma
   hominis. Can. J. Microbiol. 18:1971-2.

Rodwell, A.W. 1969. The supply of cholesterol and fatty acids for
   the growth of mycoplasmas. J. Gen. Microbiol. 58(1):29-37.

Rothblat, G.H. 1961. Sterol physiology of pleuropneumonia-like
   organisms. Diss. Abstr. 21(12):3616-7.

Rottem, S. and S. Razin. 1964. Lipase activity of mycoplasma. J.
   Gen. Microbiol. 37(1):123-34.

Rottem, S. and S. Razin. 1966. Adenosine triphosphatase activity
of mycoplasma membranes. J. Bact. 92(3):714-22.

Ruffo, G., S. Nani, and A. Podesta. 1969. Survival of Mycoplasma
agalactiae var. bovis in several materials and at different
temperatures. Arch. Vet. Italiano 20(6):459-64.

Sakamoto, H. and M. Nakamura. 1968. Stability of human strains of
mycoplasma. Influence of various physical and chemical treatments.
Jap. J. Bact. 23(2):132-6.

Schimke, R.T. 1967. Studies metabolism of arginine of mycoplasma.
Ann. N.Y. Acad. Sci. 143(1):573-7.

Schimke, R.T., C.M. Berlin, E.W. Sweeney and W.R. Carroll. 1966.
The generation of energy by the arginine dihydrolase pathway
in Mycoplasma hominis 07. J. Biol. 241(10):2228-36.

Schimke, R.T. and M.F. Barile. 1963. Arginine breakdown in
mammalian cell culture contaminated with pleuropneumonia-like
organism. Exp. Cell Res. 30(3):593-6.

Schimke, R.T. and M.F. Barile. 1963. Arginine metabolism in
pleuropneumonia-like organism isolated from mammalian
cell culture. 86(2):195-206.

Schimmel, D. 1963. Study of growth and oxygen consumption of
mycoplasma using vitamins of the B group and amino acids.
Arch. Exp. Vet. Med. 17:1161-7.

Schimmel, D., W. Ahlendorf and E. Burger. 1974. The radiation
sensitivity of mycoplasmas in broth and colostrum. Z. Ver-
suchstierkd. 16(1):36-40.

Schimmel, D. and L. Stipkovits. 1972. Proposals for the stan-
darization, isolation, preservation and serological typing
of mycoplasmas. Arch. Exp. Vet. Med. 26(1):75-95.

Sethi, K.K. and H.E. Muller. 1970. Enzymatic degradation of human
lipoproteins by mycoplasmas. Experientia 26:804-5.

Sethi, K.K. and H. Brandis. 1971. Killing of mycoplasmas by the
antibodies to foreign antigens acquired by the organisms
from the growth medium. Med. Microbiol. Immunol. 157:113-9.

Sethi, K.K. and H.E. Muller 1972. Neuraminidase activity in M.
gallisepticum. Infect.Immun. 5(2):260-2.

Shepard, M.C. 1956. T-form colonies of pleuropneumonia-like organisms. J. Bact. 71(3):362-9.

Shepard, M.C and C.D. Lunceford. 1965. Effect of pH on human mycoplasma strains. J. Bact. 89(2):265-270.

Slater, M.L. and C.E. Folsome. 1971. Induction of alpha-glyco-sidase in Mycoplasma laidlawii A. Nature New Biol. 229:117-8.

Schmidt, P.J. and H.M. McGinnis. 1967. Cell surfaces, blood groups and microorganisms (human). Nature 214(5095):1363.

Smith, P.F. 1957. Amino acid metabolism by pleuropneumonia-like organisms. II. Glutamine. J. Bact. 73(1):91-5.

Smith, P.F. 1957. Conversion of citrulline to ornithine by pleuropneumonia-like organisms. J. Bact. 74(6):801-6.

Smith, P.F. 1957. Amino acid metabolism by pleuropneumonia-like organisms. III. Glutamic acid. J. Bact. 74(1):75-8.

Smith, P.F. and C.V. Henrikson. 1965. Glucose-containing phos-pholipids in Mycoplasma laidlawii, strain B. J. Lipid Res. 6 (1):106-11.

Smith, S.C., W.R. Dunlop and R.G. Strout. 1966. Effect of culture medium on antigenic structure of mycoplasma. Avian Dis. 10(2): 173-6.

Sobeslavsky, O. and R.M. Chanock. 1968. Peroxide formation by mycoplasmas which infect man. Proc. Soc. Exp. Biol. Med. 129 (2):531-5.

Sprossig, M., P. Wutzler, H. Schweizer, H. Mucke. 1976. Cold sterilization of serums with peracetic acid. J. Hyg. Epidemiol. Microbiol. Immunol. (Praha) 20(2):157-63.

Stanbridge, E.J., L. Hayflick and F.T. Perkins. 1971. Modification of amino-acid concentrations induced by mycoplasmas in cell culture medium. Nature New Biol. 232(34):242-4.

Stopkie, R.J. and M.M. Weber. 1967. Control of NADH oxidation by ADP in membranes from mycoplasma (NADH oxidase, osmotic shock spectrophometry). Biochem. Biophys. Res. Commun. 28(6): 1034-9.

Sussman, M., J.H. Jones, J.D. Almeida and P.J. Lachmann. 1973.
Deficiency of the second component of complement associated
with anaphylactoid purpura and presence of mycoplasma in the
serum. Clin. Exp. Immunol. 14:531-9.

Sussman, M., et al. 1974. Mycoplasma-like particles in patients
with anaphylactoid purpura. J. Urol Neprol. (Paris) 80(12):
985-986.

Tallgren, L.G., R. Wegelius, L.C. Andersson, E. Jansson. 1974.
Eosinophilic leukaemia--recovery of Mycoplasma orale from the
bone marrow. Acta Med. Scand. 195(1):87-92.

Taylor-Robinson, D. and R.J. Manchee. 1967. Spermadsorption and
spermagglutination by mycoplasmas. Nature 215(5100):484-7.

Taylor-Robinson, D. 1974. T-mycoplasmas and infertility. Nature
248-67.

Tedeschi, G.G., D. Amici and M. Paparelli. 1970. The uptake of
radioactivity of thymidine, uridine, formate, glycine and
lysine into cultures of blood of normal human subjects. Relationship with mycoplasma infection. Haematologia 4(1):27-47.

Trung, P.H., et al. 1968. Ultrastructure of Mycoplasma salivarium
and of Mycoplasma orale in tissue culture. The problem of the
differentiation because of the similarities in the cellular
surfaces. Eur. J. Cancer. 4:429-35.

Tully, J.G. and S. Razin. 1968. Physiological and serological
comparisons among strains of Mycoplasma granularium and Mycoplasma laidlawii. J. Bacteriol. 95:1504-12.

Tully, J.G. 1973. Biological and serological characteristics
of the Acholeplasmas. Ann. N.Y. Acad. Sci. 225:74-93.

Tully, J.G., R.F. Whitcomb, H.F. Clark and D.L. Williamson. 1977.
Pathogenic mycoplasmas: cultivation and vertebrate pathogenicity
of a new spiroplasma. Science 195:892-894.

Veber, P., K. Jurmanova, J. Lesko, L. Hana. 1975. Drying and
irradiation of calf and horse serum. I. influence on the
growth of cell cultures and mycoplasmas. Zentralbl. Bakteriol.
(Orig. A)231(4):508-13.

Watanabe, T, K. Mishima and T. Horikawa. 1973. Proteolytic activities of human mycoplasmas. Jap. J. Microbiol. 17(2):151-3.

Watanabe, T. 1975. Proteolytic activity of Mycoplasma salivarium and Mycoplasma orale 1. Med. Microbiol. Immunol. (Berl.) 161(2):127-32.

Weber, M.M. and S.C. Kinsky. 1965. Effect of cholesterol on the sensitivity of Mycoplasma laidlawii to the polyene antibiotic filipin. J. Bact. 89(2):306-12.

Whitcomb, R.F., J.G. Tully, J.M. Bove' et al. 1973. Spiroplasmas and acholeplasmas: multiplication in insects. Science 182: 1251-3.

Whitescarver, J., M. Trocola, T. Campana, R. Marks, and G. Furness. 1976. A study of the amino acids and proteins of some human T-mycoplasma membranes. Proc. Soc. Exp. Biol. Med. 151:68-71.

Williams, C.O., et al. 1969. DNA base compositions of selected mycoplasmas and L-phase variants. J. Bact. 99:341-3.

Williams, M.H. 1970. Mycoplasma and rheumatoid arthritis. Clin. Sci. 38(4):24P.

Wright, D.N., G.D. Bailey and L.J. Goldberg. 1968. Effect of temperature on survival of airbrne Mycoplasma pneumoniae. J. Bact. 99(2):491-5.

Wright, D.N., G.D. Bailey and M.T. Hatch. 1968. Role of relative humidity in the survival of airborne Mycoplasma pneumoniae. J. Bact. 96(4):970-4.

Wright, D.N., G.D. Bailey and M.T. Hatch. 1968. Survival of airborne mycoplasma as affected by relative humidity. J. Bact. 95(1):251-2.

Wright, D.N. and G.D. Bailey. 1969. Effect of relative humidity on the stability of Mycoplasma pneumoniae exposed to simulated solar ultraviolet and to visible radiation. Can. J. Microbiol. 15(12):1449-52.

Zeigel, R.F. and H.F. Clark. 1969. Electron microscope observations on a mycoplasma-like agent associated with pathologic changes in eyes of suckling mice and rats. J. Cell Biol. 43: 163a.

Zgorniak-Nowosielska, I. and J. Branny. 1970. Mycoplasma in the semen of bulls. I. isolation and some properties of mycoplasma from bovine semen. Med. Wet. 26:51-3.

3. INCIDENCE, DETECTION AND IDENTIFICATION

Al-Aubaidi, J.M. and J. Fabricant. 1971. The practical application
of immunofluorescence (agar block technic) for the identification of mycoplasma. Cornell Vet. 61(3):519-42.

Al-Aubaidi, J.M. and J. Fabricant. 1971. Methods for purification
of mixed cultures of mycoplasma. Cornell Vet. 6(4):559-72.

Alexander-Jackson, E. 1966. Mycoplasma (PPLO) isolated from Rous
sarcoma virus. Growth 30(2):199-228.

Altucci, P., et al. 1966. Correlations between the behavior of
the arginine deiminase enzymatic test and the possibility of
isolation of mycoplasma in acellular media. Boll. Soc. Ital.
Biol. Sper. 42:1324-8.

Altucci, P., et al. 1966. The arginine deiminase enzymatic test
for the diagnosis of the presence of mycoplasma in cell cultures. Boll. Soc. Ital. Biol. Sper. 42:1321-4.

Anderson, D.R. 1965. Subcellular particles associated with human
leukemia as seen with the electron microscope. Wistar Inst.
Symp. Monog. 4:113-46.

Anderson, D.R., R.A. Manaker. 1966. Electron microscopic studies
of Mycoplasma (PPLO strain 880) in artificial medium and in
tissue culture. J. Natl. Cancer Inst. 36(1):139-54.

Baas, E.J. and D.E. Jasper. 1972. Agar block technique for
identification of mycoplasmas by use of fluorescent antibody.
Appl. Microbiol. 23(6):1097-1100.

Barile, M.F. and D.B. Riggs. 1961. Immunofluorescence of pleuor-
pneumona-like organisms in tissue cultures. Bact. Proc. 61:83.

Barile, M.F., W.F. Malizia and D.B. Riggs. 1962. Incidence and
detection of pleuropneumonia-like organisms in cell cultures
by fluorescent antibody and cultural procedures. J. Bact.
84(1):130-6.

Barile, M.F. and R.T. Schimke. 1963. A rapid chemical method
for detecting PPLO contamination of tissue cell cultures.
Proc. Soc. Exp. Biol. Med. 114(3):676-9.

Barile, M.F., G.P. Bodey, J. Synder, D.B. Riggs and M.W.
Grabowski. 1966. Isolation of Mycoplasma orale from leukemic
bone marrow and blood by direct culture. J. Nat. Cancer Inst.
36(1):155-9.

Barile, M.F. and R.A. DelGiudice. 1968. Isolation and characterization of Mycoplasma arginini spec. nov. Proc. Soc. Exp.
Biol. Med. 129(2):489-94.

Barile, M.F. 1968. Mycoplasma and cell cultures. In: NCI Monograph 29 (Cell Cultures for Virus Vaccine Production):201-4.

Barile, M.F., R.A. DelGiudice, T.R. Carski, H.M. Yamashiroya,
J.A. Verna. 1970. Isolation and rapid identification of
Mycoplasma species from canine tissues by plate immunofluor-
escence. Proc. Soc. Exp. Biol. Med. 134(1):146-8.

Barile, M.F. and J. Kern. 1971. Isolation of Mycoplasma arginini
from commercial bovine sera and its implication in contaminated cell cultures. Proc. Soc. Exp. Biol. Med. 138(2):432-7.

Barile, M.F. and R.A. DelGiudice. 1972. Isolation of mycoplasmas
and their rapid identification by plate epi-immunofluoresence.
In: Pathogenic Mycoplasmas. A Ciba Found. Symp. ASP, Amsterdam.

Barile, M.F. 1973. Mycoplasmal contamination of cell cultures:
mycoplasma-virus-cell culture interations. In: Contamination
in Tissue Culture. J. Fogh (ed.) Academic Press, 131-72.

Barile, M.F., H.E. Hopps, M.W. Grabowski, D.B. Riggs and R.A.
DelGiudice. 1973. The identification and sources of myco-
plasmas isolated from contaminated cell cultures. Ann. N.Y.
Acad. Sci. 225:251-64.

Barile, M.F., et al. 1974. Media for the isolation of mycoplasma from biologic materials. Dev. Biol. Stand. 23:128-33.

Bashmakova, M.A. and V.A. Soldatova. 1971. Use of placental
media for isolating M. hominis. Lab. Delo. 9:561-3.

Benton, W.J., M.S. Cover and F.W. Melchior. 1967. Mycoplasma
gallisepticum in a commercial laryngotracheitis vaccine.
Avian Dis. 11(5):426-9.

Black, F.T. 1973. Modifications of the growth inhibition test
and its application to human T-mycoplasmas. Appl. Microbiol.
25(4):528-33.

Boam, G.W., et al. 1970. Histochemical staining of normal
and mycoplasma-infected turkey sinus epithelial cells.
Avian Dis. 14:514-20.

Branny, J. 1974. Viruses and mycoplasmas in bull semen. Acta
Agrar. Silvestria. Ser. Zootech. 14(2):3-22.

Bredt, W., P.S. Lam, P. Fiegel and D. Hoffler. 1974.
    Demonstration of mycoplasma in suprapubic vesical puncture
    urine. Deut. Med. Wochenschr. 99:1553-6.

Brown, S., M. Teplitz, J.P. Revel. 1974. Interaction of myco-
    plasmas with cell cultures, as visualized by electron
    microscopy. Proc. Natl. Acad. Sci. USA 71(2):464-8.

Butler, M. 1969. Isolation and growth of mycoplasma in human
    embryo trachea cultures. Nature (London) 224:605-6.

Campbell, L.H., H.K. Okuda. 1975. Cultivation of mycoplasma
    from conjunctiva and production of corneal immune response
    in guinea pigs. Am. J. Vet. Res. 36(7):893-7.

Chen, T.R. 1977. In situ detection of mycoplasma contamination
    in cell cultures by fluorescent Hoechst 33258 stain. Exp. Cell
    Res. 104:255-62.

Clyde, W.A., Jr. 1961. Demonstration of Eaton's agent in
    tissue culture. Proc. Soc. Exp. Biol. Med. 107(4):715-8.

Clyde, W.A. 1963. Studies on growth of Eaton's agent in
    tissue culture. Proc. Soc. Exp. Biol. Med. 112:905-9.

Clyde, W.A., Jr. 1963. Studies on Eaton agent in tissue
    culture. In: Conference on Newer Respiratory Disease
    Viruses. 1962. Amer. Rev. Resp. Dis. 88(3Pt2):212-17.

Crawford, Y.E. and W.H. Kraybill. 1967. The mixtures of Myco-
    plasma species isolated from the human oropharynx Ann. N.Y
    Acad. Sci. 143(1):411-21.

Cross, G.F., M.R. Goodman and E. J. Shaw. 1967. Detection and
    treatment of contaminating mycoplasmas in human cell culture.
    Aust. J. Exp. Biol. Med. Sci. 45(2):201-12.

Cuccurullo, L. and A. Violante. 1968, Electron microscopic
    observations on a Mycoplasma cultured in acellular media
    and in human amniotic cells. G. Mal. Infett. Parassit. 20
    (6):496-8.

deHarven, E. 1973. Identification of tissue culture contam-
    inants by electron microscopy. In: Contamination in Tissue
    Culture, J. Fogh (ed.) N.Y., London, Academic Press 205-31.

DelGiudice, R.A., N.F. Robillard and T.R. Carski. 1967. Immunofluorescence identification of Mycoplasma on agar by use of
indirect illumination. J. Bacteriol. 93:1205-9.

DelGiudice, R.A., et al. 1974. Immunofluorescent procedures for
mycoplasma identification. Dev. Biol. Stand. 23:134-37.

Douglas, W.H. 1973. A whole cell mounting technique for detecting Acholeplasma laidlawii A on the surface of cultured cells.
In Vitro (monogr.) Abstract 51, p. 413.

Draghici, D. 1969. Comparison of primary cell cultures and cell-
free media for the isolation of mycoplasma from pigs. Archiva
Vet. 6(1/2):85-110.

Draghici, D., D. Schimmel and T. Hubrig. 1969. Porcine mycoplasmata in cell cultures: I. isolation of porcine mycoplasmas in
primary cell cultures. Arch. Exp. Vet. Med. 23(1):101-34.

Draghici, D., D. Schimmel, T. Hubrig. 1969. Porcine mycoplasmata
in cell cultures. II. Adaptation of mycoplasma isolates
in cell-free media to cell cultures. Arch. Exp. Vet. Med.
23(1):135-44.

Draghici, D., D. Schimmel and T. Hubrig. 1969. Mycoplasmata from
pigs and cell cultures: III. Staining methods to demonstrate
mycoplasmata in cell cultures and methods for demonstrating
cytopathic changes. Arch. Exp. Vet. Med. 23(3):625-32.

Ebke, J., E. Kuwert. 1972. Detection of Mycoplasma orale type I
in tissue cultures by means of the acridine orange stain.
Zentralbl. Bakteriol. (Orig. A) 221(1):87-93.

Edward, D.G. 1969. Mycoplasmas as contaminants and their detection.
Prog. Immunobiol. Stand. 3:17-22, 1969.

Eveland, W.C. 1970. Fluorescent staining with labeled mycoplasma
antigen: direct reaction with antibody-producing cells. Arch.
Environ. Health 21(3):397-401.

Fogh, J. and H. Fogh. 1964. A method for direct demonstration of
pleuropneumonia-like organism in cultured (human amnion) cells.
Proc. Soc. Exp. Biol. Med. 117(3):899-901.

Fong, C.K.Y., P.A. Gross, G.D. Hsiung and N.S. Swack. 1975.
Use of electron microscopy for detection of viral and other
microbial contaminants in bovine sera. J. Clin. Microbiol.
1(2):219-24.

Fraser, K.B., P.V. Shirodaria, M. Haire and D. Middleton. 1971.
Mycoplasma in cell cultures from rheumatoid synovial membranes.
J. Hyg. 69(1):17-25.

Garrett, A.J. and D.E. Reeson, 1975. Rapid screening of tissue
culture cells for mycoplasmal contaminants. J. Biol. Stand.
3(2):181-184.

Girardi, A.J., V.V. Hamparian, N.L. Somerson, L. Hayflick. 1965.
Mycoplasma isolates from primary cell cultures and human
diploid cell strains. Proc. Soc. Exp. Biol. Med. 120(3):
760-70.

Glan, P.V. and V.V. Neustroeva. 1968. Incorporation of H^3-tagged
thymidine into cells of mycoplasma-contaminated cultures.
Zh. Microbiol. Epidemiol. Immunobiol. 45(12):21-23.

Goff, M.T. 1971. Feline panleukopenia biologics. J. Am. Vet.
Med. Assoc. 158(6):Suppl. 2:907+.

Gogichadze, G.K., A.S. Shubin and N.P. Mazurenko. 1971.
Differentiation of murine leukemia viruses from elementary
bodies of mycoplasma by electron microscopy. Vop. Virusol.
16(5):522-6.

Gois, M., F. Sisak, F. Kuksa and M. Sovadina. 1975. Incidence
and evaluation of the microbial flora in the lungs of pigs
with enzootic pneumonia. Zbl. Ved. Med. B. 22:205-19.

Goldstein, S, P.C. Sanders and I.U. Boone. 1962. Cultivation
of pleuropneumonia-like organisms from tissue cultures.
U.S. Atomic Energy Comm. Res. and Develop. Rept. Lams.
2780:224-227.

Goodwin, R.F.W. and P. Whittlestone. 1963. Production of
enzootic pneumonia in pigs with an agent grown in tissue
culture from the natural disease. Brit. J. Exp. Path. 44
(3):291-9.

Gordon, F.B., A.L. Quan, M.K. Cook, R.M. Chanock and H.H. Fox.
1960. Growth of Eaton agent of primary atypical pneumonia
in chick entodermal tissue culture. Proc. Soc. Exp. Biol.
Med. 105(2):375-7.

Gutkina, A.V. and V.V. Neustroeva. 1971. Detection of mycoplasma
in cell culture by cytochemical methods. Zh. Mikrobiol.
Epidemiol. Immunobiol 48(3):19-23.

Harnett, G.B., P.A. Phillips and E.M. Mackay-Scollay. 1974. A simple method for detecting mycoplasma infection of cell cultures. J. Clin. Path. 27(1):70-3.

Hearn, H.J., Jr., J.E. Officer, V. Elsner and A. Brown. 1959. Detection, elimination and prevention of contamination of cell cultures with pleuropneumnia-like organisms. J. Bact. 79(4):575-82.

Hendley, J.O. and W. S. Jordan. 1968. Mycoplasma pharyngeal flora in civilians. Amer. Rev. Resp. Dis. 97(4):524-32.

Hlinak, P., J. Friedemann, G. Starke. 1969. Problems of the state examination of viral vaccines in mycoplasma contaminations. Pharmazie 24(4):189-92.

House, W., et al. 1967. Detection of mycoplasma in cell cultures. J. Path. Bact. 93:125-132.

Hung, M.H., et al. 1965. Studies on pleuropneumonia-like organisms (PPLO) I. Isolation of PPLO from established cell lines and cell strains used in Taiwan. J. Formosan Med. Ass. 64:698-706

Hung, M.H. 1971. Studies on PPLO (mycoplasma). III. Mycoplasmas in human saliva and their relation to dentition. J. Formosan Med. Assoc. 70:242-250.

Jansson, E., U. Vainino and S. Tuuri. 1971. Cultivation of a mycoplasma from the bone marrow in systemic lupus erythematosus disseminatus. Acta Rheum. Scand. 17:223-6.

Jansson, E., et al. 1972. Scanning electron microscopy of mycoplasma isolated from systemic lupus erythematosus disseminatus. Schriftner. Ver. Wasser. Boden. Lufthyg. 1:113-6.

Jagielski, M., M. Zaleska, S. Kaluzewski, I. Polna. 1976. Applicability of DAPI for the detection of Mycoplasmas in cell cultures. Med. Dows. Mikcrobiol. 28(2):161-73.

Jones, D.M. and P.J.I. Sequeira. 1966. The distribution of complement fixing antibody and growth inhibiting antibody to Mycoplasma hominis. J. Hyg. 64:441-9.

Kaklamanis, E., et al. 1969. Mycolasmacidal action of normal tissue extracts. Nature (London) 221:860-2.

Kaluzewski, S., M. Jagielski. 1972. Studies on the contamination
of cell cultures with mycoplasma. I. conditions for mycoplasma
isolation. Med. Dows. Mikrobiool. 24(2):103-13.

Keller, R. and H.E. Morton. 1954. The growth of pleuropneumonia-
like organisms of human origin: Cultivation in the developing
chick embryo and in vitro growth cycle. J. Bact. 67(2):129-34.

Kihara, K., et al. 1971. Effect of yeast extracts and autolysates
on the growth of mycoplasma. Med. Biol. (Tokyo) 84:297-302.

Kihara, K., et al. 1972. Conditions of yeast autolysis for mycoplasma culture. Med. Biol. (Tokyo) 84:231-6.

Klodnitskaya, S.N. 1974. Mycoplasma isolation from the blood of
patients with various forms of leukemia. Zh. Mikrobiol.
Epidemiol. Immunobiol. 12:76-9.

Klushina, T.N. 1967. Biological properties of pleuropneumonia-
like organism (mycoplasma) isolated from tissue culture and
normal bovine serum. Zh. Microbiol. Epidemiol. Immunobiol.
44(3):16-19.

Kraybill, W.H. and Y.E. Crawford. 1967. Comparison of two agar
media for the isolation of mycoplasma from the human oro-
pharynx. Ann. N.Y. Acad. Sci. 143:401-10.

Krogsgaard-Jensen, A. 1972. Mycoplasma: growth precipitation as a
serodiagnostic method. Appl. Microbiol. 23(3):553.

Kumagai, K., et al. 1971. Incidence, species and significance of
mycoplasma species in the mouth. J. Infect. Dis. 123:16-21.

Kundsin, R.B. and J. Praznik. 1967. Pharyngeal carriage of Mycoplasma species in healthy young adults. Amer. J. Epidemiol. 86:
579-83.

Kunze, M., I. Schwanz-Pfitzner, M. Ozel, G. Laber. 1972. Mycoplasma
(Acholeplasma laidlawii) from cold blood cell cultures. Zentralbl.
Bakteriol (Orig. A) 222(4):520-34.

Kurzepa, H., et al. 1969. Growth of parasitic mycoplasma without
serum or serum fraction. J. Bact. 99:908-9.

Leach, R. H. 1970. The occurrence of Mycoplasma arginini in
several animal hosts. Vet. Rec. 87:319-20.

L'Ecuyer, C. 1969. Enzootic pneumonia in pigs: propagation of a
    causative mycoplasma in cell cultures and in artificial medium.
    Can. J. Comp. Med. 33(1):10-19.

L'Ecuyer, C. and P. Boulanger. 1970. Enzootic pneumonia of pigs:
    identification of a causative mycoplasma in infected pigs and
    in cultures by immunofluorescent staining. Can. J. Comp. Med.
    34(1):38-46.

Lee, Y.-H., A. Donner, P.E. Bailey, S. Alpert and W.M. McCormack.
    1974. Effect of agar volume, inoculum size, and hepes buffer
    on the size of T-mycoplasmal colonies. J. Lab. Clin. Med. 84(5):
    766-70.

Lehmkuhl, H.D. and M.L. Frey. 1974. Immunofluorescent identifi-
    cation of mycoplasma colonies grown on agar-covered glass
    slides. Appl. Microbiol. 27(6):1170-71.

Lemcke, R.M. 1964. The relationship of a type of mycoplasma iso-
    lated from tissue cultures to a new human oral mycoplasma.
    J. Hyg. 62(3):351-2.

Levashov, V.S. and V.Y. Shevlyagin. 1963. Isolation of micro-
    organisms (PPLO) causing pleuropneumonia-like diseases from
    tissue cultures. Byul. Eksptl. Biol. Med. 55(4):70-2.

Levine, E.M. 1972. Mycoplasma contamination of animal cell
    cultures: a simple, rapid detection method. Exp. Cell Res.
    74(1):99-109.

Levine, E.M. 1974. A simplified method for the detection of
    mycoplasma. Methods. Cell Biol. 8:229-48.

Lind, K. 1970. A simple test for peroxide secretion by myco-
    plasma. Acta. Path. Microbiol. Scand. Sect. B 78:256-7.

Low, I.E. 1974. Isolation of Acholeplasma laidlawii from commer-
    cial, serum-free tissue culture medium and studies on its
    survival and detection. Appl. Microbiol. 27(6):1046-52.

Low, I.E. 1976. Mycoplasma in tissue culture: overview of
    detection methods. Health Lab. Sci. 13(2):129-36.

Lozinskii, T.F., B.V. Gushchin, A.V. Astakhova, S.M. Klimenko,
    V.M. Zhdanov. 1974. Detection of latent viruses and myco-
    plasma by the methods of molecular biology. Vopr. Virusol.
    (4):474-9.

Lynn, R.J. and H.E. Morton. 1956. The inhibitory action of
agar on certain strains of pleuropneumonia-like organisms.
Appl. Microbiol. 4(6):339-341.

MacMorine, H.C., N. Rankin and S. Teleki. 1973. Test for mycoplasma on tissue culture vaccines. Develop. Biol. Standard
23:120-7.

Malizia, W.F., M.F. Barile and D.B. Riggs. 1961. Immunofluorescence of pleuropneumonia-like organisms isolated from tissue
cell cultures. Nature 191(4784):191-1.

Mardh, P.A. and D. Taylor-Robinson. 1973. New approaches to the
isolation of mycoplasmas. Med. Microbiol. Immunol. 158:259-266.

Mardh, P.-A. and L. Westrom. 1970. Antibodies to Mycoplasma hominis
in patients with genital infections and in healthy controls.
Brit. J. Vener. Dis. 46(5):390-7.

Markow, G.G., I. Bradvarova, A. Mintcheva, P. Petrov, N. Shiskov,
R.G. Tsanev. 1969. Mycoplasma contamination of cell cultures:
interference with 32P-labelling pattern of RNA.   Exp. Cell Res.
57(2):374-84.

Martin Bourgon, C., et al. 1973. Determination of the presence of
mycoplasma in cellular cultures by direct isolation. Rev. Sanid.
Hig. Publica. (Madrid) 46:477-84.

McGarrity, G.J. and L.L. Coriell. 1973. Detection of anaerobic
mycoplasmas in cell cultures. In Vitro 9(1):17-18.

McGarrity, G.J. 1975. Detection of mycoplasma in cell cultures.
TCA Manual 1:113-16.

Midulla, M., et al. 1968. Isolation of mycoplasmas from the
pharynx of 257 children. G. Mal. Infett. 20:573-6.

Millian, S.J. and I. Spigland. 1966. Antibodies for mycoplasmas
in normal individuals and patients with neoplasias. Cancer
19(12):1820-4.

Morris, J.E.W. and R.J. Fallon. 1973. Studies on the microbial
flora in the air of submarines and the nasopharyngeal flora
of the crew. J. Hyg. 71:761-70.

Muelas, J.M. and J.M. Ales. 1973. Method for detecting mycoplasma and bacterial L-form colonies in relief with an
ordinary light microscope by means of oblique light. Appl.
Microbiol. 25(3):484-8.

Murphy, W.H., C. Bullis, I.J. Ertel and C.J.D. Zarafonetis.
  1967. Mycoplasma studies of human leukemia. Ann. N.Y. Acad
  Sci. 143:544-56.

Murphy, W.H., C. Bullis, L. Dabich, R. Heyn, C.J. Zarafonetis.
  1970. Isolation of mycoplasma from leukemic and nonleukemic
  patients. J. Natl. Cancer Inst. 45(2):243-51.

Nigro, N., et al. 1968. Mycoplasma pneumoniae: compliment-fixing
  serum antibodies in healthy and leukemic children. Minerva
  Pediat. 20:694-9.

Ogata, M., K. Koshimizu. 1967. Isolation of mycoplasmas from
  tissue cell lines and transplantable tumor cells. Jap. J.
  Microbiol. 11(4):289-303.

Organick, A.B. 1966. Colonylike bodies associated with epithelial
  cells in streaks of pharyngeal swabs on serum enriched PPLO
  agar plates. Amer. Rev. Resp. Dis. 94:595-9.

Page, L.A., et al. 1972. Isolation of a new serotype of mycoplasma from a bovine placenta. J. Am. Vet. Med. Assoc. 161:
  919-25.

Panem, S., W.H. Kirsten. 1975. Secondary scanning electron microscopy of cells infected with murne oncornaviruses. Virology 63(2):
  447-58.

Papageorgiou, C. 1970. Medium for the isolation and culture
  of mycoplasmas from pathological products, cell cultures
  and contaminated biological products. Bull. Acad. Vet. Fr.
  43:357-61.

Peden, K.W. 1975. A rapid and simple method for the detection
  of mycoplasma and other intracellular contaminants. Experientia 31(9):1111-2.

Perez, A.G., J.H. Kim, A.S. Gelbard, B. Djordjevic. 1972.
  Altered incorporation of nucleic acid precursors by mycoplasma-infected mammalian cells in culture. Exp. Cell Res.
  70(2):301-10.

Pollock, M.E., G.E. Kenny and J. T. Syverton. 1960. Isolation
  and elimination of pleuropneumonia-like organism from mammalian
  cell cultures. Proc. Soc. Exp. Biol. Med. 105(1)10-15.

Pollock, M.E. 1965. Use of dialyzing culture technique for high
  yield of mycoplasma. J. Bact. 90(6):1682-5.

Pospisil, Z., M. Gois, M. Cerny and J. Mesnik. 1971. Demonstration
of M. hyorhinis in tissue cultures and pig lungs by means of
immunofluorescence. Acta Vet. Brno 40(1):99-104.

Potgieter, L.N.D. and R.F. Ross. 1972. Identification of M.
hyorhins and M. hyosynoviae by immunofluorescence. Vet.
Res. 33(1):91-8.

Prozorovckii, S.V., G.M. Bochko, I.V. Rakovskaya, T.I. Mitkina.
1967. Features specific to the cultivation and antigenic
properties of mycoplasma isolated from the oral cavity. Stom-
atologia (Mosk) 46:34-8.

Purcell, R.H., N.L. Somerson, H. Fox, D.C. Wong, H.C. Turner,
R.M. Chanock. 1966. Identification of acid-inducing agent and
related mycoplasma as Mycoplasma hyorhinis. J. Natl. Cancer
Inst. 37(2):251-3.

Rakovskaya, I.V., G.Y. Kagan, V.I. Gavrilov, A.I. Soloveva
and V.N. Petrosova. 1969. Isolation and biological characteristics of mycoplasma from chronically infected pulmonary cells
of human embryo. Vestnik. Acad. Med. Nauk. SSSR 24(5):63-9.

Randall, J.H., R.J. Stein and J.C. Ayres. 1950. Pleuropneumonia-
like organisms of the female genital tract. Amer. J. Obstet.
Gynec. 59-404.

Razin, S., J. Michmann and Z. Shimshani. 1964. The occurrence of
mycoplasma (PPLO) in the oral cavity of dentulous and edentu-
lous subjects. J. Dent. Res. 43(3):402-5.

Razin, S. and S. Rottem. 1967. Identification of mycoplasma and
other microorganisms by polyacrylamide-gel electrophoresis
of cell proteins. J. Bact. 94(6):1807-10.

Romano, N., et al. 1967. Isolation of mycoplasmas from products
of abortion and internal organs of malformed fetuses. G. Mal.
Infett. 19:985-90.

Rothblat, G.H. and H.E. Morton. 1958. The detection of contaminating pleuropneumonia-like organisms (PPLO) in cultures
of tissue cells. Bact. Proc. 58:73.

Russell, W.C., C. Newman, and D.H. Williamson. 1975. A simple
cytochemical technique for demonstration of DNA in cells
infected with mycoplasmas and viruses. Nature 253(5491):461-2.

Rybicka, I. 1972. Detection of microorganisms of the genus Mycoplasma (PPLO) in biological preparations. I. viability of
mycoplasmas under various conditions of storage. Epidemiol.
Rev. 26(3):323-32.

Sabin, A.B. 1938. Identification of the filterable, transmis-
sible neurolytic agent isolated from toxoplasma-infected
tissue as a new pleuropneumonia-like microbe. Science 88:575.

Sabin, A.B. 1967. Nature and source of mycoplasma in various
tissue cultures. Ann. N.Y. Acad. Sci. 143(1):628-34.

Scarlata, G. et al. 1972. Isolation of mycoplasma from the
oropharyngeal cavity of apparently healthy subjects. Ann.
Sclavo 14:274-83.

Schaub, I.G. and J.N. Guilbeau. 1949. The occurrence of
pleuropneumonia-like organism in a material from the
postpartum uterus: simplified methods for isolation and
staining. Bull. John Hopkins Hosp. 84:(1):1-10.

Schimmel, D., et al. 1966. Contamination of cell cultures
by mycoplasma. I. on the isolation and morphology of
mycoplasma from permanent cell cultues. Munchen. Vet.
Med. 21:64-9.

Schneider, E.L., C.J. Epstein, W.L. Epstein, M. Betlach
and G. Abbo Halbasch. 1973. Detection of mycoplasma
contamination in cultured human fibroblasts: comparison
of biochemical and microbiological techniques. Exp. Cell
Res. 79(2):343-9.

Schneider, E.L., E.J. Stanbridge and C.J. Epstein. 1974.
Incorporation of ^{3}H-uridine and ^{3}H-uracil into RNA: A
simple technique for the detection of mycoplasma contamination of cultured cells. Exp. Cell. Res. 84(1):311-18.

Schneider, E.L. 1975. Detection of mycoplasma contamination
in cultured cells: comparison of biochemical, morphological,
and microbilogical techniques. Methods Cell Biol. 10:261-75.

Schneider, E.L. and E.J. Stanbridge. 1975. Comparison of
methods for the detection of mycoplasmal contamination of
cell cultures. In Vitro 11(1):20-34.

Schneider, E.L., E.J. Stanbridge. 1975. A simple biochemical
technique for the detection of mycoplasma contamination of
cultured cells. Methods Cell Biol. 10:227-90.

Schwanz-Pfitzner, I., M. Ozel. 1973. Electron microscopy
studies of cell cultures: demonstration of a mixed infection
by Egtved virus of the rainbow trout and mycoplasma
(Acholeplasma laidlawii) (author's transl.). Zentralbl.
Bakteriol (Orig. A) 225(2):431-7.

Schwobel, W., R.H. Leach. 1970. Isolation of a mycoplasma strain similar to Mycoplasma laidlawii from primary calf kidney cell cultures. Zentralbl. Bakteriol. (Orig.) 14(4):495-506.

Seman, G., C. Rosenfeld, C. Jasmin, R. Camain. 1968. Notice of two cultures and a biopsy of Burkitt's tumor seen under the electron microscope. Rev. Fr. Etud. Clin. Biol. 13(1): 83-7.

Serene, T.P. and D.L. Anderson. 1967. Isolation of mycoplasma from human root canals. J. Dent. Res. 46(2):395-9.

Shedden, W.I.H. and B.C. Cole. 1966. Rapid method for demonstrating intracellular pleuropneumonia-like organism in a strain of hamster kidney cell (BHK 21 C^{13}) Nature 210 (5038):868

Shepard, M.C. 1973. Differential methods for identification of T-mycoplasmas based on demonstration of urease. J. Infect. Dis. 127:suppl:22-25.

Simmons, D.G., P.D. Lukert. 1972. Isolation of an anaerobic mycoplasma from avian cell cultures and some of its effects on Marek's disease virus. Avian Dis. 16(3):521-8.

Skalka, B. and M. Svojanovska. 1963. Microflora of genital organs of cattle (Mycoplasma sp.) Sb. Vys. Sk. Zemedelsk. (Brno Ser. B) 11:387-93.

Soldatova, V.M., M.A. Bashmakova and G.N. Stepanova. 1972. Incidence of mycoplasma isolation in different forms of pregnancy pathology. Akush. Ginekol. (Mosk.) 48:61-3.

Stanbridge, E. and L. Hayflick. 1967. Growth inhibition test for identification of Mycoplasma species utilizing dried antiserum impregnated paper discs. J. Bact. 93(4):1392-6.

Stewart, S.M., et al. 1968. Isolation of mycoplasmas from the human respiratory tract. J. Path. Bact. 95:580-6.

Steytler, J.G. 1970. Statistical studies on mycoplasma-positive human umbilical cord blood cultures. S. Afr. J. Obstet. Gynecol. 8(1):10-13.

Steytler, J.G. 1970. Studies on endogenous infection by vaginal mycoplasma based on positive cord-blood cultures. S. Afr. J. Obstet. Gynaecol. 8(1):14-22.

Steytler, J.G. 1970. Isolation of mycoplasmas from human
    cord-blood or serum: micro-anaerobic diphasic culture
    method. S. Afr. Med. J. 44 suppl:8-13.

Stipkovits, L., L. Bodon, J. Romvary, L. Varga. 1975. Direct
    isolation of mycoplasmas and acholeplasmas from sera, kidneys
    of calves. Acta. Microbiol. Acad Sci. Hung. 22(1):45-51.

Stone, S.S. and J. Tessler. 1974. Fluorescent labeling of
    antibody for identifying mycoplasma colonies by incident
    ultraviolet light. Am. J. Vet. Res. 35(1):107-10.

Studzinski, G.P., J.F. Gierthy and J.J. Cholon. 1973. An
    auto radiographic screenng test for mycoplasma contam-
    ination of mammalian cell cultures. In Vitro 8(6):466-72.

Swartzendruber, D.C., J. Clark and W.H. Murphy. 1967. Detection
    of phage-like particle by electron microscopy in a human
    strain of mycoplasma. Bact. Proc. 1967:151.

Tallgren, L.G., R. Wegelias, L.C. Andersson and E. Jansson. 1974.
    Eosinophilic leukaemia: recovery of Mycoplasma orale from
    the bone marrow. Acta. Med. Scand. 195:87-92.

Tedeshi, G.G., D. Amici and M. Paparelli. 1969. A study of
    the ultrastructure of bodies resembling mycoplasma in
    cultures of erythrocytes from normal human blood. Microscope
    17(2):149-52.

Tessler, J. 1973. Incident light immunofluorescence of alcohol-
    fixed colonies of ruminant mycoplasma. Can. J. Comp. Med.
    37:207-9.

Theodore, T.S., J.G. Tully and R.M. Cole. 1971. Polyacrylamide
    gel identification of bacterial L forms and mycoplasma species
    of human origin. Appl. Microbiol. 21:272-7.

Todaro, G.J., S.A. Aaronson and E. Rands. 1971. Rapid detection
    of mycoplasma-infected cell cultures. Exp. Cell Res. 65(1):
    256-7.

Tompkins, A., A. MacGregor, D. Pye, M. Atkinson. 1975. Rapid
    detection and isolation of mycoplasmas from cell cultures.
    Aust. J. Exp. Biol. Med. Sci. 53(4):257-63.

Tram, C., et al. 1970. Isolation of mycoplasma from rat fetus
    by aseptic cesarean section. C.R. Soc. Biol. (Paris) 164:
    2470-1.

Tully, J.G., R.F. Whitcomb, D.L. Williamson et al. 1976.
    Suckling mouse cataract agent is a helical, wall-free
    prokaryote (Spiroplasma) pathogenic for vertebrates.
    Nature 259:117-20.

Tully, J.G., R.F. Whitcomb, H.F. Clark, D.L. Williamson.
    1977. Pathogenic mycoplasmas: cultivation and vertebrate
    pathogenicity of a new spiroplasma. Science 195:892-4.

VanHerick, W. and M.D. Eaton. 1945. An unidentifed pleuro-
    pneumonia-like organism isolated during passages in chick
    embryos. J. Bact. 50(1):47-55.

vonBonsdorff, C.H., et al. 1973. Ultrastructure of a myco-
    plasma recovered from the bone marrow to systemic lupus
    erythematosus. Ann. Rheum. Dis. 32:25-8.

Watanabe, T., et al. 1971. The occurrence of T-mycoplasma
    in oral cavities. J. Jap. Stomatol. Soc. 38:324-32.

Weiss, L.J. 1944. Pleuropneumonia-like organisms as seen by
    the electron microscope. J. Bact. 48:119.

Windsor, R.S. and C.D.H. Boarer. 1972. A method for the rapid
    enumeration of mycoplasma species growing in broth culture.
    J. Appl. Bact. 35(1):37-42.

Witzleb, W., T. Blumohr, H. Dziambor, H. Schweizer. 1970.
    On contamination of tissue cultures with mycoplasmas.
    II. detection and serological identification of mycoplasmas.
    Arch. Gesamte Virusforsch 30(2):121-9.

Wolanski, B., K. Maramorosch. 1970. Negatively stained myco-
    plasmas: fact or artifact: Virology 42(2):319-27.

Yamamoto, H., N. Ogawa and Y. Nishimura. 1969. Isolation of
    mycoplasma from fowl pox vaccine. A Rep. Natl. Vet. Assay
    Lab., Tokyo 6:169-74.

Zeigel, R.F. and H.F. Clark. 1969. Electron microscope obser-
    vations on a mycoplasma-like agent associated with pathologic
    changes in eyes of suckling mice and rats. J. Cell Biol. 43:
    163a.

Zgorniak-Nowosielska, I., W.D. Sedwick, K. Hummeler and H.
    Koprowski. 1967. New assay procedure for separation of myco-
    plasmas from virus pools and tissue culture systems. J. Virol.
    1(6):1227-37.

Zgorniak-Nowosielska, I. and J. Branny. 1970. Mycoplasma in the
    semen of bulls. I. isolation and some properties of mycoplasma
    from bovine semen. Med. Wet. 26:51-3.

Zgorniak-Nowosielska, I. 1970. Detection of mycoplasma in cell
    cultures and the antibiotic resistance of the isolated strains.
    Med. Dosw. Mikrobiol. 22(3):195-203.

Zhdanov, V.M., A.F. Bykovskii, T. A. Bektemirov, K.V. I'lin, N.P.
    Mazurenko and A.K. Astakhova. 1974. Biochemical methods for
    demonstrating latent oncornaviruses and mycoplasmas. Vop. Med.
    Khim. 20(4):396-400.

4. EFFECTS ON CELL CULTURES

A. Growth, Morphology and General Characteristics

Abenova, U.A., B.V. Guschchin, K.V. Lil'in and V.M. Zhdanov.
    1974. Isolation of oncornavirus type B from a continuous
    line of human amnion cells. Vop. Virusol. 2:216-23.

Afshar, A. 1967. The growth of Mycoplasma bovigenitalium in
    cell cultures. J. Gen. Microbiol. 47(1):103-10.

Ahuja, K.L. and N.K. Chandiramani. 1975. Behavior of Myco-
    plasma gallisepticum and M. gallinarum in cell culture.
    Nat. Inst. Anim. Health Q. (Tokyo) 15(2):103-4.

Aldridge, K.E. 1975. Growth and cytopathology of Mycoplasma
    synoviae in chicken embryo cell cultures. Infect. Immun.
    12(1):198-204.

Alexander -Jackson, E. 1966. Mycoplasma (PPLO) isolated from
    Rous sarcoma virus. Growth 30(2):199-228.

Allen, G.P., J. T. Bryans. 1974. Studies of an established
    equine cell line derived from a transitional cell carcinoma.
    Am. J. Vet. Res. 35(9):1153-60.

Anderson, D.R., H.E. Hopps, M.F. Barile, B.C. Bernheim. 1965.
    Comparison of the ultrastructure of several rickettsiae,
    ornithosis virus, and mycoplasma in tissue culture. J. Bac-
    teriol. 90(5):1387-1404.

Armstrong, D., G. Henle, N.L. Somerson and L. Hayflick. 1965.
    Cytopathogenic mycoplasmas associated with two human tumors.
    J. Bact. 90(2):418-24.

Balducci, L, et al. 1968. Peculiarities of a strain of Mycoplasma hominis, type I isolated by tissue culture. Boll.
Soc. Ital. Biol. Sper. 44:856-8.

Balduzzi, P. and R.J. Charbonneau. 1964. Decontamination of
PPLO infected tissue cultures. Experientia 20(11):651-2.

Barbuti, S. 1968. Research on the presence of mycoplasmas in
cell cultures and virus strains. Ann. Sclavo. 10(2):167-83.

Barile, M.F., W.F. Barile and D. B. Riggs. 1962.
Incidence and detection of pleuropneumonia-like organisms
in cell cultures by fluorescent antibody and cultural
procedures. J. Bact. 84(1):130-6.

Barile, M.F. 1968. Mycoplasma and cell cultres. In: Cell
Cultures for Virus Vaccine Production. J. Nat. Cancer Inst.
Monogr. 29:201-4.

Barile, M.F., and J. Kern. 1971. Isolation of Mycoplasma
arginini from commercial bovine sera and its implication
in contaminated cell cultures. Proc. Soc. Exp. Biol. Med.
138(2):432-7.

Boatman, E., F. Cartwright and G. Kenny. 1976. Morphology,
morphometry and electron microscopy of HeLa cells infected
with bovine mycoplasma. Cell Tissue Res. 170:1-16.

Bothig, B., et al. 1970. Influence of mycoplasma infections
in permanent cell cultures on the propagation of enteroviruses
and the elimination of mycoplasma infections using antibiotic
therapy. Deut. Gesundheitsw. 25:1278-82.

Brown, A. and J.E. Officer. 1968. Contamination of cell cultures
by mycoplasma (PPLO). In: Methods in Virology. K. Maramorosch
and H. Koprowski, eds. 4:531-64. Academic Press, N.Y.

Brown, A., M. Teplitz and J.P. Revel. 1974. Interaction of mycoplasmas with cell cultures, as visualized by electron microscopy. Proc. Natl. Acad. Aci. 71(2):464-8.

Butler, M. and R.H. Leach. 1964. A mycoplasma which induces acidity
and cytopathic effect in tissue culture. J. Gen. Microbiol. 34(2):
285-94.

Butler, M. and R.H. Leach. 1966. Mycoplasma associated with tissue
cultures, leukaemia and human tumours. Proc. Roy. Soc. Med.
59:1116-7.

Cailleau, R., R. Young, M. Olive and W.J. Reeves, Jr. 1974.
    Breast tumor cell lines from pleural effusions. J. Natl.
    Cancer Inst. 53(3):661-74.

Carp, R.I., G.S. Merz, P.C. Licursi. 1974. Reduced cell yields of
    mouse cell line cultures after exposure to homogenates of mul-
    tiple sclerosis tissues. Infect. Immun. 9(6):1011-5.

Carp, R.I., P.C. Licursi, G.S. Merz. 1975. Multiple sclerosis-
    induced reduction in the yield of a mouse cell line. Infect.
    Immun. 11(4):737-41.

Castrejon-Diez, J., T.N. Fisher and E. Fisher, Jr. 1963. Exper-
    imental infection of tissue cultures with certain mycoplasma
    (PPLO). Proc. Soc. Exp. Biol. Med. 112(3):643-7.

Chao, F.C., G. Freeman, J.G. Cummings, B.J. Berridge, Jr. 1967.
    Amino acids of the ornithine cycle in transformed hamster
    fibroblasts carrying pleuropneumonia-like organisms. Cancer
    Res. 27(8):1474-81.

Chanock, R.M., H.H. Fox, W.D. James, H.H. Bloom and M.A.
    Mufson. 1960. Growth of laboratory and naturally occurring
    strains of Eaton agent in monkey kidney tissue culture.
    Proc. Soc. Exp. Biol. Med. 105(2):371-5.

Chapman, A.L., W.J. Bopp, A.S. Brightwell, H. Cohen, A.H. Nielson,
    C.R. Gravelle and A.A. Werder. 1967. Preliminary report on
    virus-like particles in canine leukemia and derived cell cul-
    tures. Cancer Res. 27:18-25.

Clyde, W.A., Jr. 1961. Demonstration of Eaton's agent in tissue
    culture. Proc. Soc. Exp. Biol. Med. 107(4):715-8.

Clyde, W.A., Jr. 1963. Studies on Eaton agent in tissue culture.
    In: Conference on newer respiratory disease viruses, 1962.
    Amer. Rev. Resp. Dis. 88(3Pt2):212-17.

Collier, L.H. 1957. Contamination of stock lines of human car-
    cinoma cells by pleuropneumonia-like organisms. Nature,
    London 180-757.

Coriell, L.L., D.P. Fabrizio and S.R. Wilson. 1960. Comparison
    of pleuropneumonia-like organism strains from tissue culture
    by complement-fixation. Ann. N.Y. Acad. Sci. 79(10):686-95.

Coriell, L.L. 1968. Tissue and medium antigens in vaccines.
    Natl. Cancer Inst. Monogr. 29:179-91.

Crandell, R.A., C.G. Fabricant, W.A. Nelson-Rees. 1973. Development, characterization, and viral susceptibility of a
feline (Felis catus) renal cell line (CRFK). In Vitro 9(3):
176-85.

Cross, G.F., M.R. Goodman and E.J. Shaw. 1967. Detection and
treatment of contaminating mycoplasmas in human cell culture.
Aust. J. Exp. Biol. Med. Sci. 45(2):201-12.

Cuccurollo, L., and A. Violante. 1968. Electron microscopic
observations on a Mycoplasma cultured in acellular media and
in human amniotic cells. G. Mal. Infett. Parassit. 206:496-8.

Demidova, S.A. and N.M. Ritova. 1974. Cell culture contaminants.
Vop. Virusol. 5:521-7.

Demidova, S.A., B.V. Gushchin, T., F. Lozinskii, V.V. Perekrest,
N.M. Ritova, S.M. Klimenko, I.S. Shushkov and V.M. Zhdanov.
1974. Viral contaminants of cell cultures in the aspect of
persistent infections. Vestn. Akad. Med. Nauk. SSSR 9:27-35.

DeVries, J.E., M. Meyering, A. Van Dongen and P. Rumke. 1975.
The influence of different isolation procedures and the use
of target cells from melanoma cell lines and short-term
cultures on the non-specific cytotoxic effects of lymphocytes from healthy donors. Int. J. Cancer 15(3):391-400.

Dewey, W.C., R.M. Humphrey, B.A. Sedita. 1968. Variations in
rates of thymidine incorporation into DNA and conversion
to thymine in mammalian cells grown in culture. Exp. Cell
Res. 50(2):349-54.

Draghici, D., D. Schimmel and T. Hubrig. 1969. Procine mycoplasmata in cell cultures: I. isolation of porcine mycoplasmata in
primary cell cultures. Arch. Exp. Vet. Med. 23(1):101-34.

Draghici, D., D. Schimmel and T. Hubrig. 1969. Porcine mycoplasmata in cell cultures: II. adaptation of mycoplasma isolates
in cell-free media to cell cultures. Arch. Exp. Vet. Med. 23
(1):135-44.

Draghici, D., D. Schimmel and T. Hubrig. 1969. Mycoplasmata
from pigs and cell cultures: III. staining methods to demonstrate mycoplasmata in cell cultures and methods for demonstrating cytopathic changes. Arch. Exp. Vet. Med. 23(3):615-32.

Dunlop, W.R., S. D. Kottaridis and S.C. Smith. 1966. The influence of tissue culture mycoplasma on transovarian transmission
of M. gallisepticum. Poult. Sci. 45:1081.

D'Yakonova, E.V. 1968. Biological properties of laryngotracheitis
  virus when it is grown together with the causative agent of
  mycoplasmosis in chick embryos. Byull. Vses. Inst. Eksp.
  Vet. 4:19-21.

Dzhikidze, E.K., G. Ya. Kagan and E. Ya. Balaeva. 1973.
  Isolation of mycoplasma during leukemia in sacred baboons.
  Vestn. Akad. Med. Nauk. SSSR 28(4):48-50.

Eaton, M.D., A.E. Farnham, J.D. Levinthal and A.R. Scala.
  1962. Cytopathic effect of the atypical pneumonia organism
  in cultures of human tissue. J. Bact. 84:1330-7.

Edward, D.G. 1969. Mycoplasmas as contaminants and their detection. Prog. Immunobiol. Stand 3:17-22.

Edwards, G.A. and J. Fogh. 1960. Fine structure of pleuropneumonia-like organisms in pure culture and in infected
  tissue culture cells. J. Bact. 79(2):267-76.

Fallon, R.J. and D.K. Jackson. 1967. The relationship between
  a rodent mycoplasma Mycoplasma pulmonis, and certain mycoplasmas isolated from tissue cultures inoculated with material
  from patients with leukaemia. Lab. Anim. 1(1):55-64.

Fleer, G.P., et al. 1969. The effect of certain mycoplasma on
  the formation of plaques by Langat virus in a primary culture
  of chick embryo cells. Vestn. Akad. Med. Nauk. SSSR. 24:68-72.

Fogh, J., E. Hahn, 3rd, H. Fogh. 1965. Effects of pleuropneumonia-like organisms on cultured human cells. Exp. Cell
  Res. 39(2):554-66.

Fogh, J. 1969. Reduced tumor-producing capacity of mycoplasma
  modified lines of FL human amnion cells in the cheek pouch
  of cortisonized hamsters. Cancer Res. 29(9):1721-31.

Fogh, J. 1970. Mycoplasma effects on SV40 transformation of
  human amnion cells. Proc. Soc. Exp. Biol. Med. 134(1):217-24.

Fogh, J. 1973. Reversible and irreversible alterations of cultured FL human amnion cells after experimental mycoplasmal
  infection. In: Contamination in Tissue Culture, 175-94 pp.

Fogh, J. 1973. Increased mycoplasma-cell association in transformed human amnion cells. J. Infect. Dis. 127:Suppl:77-81.

Fogh, J. and H. Fogh. 1965. Chromosome changes in pleuropneumonia-like organism-infected FL human amnion cells.
Proc. Soc. Exp. Biol. Med. 119(1):233-38.

Fogh, J., H. Fogh, and L. Ramos. 1971. Growth in vitro of mycoplasma infected human amnion cells, FI amnion cells, and mycoplasma modified FL cells. Proc. Soc. Exp. Biol. Med. 136(3):
809-18.

Fraser, K.B., P.V. Shirodaria, M. Haire and D. Middleton. 1971.
Mycoplasma in cell cultures from rheumatoid synovial membranes.
J. Hyg. 69(1):17-25.

Friend, C., M.C. Patuleia and J.B. Nelson. 1966. Antibiotic
effect of tylosin on a mycoplasma contaminant in a tissue
culture leukemia cell line. Proc. Soc. Exp. Biol. Med.
121(4):1009-10.

Furness, G., et al. 1975. Adaptation of Mycoplasma hominis to
an obligate parasitic existence in monkey kidney cell culture
(BSC-1). Proc. Soc. Exp. Biol. Med. 149(2):427-32.

Gabridge, M.G., D.D. Gamble. 1974. Independence of leukemoid
potential and toxigenicity of Mycoplasma fermentans. J. Infect.
Dis. 130(6):664-8

Gabridge, M.G. and P.R. Schneider. 1975. Cytotoxic effect of
Mycoplasma fermentans on mouse thymocytes. Infect. Immun. 11
(3)460-5.

Gabridge, M.G., D.M. Yip and K. Hedges. 1975. Levels of lysosomal
enzymes in tissues of mice infected with Mycoplasma fermentans.
Infect. Immun. 12(2):233-9.

Gaffney, E.V., J. Fogh. 1970. DNA content of mycoplasma-modified
FL human amnion cells. Proc. Soc. Exp. Biol. Med. 133(2):607-8.

Gaffney, E.V., J. Fogh, L. Ramos, J.D. Loveless, H. Fogh and A.M.
Dowling. 1970. Established lines of SV-40 transformed human
amnion cells. Cancer Res. 30(6):1668-76.

Gill, P. and J. Pan. 1970. Inhibition of cell division in L5178Y
cells by arginine degrading mycoplasmas: the role of arginine
deiminase. Can. J. Microbiol. 16(6):415-19.

Girardi, A.J., V.V. Hamparian, N.L. Somerson, L. Hayflick. 1965.
Mycoplasma isolates from primary cell cultures and human diploid
cell strains. Proc. Soc. Exp. Biol. Med. 120(3):760-70.

Goldstein, S., P.C. Sanders and I.U. Boone. 1962. Cultivation of pleuropneumonia-like organisms from tissue cultures. U.S. Atomic Energy Comm. Res. and Develop. Rept. Lams. 2780:224-7.

Goodwin, R.F.W. andf P. Whittlestone. 1963. Production of enzootic pneumonia in pigs with an agent grown in tissue culture from the natural disease. Brit. J. Exp. Path. 44(3):291-99.

Grumbles, L.C., C.F. Hall and G. Cummings. 1964. Characteristics of avian mycoplasma (PPLO) in tissue cultures of human and avian cells. Avian Dis. 8(2):274-80.

Gupta, R.K.P. 1973. Studies on the development of pathological changes in chick embryos experimentally infected with virulent and avirulent strains of Mycoplasma caprae. Agra Univ. J. Res. 22(1):101-2.

Hargreaves, F.D., et al. 1970. The influence of mycoplasma infection on the sensitivity of HeLa cells for growth of viruses. J. Med. Microbiol. 3:259-65.

Hayflick, J. and W.R. Stinebring. 1955. Intracellular growth of pleuropneumonia-like organisms. Anat. Rec. 121:477-8.

Hayflick, L. W.R. Stinebring, F.C. Breckenridge and C.M. Pomerat. 1956. Some effects of human pleuropneumonia-like organisms on tissue cultures of human synovial cells. Bact. Proc. p. 83.

Hayflick, L., and W.R. Stinebring. 1960. Intracellular growth of pleuropneumonia-like organisms in tissue culture and in ovo. Ann. N.Y. Acad. Sci. 79(10):433-49.

Herderschee, D., A.C. Ruys and G.R. van Rhijn. 1963. Pleuro-pneumonia-like organisms in tissue cultures. A.V.L.J. Microbiol., Serol. 29:368-76.

Hollingdale, M.R., R.J. Manchee. 1972. The role of mycoplasma membrane proteins in the adsorption of animal cells to Mycoplasma hominis colonies. J. Gen. Microbiol. 70(2):391-3.

Holmgren, N.B. and W.E. Campbell, Jr. 1960. Tissue cell culture contamination in relation to bacterial pleuropneumonia-like organisms. L-form conversion. J. Bact. 79(6):869-74.

Holmgren, N.B. and F.E. Payne. 1966. Some intraspecies of differences in antigens on the surface of certain living human cells. J. Nat. Cancer Inst. 36(3):355-74.

Hopps, H.E., B.C. Meyer, M.F. Barile and R.A. DelGiudice. 1973.
   Problems concerning "noncultivable" mycoplasma contaminants
   in tissue cultures. Ann. N.Y. Acad. Sci. 225-265-76.

House, W., et al. 1967. Detection of mycoplasma in cell
   cultures. J. Path. Bact. 93:125-32.

Hummeler, K., D. Armstrong and N. Tomassini. 1965. Cytopathogenic mycoplasmas associated with two human tumors. II. morphological aspects. J. Bact. 90(2):511-16.

Hummeler, K., N. Tomassini and L. Hayflick. 1965. Ultrastructure
   of a mycoplasma (negroni) isolated from human leukemia. J. Bact.
   90(2)517-23.

Hummeler, K., D. Armstrong. 1967. Observations on mycoplasma
   strains in tissue cultures. Ann. N.Y. Acad. Sci. 143(1):622-5.

Hung. M.H., et al. 1965. Studies on pleuropneumonia-like organisms
   (PPLO) I. isolation of PPLO from established cell lines and cell
   strains used in Taiwan. J. Formosan Med. Ass. 61:698-706.

Hung, M.H. and C. Yang. 1968. Studies on pleuropneumonia-like
   organsisms (mycoplasma): II. identification of mycoplasmas
   isolated from cell lines and human specimens by growth inhibition test. Chinese J. Microbiol. 1(3/4):106-16.

Jagielski, M., S. Kaluzewski. 1972. Contamination of cell cultures
   with mycoplasma. II. properties of isolated mycoplasma. Med.
   Dosw. Mikrobiol. 24(4):323-31.

Jasmin, G. and C.L. Richer. 1959. On the contamination of the
   Murphy-Sturm lymphosarcoma with a pleuropneumonia-like organism.
   Experientia 15(9):329-31.

Jeffreys, A.J., I.W. Craig. 1976. Analysis of proteins synthesized
   in mitochondria of cultured mammalian cells. An assessment of
   current approaches and problems in interpretation. Eur. J.
   Biochem. 68(1):301-11.

Jentzsch, K.D., J. Zipper, W. Halle. 1974. Current problems in
   active-substance research. 5. utilization of animal cell- and
   tissue cultures for the comprehension and clarification of
   biological effects of substances -- general aspects. Pharmazie
   29(6):369-73.

Joncas, J., A. Chagnon, G. Lussier and V. Pavilanis. 1969.
Characteristics of a Mycoplasma hyorhinis strain contaminating a human fetal diploid cell line. Can J. Microbiol.
15(5):451-4.

Kagan, G.Y., I.V. Rakovskaya, E.I. Koptelova, S.V. Prozorovskii,
B.V. Zhiv, S.G. Komm. 1965. Comparison of the cytopathopatho-
genic effect of the L-forms of various species of bacteria
and mycoplasmas in tissue cultures. Vestnik. Akad. Med.
Nauk. SSSR 20 (8):66-74.

Kagan, G.Y. 1966 and 1967. Mycoplasma: infections of man,
animals, and tissue cultures. Genetics of microorganisms
53-67, 1966. Ref. Zh. Biol. 1967. No. 10B774.

Kagan, G.Y., F.I. Lershov., I.V. Rakovskaya, A.A. Tsareva and
V.M. Zhdanov. 1967. Effect of mycoplasma infection on the
replication of some ribonucleic acid-containing viruses. Vop.
Virusol. 12(4):478-85.

Kagan, G.Y., K.S. Kulikova, V.V. Neustroeva, A.I. Rezepova and
Z.D. Sultanova. 1968. Effect of mycoplasma infection of culture
cells on replication, cytopathic action, and hemagglutinating
capacity of some viruses. Vop. Virusol. 13(5):600-5.

Kagan, G.Y. and I.V. Rakovskaya. 1969. Mycoplasma infection
in tissue cultures. Ref. Zh. Biol. 1969. No. 8B884K:1-173.

Kagan, G.Y. 1969. Mycoplasma infection of cellular cultures.
Vestn. Akad. Med. Nauk. SSSR 24(5):46-57.

Kaklamanis, E., L. Thomas, K. Stavropoulos, I. Borman, C.
Boshwitz. 1969. Mycoplasmacidal action of normal tissue extracts
Nature 221(183):860-2.

Kaluzewski, S., M. Jagielski. 1972. Studies on the contamination
of cell cultures with Mycoplasma. I. conditions for Mycoplasma
isolation. Med. Dosw. Mikrobiol. 24(2):103-13.

Kawamura, H., S. Sato, F. Shimizu and H. Tsubahara. 1964.
Cytopathic effect and plaque formation of avian mycoplasma
in chicken kidney cell cultures. Nat. Inst. Anim. Health
Quart. (Tokyo) 4:28.

Keller, R. and H E. Morton. 1954. The growth of pleuropneumonia-
like organisms of human origin: cultivation in the developing
chick embryo and in vitro growth cycle. J. Bact. 67(2):129-34.

Kenny, G.E., M.E. Pollock and J.T. Syverton. 1961. Effect of
pleuropneumonia-like organisms on a mammalian cell culture
growth. Bact. Proc. 61:153.

Kenny, G.E. and M.E. Pollock. 1963. Mammalian cell cultures contaminated with pleuropneumonia-like organism. I. Effect of
pleuropneumonia-like organism. I. effect of pleuropneumonia-
like organism on growth of established cell strains. J. Infect.
Dis. 112(1):7-16.

Kenny, G.E. 1973. Contamination of mammalian cells in culture by
mycoplasmata. In: Contamination in Tissue Culture. Jorgen Fogh,
Ed. Academic Press. 107-29.

Klushina, T.N. 1967. Biological properties of pleuropneumonia-
like organism (mycoplasma) isolated from tissue cultures and
normal bovine serum. Zh. Microbiol. Epidemiol. Immunobiol.
44(3):16-19.

Kottaridis, S.D., W.R. Dunlop, S.C. Smith. 1967. Tissue-culture-
propagated mycoplasma for the control of chronic respiratory
disease. Avian Dis. 11(4):528-31.

Kraemer, P.M., V. Defendi, L. Hayflick and L.A. Manson. 1963.
Mycoplasma (PPLO) strains with lytic activity for murine
lymphoma cells in vitro. Proc. Soc. Exp. Biol. Med. 112(2):
381-7.

Kraemer, P.M. 1964. Mycoplasma with lytic activity for murine
lymphoma cells grown in vitro. Diss. Abstr. 25(6):3213.

Kunze, M., I. Schwanz-Pfitzner, M. Ozel, G. Laber. 1972.
Mycoplasma (Acholeplasma laidlawii) from cold blood cell
cultures. Zentralbl. Bakteriol (Orig. A) 222(4):520-34.

Kuzmina, S.V., L.K. Glazkova, L.I. Kalinina, F.B. Levin, V.V.
Neustroeva. 1972. New lines of mice fibroblasts. Tsitologiia
14(3):369-78.

Kuzmina, S.V., I.V. Rakovskaya, L.K. Glazkova and V.N.
   Petrosova. 1972. Biological characteristics of mycoplasmas
   isolated from transplantable lines of mouse fibroblasts.
   Z. Mikrobiol. Epidemiol. Immunobiol. 7:61-4.

Larin, N.M., N.V. Saxby, Buggey, D. 1969. Quantitative aspects
   of Mycoplasma pneumoniae-cell relationships in cultures of
   lung diploid fibroblasts. J. Hyg. (Camb.) 67(3):375-85.

Leach, R.H. and M. Butler. 1966. Comparison of mycoplasmas
   associated with human tumors, leukemia and tissue cultures.
   J. Bact. 91(3):934-41.

L'Ecuyer, C. 1969. Enzootic pneumonia in pigs: propagation of
   a causative mycoplasma in cell cultures and in artificial
   medium. Can. J. Comp. Med. 33(1):10-19.

Lemcke, R.M. 1964. The relationship of a type of mycoplasma
   isolated from tissue cultures to a new human oral mycoplasma.
   J. Hyg. 62(3):351-2.

Levashov. V.S. and V.Y. Shevlyagin. 1963. Isolation of microorganisms (PPLO) causing pleuropneumonia-like diseases from
   tissue cultures. Byul. Eksptl. Biol. Med. 55(4):70-2.

Levashov. V.S. and Y.Y. Tsilinskii. 1964. The degree of contamination of tissue cultures by pleuropneumonia-like organism and
   a technique for purifying these cultures. TR Inst. Poliomelita
   Virusn. Entsefalitov. 5:150-3.

Levashov, V.S. and Y.Y. Tsilinskii. 1964. Contamination of tissue
   cultures with the pleuropneumonia-like organism. Zh. Mikrobiol.
   Epidemiol. Immunobiol. 41(4):115-18.

Levashov, V.S. and T.N. Klushina. 1969. Biological properties
   of reversed cultures from some mycoplasma isolated from
   tissue cultures and normal bovine serum. Zh. Mikrobiol.
   Epidemiol. Immunobiol. 46(6):107-10.

Mackay, J.M. 1969. Tissue culture studies of sheep pulmonary
   adenomatosis (Jaagsiekte). I. direct cultures of affected
   lungs. J. Comp. Path. 79:141-6.

MacPherson, I. 1966. Mycoplasma in tissue culture. J. Cell
   Sci. 1:145-67.

MacPherson, I. and W. Russell. 1966. Transformation in hamster
cells mediated by mycoplasmas. Nature 210(5043):1343-5.

MacPherson, I. 1968. Neoplastic properties of animal cell lines --
general comments. Natl. Cancer Inst. Monogr. 29:295-6.

Maillet, P.L. 1970. Simultaneous infection by particles of the
PLT type (Rickettsial) and of the PPLO type (Mycoplasmatales)
in an insect vector of clover phyllody, Euscelis lineolatus.
Brulle (Homoptera Jassidae). J. Microsc. (Paris) 6(6):
827-32.

Manchee, R.J. and D. Taylor-Robinson. 1969. Studies on the nature
of receptors involved in attachment of tissue culture cells to
mycoplasmas. Br. J. Exp. Pathol. 50:66-75.

Manchee, R.J. and D. Taylor-Robinson. 1970. Lysis and protection of erythrocytes by T-mycoplasmas. J. Med. Microbiol.
3(3):539-46.

Martin, R.R., G.A. Warr, R.B. Couch, H. Yeager and V. Knight.
1974. Effects of tetracycline on leukotaxis. J. Infec. Dis.
129(2):110-16.

Maruyama, K., L. Dmochowski, J.M. Bowen and R.L. Hales. 1968.
Studies of human leukemia and lymphoma cells by membrane
immunofluorescence and mixed hemabsorption tests. Tex. Rep.
Biol. Med. 26(4):545-63.

Mazzali, R., D. Taylor-Robinson. 1971. The behaviour of
T-mycoplasmas in tissue culture. J. Med. Microbiol. 4(1):
125-38.

Meloni, G.A., D. Rizzu and S. Addis. 1969. Studies on the reproduction of four strains of Mycoplasma hominis type 1 isolated
from cell cultures in vitro. Boll. Ist. Sieroterap., Milan
48(1):23-38.

Milligan, W.H. III. 1973. Effect of Mycoplasma pneumoniae on
rhinovirus replication in cell culture. Diss. Abstr. 34(4):
1652-1653-B.

Moorhead, P.S. 1968. Identification of established cell lines
with reference to karyology. Natl. Cancer Inst. Monogr. 29:
45-50.

Naglic, T., E. Topolnik and N. Fijan. 1974. Mycoplasmal contamination of cell cultures: Acholeplasma laidlawii isolated from
fish cell lines. Veterinarski Arhiv. 45(9/10):228-34.

Nakamura, M. and S. Hiroaki. 1969. Modification of the growth of
human mycoplasmas in tissue culture by infection with influenza
virus and Japanese encephalitis (JE) virus. Proc. Soc. Exp.
Biol. Med. 131(2):345-8.

Nasemann, T. and H. Rockl. 1960. Pleuropneumonia-like organisms:
their effect on chicken chorioallantoic membrane and the resistance to antibiotics. Ann. N.Y. Acad. Sci. 79(10):588-92.

Nelson, J.B. 1936. Studies onb an uncomplicated coryza of the
domestic fowl. VII. Cultivation of the coccobacilliform bodies
in fertile eggs and in tissue culture. J. Exp. Med. 64-749.

Nelson, J.B. 1936. Studies on an uncomplicated coryza of the
domestic fowl. VIII. the infectivity of fetal membrane and
tissue culture suspensions of the coccobacilliform bodies.
J. Exp. Med. 64:759.

Nelson, J.B. 1939. Growth of the fowl coryza bodies in tissue
culture and in blood agar. J. Exp. Med. 69:199.

Nelson, J.B. 1960. The behaviour of murine pleuropneumonia-like
organism in HeLa cell cultures. Ann. N.Y.Acad. Sci. 79(10):
450-7.

Neustroeva, V.V., I.V. Vulfovich, G.Y. Kagan. 1976. Localization
and possible development cycle of mycoplasmas and bacterial
L-forms in cell cultures. Biull. Eksp. Biol. Med. 81(4):
439-40.

Norval, M. A. Graham, B.P. Marmion. 1976. Cytology of rheumatoid
synovial cells in culture. IV. further investigations of cell
lines cocultivated with rheumatoid synovial cells. Ann. Rheum.
Dis. 35(4):297-305.

O'Connell, R.C. 1964. A study of factors contributing to wide
spread contamination of tissue cultures with pleuropneumonia-
like organism. Diss. Abstr. 24(12 Pt.) 1:4922.

O'Connell, R.C., R.G. Wittler and J.E. Faber. 1964. Aerosols
as a source of wide spread mycoplasma contamination of tissue
cultures. Appl. Microbiol. 12(4):337-42.

Ogata, M. and K. Koshimizu. 1967. Isolation of mycoplasmas from
tissue cell lines and transplantable tumor cells. Jap. J.
Microbiol. 11(4):289-303.

Ogata, M., K. Koshimizu. 1971. Contamination of the BAT cells
with Mycoplasma. Jap. J. Clin. Med. 29(2):750-2.

Ohllsson-Wilhelm, B.M., J.J. Freed, R.P. Perry. 1976. Selective
isolation of revesible cold sensitive variants from Chinese
hamster ovary cell cultures. J. Cell Physiol. 89(1):77-88.

O'Reilly, K.J. and A.M. Whitaker. 1969. The development of feline
cell lines for the growth of feline infectious enteritis
(panleucopaenia) virus. J. Hyg. 67(1):115-24.

O'Toole, C., S. Nayak, Z. Price, W.H. Gilbert, J. Waisman. 1976.
A cell line (SCABER) derived from squamous cell carcinoma of
the human urinary bladder. Int. J. Cancer 17(6):707-14.

Pijoan, C. 1975. The effects of Mycoplasma hyorhinis and of
Mycoplasma hyopneumoniae on pig kidney primary tissue culture.
Br. Vet. J. 131(5):586-94.

Pollock, M.E. 1963. Pleuropneumonia-like organism in mammalian
cell cultures: their significance. Diss. Abstr. 24(1):34.

Pollock, M.E., P.E. Treadwell and G.E. Kenny. 1963. Mammalian
cell cultures contaminated with pleuropneumonia-like organism.
II. effect of pleuropneumonia-like organism on cell morphology
in established monolayer cultures. Exp. Cell Res. 31(2):321-8.

Potgieter, L.N., M.L. Frey, R.F. Ross. 1972. Chronological development of Mycoplasma hyorhinis and Mycoplasma hyosynoviae infections in cultures of a swine synovial cell strain. Can. J. Comp.
Med. 36(2):145-9.

Powelson, D. 1959. Pleuropneumonia-like organism in tissue cultures. Proc. Indiana Acad. Sci. 69:99.

Powelson, D.M. 1961. Metabolism of animal cells infected with
mycoplasma. J. Bact. 82(2):288-97.

Prozorovskii, S.V. and G.A. Levina. 1973. A comparative analysis
of behavior in cell cultures of L-form bacteria and mycoplasmas.
Zh. Mikrobiol. Epidemiol. Immunobiol. 50(1):77-82.

Rakovskaya, I.V. 1965. Contamination of tissue cultures by pleuropneumonia-like organism. Vop. Virusol. 10(2):233-5.

Rakovskaya, I.V. 1965. Biological properties of mycoplasmas contaminating tissue cultures. Vestn. Akad. Med. Nauk. SSSR 20(8):
50-4.

Reis, R., N. Matzer and R. Yamamoto. 1971. Pathogenesis of M. mel-
eagridis in diethylstilboesterol treated turkey embryos and
poults. J. Comp. Path. 81(2):235-42.

Robinson, L.B., R.H. Wichelhausen and B. Roizman. 1956. Contamination of human cell cultures by pleuropneumonia-like organisms.
Science 124(3232):1147-8.

Rose, N.R., V. Milisauskas, J.H. Kite, Jr. 1972. Effect of mycoplasma infection on esterase activity of human FL amnion and
WI-38 cells. Proc. Soc. Exp. Biol. Med. 140(2):391-4.

Rose, N.R., V. Milisauskas, G. Zeff. 1975. Antigenic and enzymatic changes in infected and transformed human diploid cells.
Immunol. Commun. 4(1):1-16.

Rothblat, G.H. 1960. PPLO contamination in tissue cultures.
Ann. N.Y. Acad. Sci. 79(10):430-2.

Rovozzo, G.C., R.E. Luginbuhl and C.F. Helmboldt. 1963. A mycoplasma from bovine causing cytopathogenic effects in calf kidney
tissue culture. Cornell Vet. 53(4):560-6.

Russell, W.C., J.S.F. Niven and L.D. Berman. 1968. Studies on the
biology of the mycoplasma-induced "stimulation" of BHK (baby
hamster kidney) 21-C13 cells. Int. J. Cancer 3(2):191-202.

Sabin, A.B. 1938. Identification of the filterable, transmissable
neurolytic agent isolated from toxoplasma-infected tissue as a
new pleuropneumonia-like microbe. Science 88:575.

Sabin, A.B. 1967. Nature and source of mycoplasma in various
tissue cultures. Ann. N.Y. Acad. Sci. 143(1):628-34.

Schimmel, D., P. Hlinak. 1966. Contamination of cell cultures by
mycoplasma I. on the isolation and morphology of mycoplasma from
permanent cell cultures. Monatsh Vet. Med. 21(2):64-9.

Schimmel, D. and P. Hlinak. 1967. Mycoplasma contamination of cell
cultures. II. isolated from primary cultures or various tissues
Munchen. Vet. Med. 22:387-90.

Schneider, E.L., C.J. Epstein, W.L. Epstein, M. Betlach and
  G. Abbo Halbasch. 1973. Detection of mycoplasma contamination
  in cultured human fibroblasts: comparison of biochemifal and
  microbiological techniques. Exp. Cell Res. 79(2):343-9.

Schwobel, W. and R.H. Leach. 1970. Isolation of a mycoplasma
  strain similar to M. laidlawii from primary calf kidney cell
  cultures. Zentralbl. Bakt. Parasitnek. Infektionskrankh. Hyg.
  Abt. I. Orig. 214(4):495-506.

Scott., F.W. 1971. Comments on feline panleukopenia biologics.
  J. Am. Vet. Med. Assoc. 158(6):Suppl. 2:910-5.

Seman, G., C. Rosenfeld, C. Jasmin, R. Camain. 1968. Notice of two
  cultures and a biopsy of Burkitt's tumor seen under the electron
  microscope. Rev. Fr. Etud. Clin. Biol. 13(1):83-7.

Sethi, K.K., et al. 1970. Interaction between mycoplasmas and Ehrlich ascites tumor cells. Experimentia 26:1244-5.

Sethi, K.K. and H. Brandis. 1970. Oncolytic effect of a M. gallisepticum strain on solid Ehrlich carcinoma. Path. Microbiol.
  37(2):105-12.

Sethi, K.K. 1972. On the incidence of mycoplasma contamination in
  cell cultures. Zentralbl. Bakteriol. (Orig. A) 219(4):550-4.

Sethi, K.K. and M. Teschner. 1972. Mycoplasma interactions with
  cell cultures, uncultured living cells and the problems posed
  by their presence in tissue culture. Klin. Wochenschr. 50:
  226-33.

Shepard, M.C. 1958. Growth and development of T-strain pleuropneumonia-like organisms in human epidermoid carcinoma cells
  (HeLa). J. Bact. 75(3):351-5.

Simmons, D.G. 1972. Some characteristics of a biological inhibitor (mycoplasma sp.) of Marek's disease virus. Diss. Abstr.
  32(7):4107-B.

Simmons, D.G. 1972. Isolation of an anaerobic mycoplasma from
  avian cell cultures and some of its effects on Marek's disease
  virus. Avian Dis. 16(3):521-8.

Smirnova., T.D. and G. Y. Kagan. 1972. Stimulating effect
  of Langat virus on reproduction of Mycoplasma laidlawii in
  combined infection of primary chick embryo cell culture. Zh.
  Mikrobiol. Epidemiol. Immunobiol. 49(6):81-3.

Sodhi, S.S., S.S. Dhillon, K.K. Baki. 1976. Adaptation and cytopathic effects of avian mycoplasma in chicken embryo cell cultures. Zentralbl. Veterinaermed (B) 23(7):609-12.

Sokova, V.A., S.A. Vitina, L.M. Pichugin, D.F. Osidze. 1970.
Effect of mycoplasma on diploid cells. Veterinariia 7:40-3.

Somerson, N.L. and M.K. Cook. 1965. Suppression of Rous sarcoma
virus growth in tissue cultures by Mycoplasma orale. J. Bact.
90(2):534-40.

Sorodoc, G., I.Aderca, N. Stoian, C. Surdan and P. Peiulescu.
1972. Influence of mycoplama infection on the cultivation
of some viruses in cell cultures. Rev. Roum. Virol. 9(1):77-8.

Stanbridge, E. 1971. Mycoplasmas and cell cultures. Bacteriol.
Rev. 35(2):206-27.

Stewart, S.M., et al. 1971. Isolation of Mycoplasma arginini
from tissue cultures. Lancet 1:347.

Swift, H.F., 1941. Capacity of pleuropneumonia-like microorganisms to grow on chorioallantoic membranes. J. Exp. Med.
74(6):557-68.

Taylor-Robinson, D. and R.J. Manchee. 1967. Novel approach to
studying relationships between mycoplasmas and tissue culture
cells. Nature 216(5122):1306-7

Taylor-Robinson, D. and J.D. Cherry. 1972. A non-pathogenic
mycoplasma inhibiting the effect of a pathogenic mycoplasma in
organ culture. J. Med. Microbiol. 5(3):291-8.

Tedeschi, G.G., D. Amici and O. Murri. 1973. Multiplication of
mycoplasma-like organisms brought in a culture medium by inactivated bovine serum. Ann. Sclavo 14(6):765-71.

Todorov, T., L. Karaivanov, I. Todorov and Ts. Valerianov. 1967.
Metabolism of chick fibroblast infected with fowl mycoplasmas.
1st Congr. Bulg. Microbiol., Sofia 1965:447-56.

Trung, P.H., A. Boue, F. Lardemer and F. Haguenan. 1968. Ultrastructure of Mycoplasma salivarium and Mycoplasma orale in
tissue culture. The problem of their reproduction from the cell
surface. Eur. J. Cancer. 4(4):429-35.

Tully, J.G. 1966. Mycoplasma granularum of swine origin as a tissue
culture contaminant. Proc. Soc. Exp. Biol. Med. 122(2):565-8.

VanHerick, W., and M.D. Eaton. 1945. An unidentified pleuropneumonia-like organism isolated during passages in chick
embryos. J. Bact. 50(1):47-55.

Veber, P., K. Jurmanova, J. Leska and L. Hana. 1975. Drying and
irradiation of calf and horse serum. I. influence on the growth
of cell cultures and mycoplasmas. Zentrabl. Bacteriol. 231:
508-13.

Vogelzang, A.A., B. van Klingeren. 1974. Proceedings: Mycoplasmas
in cell cultures. Antonie van Leeuwenhoek 40:316-17.

Witzleb, W. 1970. On contamination of tissue cultures with mycoplasmas. I. alterations of cell physiology and effects on
virological diagnostics. (Survey of Literature). Arch. Ges.
Virusforsch. 30:113-20.

Young, R.K., R.M. Cailleau, B. Mackay and W.J. Reeves, Jr. 1974.
Establishment of epithelial cell line MDA-MB-157 from metastatic
pleural effusion of human breast carcinoma. In Vitro (Rockville)
9(4):239-45.

Zgorniak-Nowosielska, I., W.D. Sedwick, K. Hummeler and H.
Koprowski. 1967. New assay procedure for separation of mycoplasmas from virus pools and tissue culture systems. J. Virol.
1(6):1227-37.

Zgorniak-Nowosielska, I. 1969. Mycoplasma contamination of cell
culture and its significance for biological research. Posterpy.
Hyg. Med. Dosw. 23(6):837-50.

Zgorniak-Nowosielska, I., J. Borysiewicz and M. Gorczyca. 1972.
Mycoplasma in artificially infected HeLa cultures. Exp. Med.
Microbiol. 24(3):224-32.

Zucker-Franklin, D., M. Davidson and L. Thomas. 1966. The
interaction of mycoplasmas with mammalian cells. I. HeLa cells,
neutrophils and eosinophils. J. Exp. Med. 124(3):521-32.

B. Amino Acid Metabolism

Chao, F.C., G. Freeman, J.G. Cummings and B.J. Berridge, Jr.
1967. Amino acids of the ornithine cycle in transformed hamster
fibroblasts carrying pleuro-pneumonia-like organisms. Cancer Res.
27(Suppl. Part 1) 1474-81.

Kenny, G.E. and M. F. Pollock. 1962. Effect of amino acid depletion by pleuropneumonia-like organism on growth of cells
in culture. In: 46th Ann. Meeting, Atlantic City, New, Jersey,
Fed. Proc. 21(2):161.

Kraemer, P.M. 1964. Mycoplasma (PPLO) from covertly contaminated
tissue cultures: differences in arginine degradation between
strains of mouse lymphoma cells. Proc. Soc. Exp. Biol. Med.
117(3):910-18.

Kraemer, P.M. 1964. Interaction of mycoplasma (PPLO) and murine
lymphoma cell culturees: prevention of cell lysis by arginine.
Proc. Soc. Exp. Biol. Med. 115(1):206-12.

McCarty, K.S., B. Woodson, M. Amstey and O. Brown. 1964.
Arginine as a precursor of pyrimidines in strain L-929 fibro-
blasts infected with pleuropneumonia-like organism. J. Biol.
Chem. 239(2):544-9.

Miller, G., J. Emmons and D. Stitt. 1971. Susceptibility of
human lymphoblastoid cell lines to a cytopathic effect
induced by an arginine-utilizing mycoplasma strain. J. Inf.
Dis. 124(3):322-6.

Pollock, M.E., P.E. Treadwell and G.E. Kenny. 1962. Effect of
amino acid depletion by pleuropneumonia-like organism on morphology of cells in culture. Fed. Proc. 21(2):161.

Romano, N., et al 1970. Inhibition of growth of measles virus
by mycoplasma in cell cultures and the restoring effect of
arginine. Arch. Ges. Virusforsch. 29:39-43.

Rouse, H.C., V.H. Bonifas and R. W. Schlesinger. 1963. De-
pendence of adenovirus replication or arginine and inhibition
of plaque formation by pleuropneumonia-like organism. Virology
20(2):357-65.

Schimke, R.T. and M.F. Barile. 1963. Arginine metabolism
pleuropneumonia-like organism isolated from mammalian cell
culture. 86(2):195-206.

Schimke, R.T. and M.F. Barile. 1963. Arginine breakdown in
mammalian cell culture contaminated with pleuropneumonia-
like organisms. Cell Res. 30(3):593-6.

Smith, P.F. 1957. Amino acid metabolism by plueropneumonia-
like organisms. II. glutamine. J. Bact. 73(1):91-5.

Stanbridge, E.J., L. Hayflick and F.T. Perkins. 1971. Modification of amino-acid concentrations induced by mycoplasmas
in cell culture medium. Nature New Biol. 232(34):242-4.

Woodson, B.K., K.S. McCarty and M.C. Shepard. 1965. Arginine
metabolism in mycoplasma and infected strain L-929 fibroblasts. Arch. Biochem. Biophys. 109(2):364-71.

C. Nucleic Acid Metabolism

Glan, P.V., V.V. Neustroeva. 1968. Incorporation of H3-thymidine
into the cells of cultures infected with mycoplasma. Zh. Mikrobiol. Epidemiol. Immunobiol. 45(12):21-3.

Gruneisen, A., M.F. Rajewsky, I. Remmer, J. Uschkoreit. 1975.
Inhibition of 3H-thymidine incorporation by hydroxyurea: atpic
response of mycoplasma-infected cells in culture. Exp. Cell
Res. 90(2):365-73.

Hakala, M.T., J.F. Holland and J.S. Horoszewicz. 1963. Change in
pyrimidine deoxiribonucleoside metabolism in cell culture
caused by mycoplasma (PPLO) contamination. Biochem. Biophys.
Res. Commun. 11(6):466-71.

Hall, R.H. and A. Mittleman. 1964. Characterization of the nucleic
acids of a Mycoplasma (PPLO-880) isolated from extracts of human
tissue. Int. Congr. Biochem. 6(1):58.

Harley, E.H., et al. 1970. HeLa cell nucleic acid metabolism.
The effect of mycoplasma contamination. Biochim. Biophys. Acta.
213:171-82.

Harley, E.H., K.R. Rees. 1972. Mitochondrial RNA in mycoplasma
infected HeLa cells. Biochim. Biophys. Acta 259(2):228-38.

Holland, J.F., H.J. Minnemeyer, J.T. Grace, Jr., R. Block, J.
O'Malley and H. Tieckelmann. 1963. 5-allyl-2'-deoxyuridine
(AVdR) (anti-tumor agent) activity on metabolism of pyrimidine
deoxynucleosides by HeLa cells infected with mycoplasma. Proc.
Amer. Assoc. Cancer Res. 4(1):29.

Holland, J.F., R. Korn, J. O'Malley, H.J. Minnemeyer and H.
  Tieckelmann. 1967. 5-allyl-2'deoxyuridine inhibition on nucleo-
  side phosphorylase in HeLa cells containing mycoplasma (human).
  Cancer Res. 2(10 part 1):1867-73.

Jezequel, A.M., M.M. Shreeve and J.W. Steiner. 1967. Segregation
  of nucleolar components in mycoplasma-infected cells. Lab.
  Invest. 16(2):287-304.

Levine, E.M., L. Thomas, D.McGregor, L. Hayflick and H. Eagle.
  1968. Altered nucleic acid metabolism in human cell cultures
  infected with mycoplasma. Proc. Nat. Acad. Sci. USA 60(2):583-9.

Markov, G.G., I. Bradvarova, A. Mintcheva, P. Petrov, N. Shishkov,
  R.G. Tsanev. 1969. Mycoplasma contamination of cell cultures:
  interference with 32P-labelling pattern of RNA. Exp. Cell Res.
  57(2):374-84.

Nardone, R.M., J. Toldd, P. Gonzalez and E.V. Gaffney. 1965.
  Nucleoside incorporation into strain L cells: inhibition by
  pleuropneumonia-like organisms (PPLO). Science 149(3688):
  1100-1.

Perez, A.G., J.H. Kim, A.S. Gelbard, B. Djordjevic. Altered
  incorporation of nucleic acid precursors by mycoplasma-infected
  mammalian cells in culture. Exp. Cell Res. 70(2):301-10.

Pratt, W.B., S.R. Gross, L. Aronow. 1968. Endosymbionts as a
  source of cytoplasmic satellite deoxyribonucleic acid.
  J. Mol. Biol. 33(2):521-5.

Randall, C.C., L.G. Gafford, G.A. Gentry and L.A. Lawson. 1965.
  Lability of host-cell DNA in growing cell cultures due to
  mycoplasma. Science 149:1098-9.

Russell, W.C. 1966. Alterations in the nucleic acid metabolism of
  the tissue culture (hamster fibroblast) cells infected by
  mycoplasmas. Nature 212(5070):1537-40.

Smith, C.G., H.H. Buskirk and W.L. Lummis. 1965. Effect of arabin-
  ofuranosyluracil on the cytotoxicity of arabinofuranaosylcyto-
  sine in PPLO-contaminated cell cultures. Proc. Amer. Assoc.
  Cancer Res. 6:60.

Stanbridge, E.J., J.A. Tischfield and E.L. Schneider. 1975.
  Appearance of hypoxanthine guanine phosphoribosyltransferase
  activity as a consequence of mycoplasma contamination.
  Nature. 256(5515):329-31.

Tedeschi, G.G., D. Amici and M. Paparelli. 1970. The uptake of
radioactivity of thymidine, uridine, formate, glycine and
lysine into cultures of blood of normal human subjects. Relationship with mycoplasma infection. Haematologia 4(1):27-47.

VanDiggelen, O.P., D.M. Phillips and S. Shin. 1977. Endogenous
HPRT activity in a cryptic strain of mycoplasma and its effect
on cellular resistance to selective media in infected cell
lines. Exp. Cell Res. 106:191-203.

D. Cytogenetics

Allison, A.C. and G.R. Paton. 1966. Chromosomal abnormalities
in human diploid cells injected with mycoplasma and their
possible relevance to the aetiology of Down's syndrome
(mongolism). Lancet 7475. 1229-30.

Aula, P. and W.W. Nichols. 1967. The cytogenic effects of mycoplasma in human leucocyte cultures. J. Cell Physiol. 70(3):281-9.

Copperman, R., H.E. Morton. 1966. Reversible inhibition of mitosis
in lymphocyte cultures by non-viable mycoplasma. Proc. Soc. Exp.
Biol. Med. 123(3):790-5.

Fogh, J., H. Fogh. 1965. Chromosome changes in PPLO-infected FL
human amnion cells. Proc. Soc. Exp. Biol. Med. 119:233-238.

Fogh, J., H. Fogh. 1966. Irreversibility of major chromosome
changes in a mycoplasma-modified line of FL human amnion cells.
Riv. Patol. Nerv. Ment. 87(4):67-74.

Fogh, J., H. Fogh. 1967. Morphological and quantitative aspects
of mycoplasma-human cell relationships. Proc. Soc. Exp. Biol.
Med. 125(2):423-30.

Fogh, J., H. Fogh. 1967. Irreversibility of major chromosome
changes in a mycoplasma-modified line of FL human amnion cells.
Proc. Soc. Exp. Biol. Med. 126(1):67-74.

Fogh, J., H. Fogh. 1968. Karyotypic changes in mycoplasma-modified
lines of FL human amnion cells. Proc. Soc. Exp. Biol. Med. 129
(3):944-50.

Fogh, J., H. Fogh and A.M. Dowling. 1970. Chromosomes of SV40
transformed human amnion cells after mycoplasma infection.
Proc. Soc. Exp. Biol. Med. 135(2):206-11.

Fogh, J., H. Fogh. 1973. Chromosome changes in cell culture induced by mycoplasma infection. Ann. N.Y. Acad. Sci. 225:311-29.

Kundsin, R.B., M. Apolla, S. Streeter and P. Neurath. 1969.
  Chromosomal aberrations induced by T-strain mycoplasmas. Bact.
  Proc. M183.

Kundsin, R.B. 1971. Chromosomal aberrations induced by T strain
  mycoplasmas. J. Med. Genet. 8(2):181-7.

Kuzmina, S.V., V.V. Neustroeva. 1971. Comparative analysis of
  mitotic activity and chromosome aberrations in cell lines contaminated with mycoplasma and after decontamination. Biull. Eksp.
  Biol. Med. 72(11):101-3.

Kuzmina, S.V. 1972. Action of mycoplasmas on the chromosomal
  apparatus of mouse fibroblasts in tissue culture. Sov.
  Genet. 8(1):126-7.

Kuzmina, S.V. 1972. The ratio of the phases of mitosis in
  decontaminated cell lines and in cell lines contaminated with
  mycoplasma. Biull. Eksp. Biol. Med. 13(2):100-2.

Kuzmina, S.V. 1972. Effect of mycoplasmata on the chromosome
  apparatus of cells in cultured mouse fibroblasts. Genetika
  8(1):165-7.

Paton, G.R., J.P. Jacobs and F.T. Perkins. 1965. Chromosome
  changes in human diploid cell cultures infected with mycoplasma. Nature 207(4992):43-5.

Paton, G., J.P. Jacobs and F.T. Perkins. 1967. The effect of
  mycoplasma on the karyology of normal cells. Ann. N.Y. Acad.
  Sci. 143(1):626-7.

Riggs, A.D. 1966. Part I. Studies on Mycoplasma gallisepticum.
  Part II. autoradiography of chromosomal DNA fibers from
  Chinese hamster cells. Diss. Abstr. 27(1-3):85B.

Romano, N., R. Comes and L. Valentino. 1970. Chromosome changes
  in human diploid cells infected by mycoplasmata. G. Microbiol.
  13(1-4):33-46.

Schneider, E.L., E.J. Stanbridge, C.J. Epstein, M. Golbus,
  G. Abbo-Halbasch and G. Rodgers. 1974. Mycoplasma contamination of cultured amniotic fluid cells: potential hazard to
  prenatal chromosomal diagnosis. Science. 184(135):477-80.

Simberkoff, M.S., G.J. Thorbecke and L. Thomas. 1969. Studies
of PPLO infection. V. Inhibition of lymphocyte mitosis and
antibody formation by mycoplasmal extracts. J. Exp.
Med. 129(6):1163-181.

Spitler, L., K. Cochrum, H.H. Fudenberg. 1967. Mycoplasma
inhibition of phytohemagglutinin stimulation of lymphocytes. Science 161(846):1148-9.

Stanbridge, E., M. Onen, F.T. Perkins and L. Hayflick. 1969.
Karyological and morphological characteristics of human
diploid cell strain WI-38 infected with mycoplasmas. Exp.
Cell Res. 57(2/3):397-410.

E. Immunological Cells and Mechanisms

Andzhaparidze, O.G., R.I. Rapaport and G.B. Iurovskaia. 1970.
The transforming effect of blood from leukemic patients on a
culture of human diploid cells. Vopr. Virusol. 15:579-84.

Bailey, J.S., H.W. Clark, W.R. Felts, R.C. Fowler and T.
McP. Brown. 1961. Antigenic properties of pleuropneumonia-
like organisms from tissue cell cultures and the human
genital area. J. Bact. 82:542-7.

Barile, M.F. 1965. Mycoplasma (PPLO), leukemia and autoimmune
disease. Wistar Inst. Symp. Monogr. 4:171-85.

Barile, M.F., B.G. Leventhal. 1968. Possible mechanism for
mycoplasma inhibition of lymphocyte transformation induced
by phytohaemagglutinin. Nature 219(155):750-2.

Beltran, G., J.W. Northington, E. Liederman, W.J. Mogabagab
and W. J. Stuckey. 1971. Antibody to human cell lines with
and without ultrastructural evidence for Epstein-Barr virus
(EBV) infection in sera from patients with diverse viral
illness. Int. J. Cancer 7(3):375-9.

Berquist, L.M., H.S.B. Lau and C. E. Winter. 1974. Mycoplasma-
associated immunosuppression. Effect on hemagglutinin response
to common antigens in rabbit. Infect. Immun. 9(2):410-15.

Biberfeld, G., P. Biberfeld, G. Sterner. 1974. Cell-mediated
immune response following Mycoplasma pneumoniae infection in
man. I. lymphocyte stimulation. Clin. Exp. Immunol. 17(1):
29-41.

Biberfeld, G. 1974. Cell-mediated immune response following
Mycoplasma pneumoniae infection in man. II. leucocyte migration
inhibition. Clin. Exp. Immunol. 17(1):43-9

Biberfeld, G., E. Gronowica. 1976. Mycoplasma pneumoniae is a
polyclonal B-cell activator. Nature 261(5557):238-9.

Bloom, E.T. 1973. Microcytotoxicity tests on human cells in
culture: effect of contamination with mycoplasma. Proc. Soc.
Biol. Med. 143(1):244-8.

Brautbar, C., E.J. Stanbridge, M.A. Pellegrino, S. Ferrone,
R.A. Reisfeld, R. Payne, L. Hayflick. 1973. Expression of
HL-A antigens on cultured human fibroblasts infected with
Mycoplasmas. J. Immunol. 111(6):1783-9.

Campbell, L.H., H.K. Okuda. 1975. Cultivation of mycoplasma
from conjunctiva and production of corneal immune response
in guinea pigs. Am. J. Vet. Res. 36(7):893-7.

Cole, B.C. and J.R. Ward. 1973. Interaction of Mycoplasma
arthritidis and other mycoplasmas with murine peritoneal
macrophages. Infect. Immun. 7(5):691-9.

Cole, B.C., J.C. Overall, Jr., P.S. Lombardi and L.A. Glasgow.
1976. Induction of interferon in ovine and human lymphocyte
cultures by mycoplasmas. Infect. Immun. 14:88-94.

Dajani, A.S. and E.M. Ayoub. 1969. Mycoplasmacidal effect of
polymorphonuclear leucocyte extract. J. Immunol. 102(3):
698-702.

Elsbach, P. 1973. On the interaction between phagocytes and
micro-organisms. N. Engl. J. Med. 289(16):846-52.

Fernald, G.W. 1972. In vitro response of human lymphocytes to
M. pneumoniae. Infect. Immun. 5(4):552-8.

Gabridge, M.G., P.R. Schneider. 1975. Cytotoxic effect of Mycoplasma fermentans on mouse thymocytes. Infect. Immun. 11(3):
460-5.

Ginsburg, H. and J. Nicolet. 1973. Extensive transformation of
lymphocytes by a mycoplasma organism. Nature New Biol. 246:
143-6.

Howard, C.J., G. Taylor, J. Collins, R.N. Gourlay. 1976.
Interaction of Mycoplasma dispar and Mycoplasma agalactiae
bovis with bovine alveolar macrophages and bovine lacteal
polymorphonuclear leukocytes. Infect. Immun. 14(1):11-7.

Jones, T.C., J.G. Hirsch. 1971. The interaction in vitro of
Mycoplasma pulmonis with mouse peritoneal macrophages and
L-cells. J. Exp. Med. 133(2):231-59.

Jones, T.C., S. Yeh, J.G. Hirsch. 1972. Studies on attachment
and ingestion phases of phagocytosis of Mycoplasma pulmonis
by mouse peritoneal macrophages. Proc. Soc. Exp. Biol. Med.
139(2):464-70.

Leventhal, B.G., C.B. Smith, P.P. Carbone and E.M. Hersh. 1967.
Lymphocyte transformation in response to Mycoplasma pneumoniae
after experimental infection in man. In: Proc. of the 3rd Ann.
Leucocyte Culture Conference, Appleton-Century Crofts, N.Y.

Liudogovskaia, L.A., V.T. Kakiakov. 1966. A study of the
antigens of transplantable and strain cultures of human
cells by agar precipitation. Vopr. Onkol. 12(10):64-8.

Low, I.E., et al. 1973. Mycoplasmacidal activity of a
leukocytic myeloperoxidase-hydrogen peroxide-halide
system. J. Infect. Dis. 127:Suppl:72-6.

Maini, R.N., R.M. Lemcke, G.D. Windsor, L.M. Roffe, I.T.
Magrath, D.C. Dumonde. 1975. The significance of leucocyte
migration inhibition by M. fermentans. Rheumatology 6:118-30.

Manchee, R.J. and D. Taylor-Robinson. 1969. Utilization of
neuraminic acid receptors by mycoplasmas. J. Bact. 98(3):914-19.

Manchee, R.J. and D. Taylor-Robinson. 1969. Studies on the nature
of receptors involved in attachment of tissue culture cells to
mycoplasmas. Brit. J. Exp. Path. 50(1):66-75.

Martin, R.R., G. Warr, R. Couch, V. Knight. 1973. Chemotaxis of
human leukocytes: responsiveness to Mycoplasma pneumoniae.
J. Lab. Clin. Med. 81(4):520-9.

Morton, H.E., R. Copperman, G.T. Lam. 1968. Some properties of
the inhibitor(s) of lymphocyte mitosis derived from mycoplasma.
J. Bacteriol. 95(6):2418-9.

Niklasson, P.M. and R.C. Williams, Jr. 1974. Studies of per-
iferal blood T- and B-lymphocytes in acute infections.
Infect. Immun. 9(1):1-7.

Parkinson, C.F., P.B. Carter. 1975. Phagocytosis of Mycoplasma
salivarium by human polymorphonuclear leukocytes and monocytes. Infect. Immun. 11(2):405-14.

Parkinson, C.F. 1975. Histamine released from human leukocytes
when stimulated by Mycoplasma salivarium. Infect. Immun.
11(3):595-7.

Rakovskaya, I.V., Z.A. Postnikova, T.D. Morgunova and G.Ya.
Kagan. 1972. Study of immunodepressive effect of Mycoplasma
laidlawii on the formation of humoral antibodies in mice.
Bull. Eksp. Biol. Med. 74(10):60-2.

Roberts, D.H. 1972. Inhibition of lymphocyte transformation
induced by phytohaemaglutinin with porcine mycoplasma.
Brit. Vet. J. 128(11):585-90.

Rose, N.R. V. Milisauskas, G.Zeff. 1975. Antigenic and enzymatic changes in infected and transformed human diploid
cells. Immunol. Commun. 4(1):1-16.

Rothenberger, W., H.G. Thiele. 1971. Leucocyte-migration
inhibition in rheumatoid arthritis. Lancet 2(720):372.

Schendler, S., R.J. Harris. 1967. The effect of Rous sarcoma
virus (Schmidt-Ruppin strain) on the chromosomes of human
leucocytes in vitro. Int. J. Cancer 2(2):109-15.

Simberkoff, M.S., G.J. Thorbecke and L. Thomas. 1969.
Studies of PPLO infection V. inhibition of lymphocyte mitosis
and antibody formation by mycoplasma extracts. J. Exp. Med.
129(6):1163-81.

Simberkoff, M.S. and P. Elsbach. 1971. The interaction in
vitro between polymorphonuclear leukocytes and mycoplasma.
J. Exp. Med. 134(6):1417-30.

Tuomi, J. 1966. A microorganism affecting bovine platelets.
Experientia 22:458-9.

Tuomi, J. and C.H. vonBonsdorff. 1967. Some characteristics
of a bovine infection affecting platelets and of its causative
agent. Scand. J. Clin. Lab. Invest. 19:Suppl. 95-8.

Tuomi, J. and C.H. vonBonsdorff. 1967. Ultrastructure of microorganism associated with bovine platelets. Experientia 23:
111-12.

Vasileva, V.A., B.A. Lapin, L.A. Yakovleva, M.T. Ivanov, D.S.
Markaryan, A.F. Bykovskii and B. Sanguliya. 1971. Production
of a continuous cell line from a culture of leukocytes of Papino
hamadryas with leucosis-reticulosis. Vop. Virusol. 16:312-16.

Zucker-Franklin, D., M. Davidson and L. Thomas. 1966. The interaction of mycoplasmas with mammalian cells. II. monocytes and
lymphocytes. J. Exp. Med. 124(3):533-42.

F. Radiation

Pageau, R. 1971. Effects of mycoplasma contamination on the
radio-sensitivity of rat glial cells. Experientia 27:1328-9.

Pritchard, J.A.V. and J.L. Moore. 1971. The modification of
radio-sensitivity by mycoplasma. Int. J. Radiat. Biol. 20(6):
597-8.

Randall, C.C., L.G. Gafford, G.A. Gentry and L.A. Lawson. 1965.
Lability of host-cell DNA in growing cell cultures due to
mycoplasma. Science. 148(3688):1098-9.

G. Viruses

1) General

Aktan, M., M. Guley and M. Doguer. 1955. Abortion in sheep following immunization with contaminated sheep pox vaccine. Turk. Vet.
Hekim. Dern. Derg. 25:2463-77.

Anderson, D.R., H.E. Hopps, M.F. Barile, B.C. Bernheim. 1965.
Comparison of the ultrastructure of several rickettsiae,
ornithosis virus, and mycoplasma in tissue culture. J. Bacteriol. 90(5):1387-1404.

Banttari, E.E. and R.J. Zeyen. 1973. Combined virus and mycoplasma-like infections of plants and insects. Ann. N.Y. Acad.
Sci. 225:503-8.

Baizhomartov, M.S., R.S. Dreizin, S.V. Prozorovski. 1971. The
associative interrelationships of Mycoplasma pneumoniae and
respiratory-syncytial virus in cell cultures. Vopr. Virusol.
16(1):36-41.

Barbuti, S. 1968. Research on the presence of mycoplasmas in cell
cultures and virus strains. Ann. Sclavo. 10(2):167-83.

Bardell, D., T.G. Metcalf. 1972. Differential release of cellular
lactate dehydrogenase during replication of adenovirus types 5
and 12. J. Gen. Virol. 14(2):219-22.

Barile, M.F. 1968. Mycoplasma and cell cultures. In: Cell Cultures
for Virus Vaccine Production. J. Nat. Cancer Inst. Monogr. 29:
201-4.

Benton, W.J., M.S. Cover and F.W. Melchior. 1967. Mycoplasma
gallisepticum in a commercial laryngotracheitis vaccine.
Avina Dis. 11(3):426-9.

Bothig, B., et al. 1970. Influence of mycoplasma infections in
permanent cell cultures on the propagation of enteroviruses
and the elimination of mycoplasma infections using antibiotic
therapy. Deut. Gesundheitsw. 25:1278-82.

Boue, A., J.G. Boue. 1968. Human viruses and chromosomes. Pathol.
Biol. (Paris) 16(11):677-90.

Cernik, K. 1967. The possible contamination of live vaccines
against poultry diseases with mycoplasma. Veterinarstvi 17:24-5.

Cherry, J.D., D. Taylor-Robinson. 1970. Large-quantity production
of chicken embryo tracheal organ cultures and use in virus and
mycoplasma studies. Appl. Microbiol. 19(4):658-62.

Chu, H.P., et al. 1975. Single and mixed infections of avian
infectious bronchitis virus and Mycoplasma galisepticum.
Dev. Biol. Stand. 28:101-14.

Coria, M.F., J.K. Peterson. 1971. Adaptation and propagation of
avian infectious bronchitis virus in embryonic turkey kidney
cell cultures. Avian Dis. 15(1):22-7.

Coriell, L.L. 1968. Tissue and medium antigens in vaccines. Natl.
Cancer Inst Monogr. 29:179-91.

Cross, G.F., M.R. Goodman, J. Chatterji, T.S. Beswick, J.A. Chapman. 1970. Another case of mistaken identity: rubella and mycoplasma. J. Gen. Virol. 8(1):77-81.

Demidova, S.A., B.V. Gushchin, T.F. Lozinskii, V.V. Perekrest,
N.M. Ritova, S.M. Klimenko, L.S. Shushkov and V.M. Zhdanov.
1974. Viral contaminants of cell cultures in the aspect of
persistent infections. Vestn. Akad. Med. Nauk. SSSR 9:27-35.

D'yakonova, E.V. and V.A. Shubin. 1968. Experimental mixed infection with laryngotracheitis and mycoplasmosis in chicks. Byull.
Vses. Inst. Eksp. Vet. 1968(4):22-3.

D'yakonova, E.V. 1968. Biological properties of laryngotracheitis
virus when it is grown together with the causative agent of
mycoplasmosis in chick embryos. Byull. Vses. Inst. Eksp. Vet.
4:19-21.

D'yakanova, E.V. 1970. The interaction of the virus of infectious bronchitis and the pathogen of fowl mycoplasmosis when
they are cultivated together in chick embryos. Byull. Vses.
Inst. Evsp. Vet. 7:20-2.

D'yakanova., E.V. 1970. A study of the interaction of the fowl
pox virus with mycoplasmata in chick embryos. Byull. Vses.
Inst. Eksp. Vet. 7:23-5.

Edward, D G.ff. 1969. Mycoplasmas as contaminants and their
detection. Progr. Immunobiol. Stand. 3:17-22.

Ershov, F.I. and V.M. Zhdanov. 1965. Influence of pleuropneumonia-
like organisms on the production of interferon by infected
cells. Dokl. Akad. Nauk. SSSR 164(5):1165-6.

Fleer, G.P., et al. 1969. The effect of certain mycoplasma
on the formation of plaques by Langat virus in a primary culture of chick embryo cells. Vestn. Akad. Med. Nauk. SSSR.
24:68-72.

Fletcher, R.D., W.H. Milligan, III and J.N. Albertson, Jr. 1970.
Contributing factor to M. pneumoniae produced stimulation
of rhinovirus-RNA synthesis. Folia Microbiol. 15(5):325-9.

Fraser, D. and C. Fleischmann. 1974. Interaction of mycoplasma
   with viruses: I primary adsorption of virus is ionic in
   mechanism. J. Virol. 13(5):1067-74.

Gafford, L.G., F. Sinclair, C.C. Randall. 1969. Growth cycle of
   fowlpox virus and change in plaque morphology and cytopathology
   by contaminating mycoplasma. Virology 37(3):464-72

Golden, B., A.P. McKee. 1970. Enhancement of the infectivity titer
   of adenovirus type 8. Arch. Ophthalmol. 83(4):455-7.

Hargreaves, F.D., et al. 1970. The influence of mycoplasma infection on the sensitivity of HeLa cells for growth of viruses.
   J. Med. Microbiol. 3:259-65.

Hendley, J.O., A.J. Anderson. 1968. Mycoplasmal studies in infectious mononucleosis. Proc. Soc. Exp. Biol. Med. 129(2):374-6.

Hlinak, P., J. Friedemann, G. Starke. 1969. Problems of the state
   examination of viral vaccines in mycoplasma contaminations.
   Pharmazie 24(4):189-92.

Ikoev, V.N., G.M. Gonskii and S.G. Dzagurov. 1973. Ultracen-
   trifugation method used for control of live virus vaccines
   for the absence of mycoplasma. Vop. Virusol. 18(5):625-8.

Kagan, G.Y., K.S. Kulikova, V.V. Neustroeva, A.I. Rezepova
   and Z.D. Sultanova. 1968. Effect of mycoplasma infection of
   culture cells on replication cytopathic action, and hemagglutinating capacity of some viruses. Vop. Virusol. 13(5):
   600-5.

Kawamura, H., S. Sato, F. Shimizu and H. Tsubahara. 1964. Cytopathic effect and plaque formation of avian mycoplasma in
   chicken kidney cell cultures. Nat. Inst. Anim. Health Quart.
   (Tokyo) 4:28.

Keeble, S.A. 1972. Extraneous contaminants in avian live virus
   vaccines. Vet. Rec. 9(25):642.

Kikava, E.M. and L.I. Fadeeva. 1967. Special diagnostic features
   of mycoplasmas in contaminated virus cultures. Ref. Zh. Biol.
   No. 9B116.

Kikava, E.M. 1970. Study of virus cultures with regard to mycoplasma contamination and development of purification methods.
   Vopr. Virusol. 15:241-4.

Kilgore, J.M., R.W. Beck, A. Brown. 1972. Lack of interaction between Sendai virus and bacterial cells. Proc. Soc. Exp. Biol. Med. 140(2):409-13.

Kisary, J., L. Stipkovits. 1975. Effect of Mycoplasma gallinarum on the replication in vitro of goose parvovirus strain "B". Acta. Microbiol. Acad. Sci. Hung. 22(3):305-7.

Koziorowska, J., K. Wlodarski, M. Mazurowa. 1971. Transformation of mouse embryo cells by vaccinia virus. J. Natl. Cancer Inst. 46(2):225-41.

Kralj, M., M. Herceg, Z. Bombek and D. Peric. 1968. Effect of Newcastle disease on the mortality rate from chronic respiratory disease in fowls. Vet. Arh. 38:344-52.

Larson, V.M., et al. 1971. Tests for oncogenicity of viruses under conditions of altered host and virus. Proc. Soc. Exp. Biol. Med. 136:1304-13.

Lozinskii, T.F., B.V. Gushchin, A.V. Astakhova, S.M. Klimenko and V.M. Zhdanov. 1974. Detection of latent viruses and mycoplasmas by molecular biology methods. Vop. Virusol. 4:474-9.

Macpherson, I. 1968. Neoplastic properties of animal cell lines -- general comments. Natl. Cancer Inst. Monogr. 29:295-6.

Manchee, R.J., D. Taylor-Robinson. 1969. Studies on the nature of receptors involved in attachment of tissue culture cells to mycoplasmas. Br. J. Exp. Pathol. 50(1):66-75.

Manchee, R.J., D. Taylor-Robinson. 1969. Utilization of neuraminic acid receptors by mycoplasmas. J. Bacteriol. 98(3):914-9.

Manischewitz, J.E., B.G. Young and M.F. Barile. 1975. The effect of mycoplasmas on replication and plaquing ability of herpes simplex virus. Proc. Soc. Exp. Biol. Med. 148(3):859-63.

Milligan, W.H., III, R.D. Fletcher. 1969. Effect of Mycoplasma pneumoniae on rhinovirus ribonucleic acid synthesis in KB cells. Antimicrob. Agents Chemother. 9:196-9.

Milligan, W.H., III. 1973. Effect of Mycoplasma pneumoniae on rhinovirus replication in cell culture. Diss. Abstr. 34(4): 1652-3-B.

Milligan, W.H., R.D. Fletcher. 1975. Effect of Mycoplasma pneumoniae on poliovirus replication. Infect. Immun. 11(3): 607-8.

Mohadjer, S. and S. Kaftarians. 1973. The interaction between Mycoplasma hominis and poliovirus in cell culture. J. Gen. Virol. 20(3):303-10.

Muller, H.E. and K.K. Sethi. 1972. The occurrence of neuraminidase in Mycoplasma gallisepticum. Med. Microbiol. Immunol. (Berlin) 2:160-8.

Nakamura, M. and S. Hiroaki. 1969. Modification of the growth of human mycoplasmas in tissue culture by infection with influenza virus and Japanese encephalitis (JE) virus. Proc. Soc. Exp. Biol. Md. 131(2):343-5.

Netter, R., et al. 1968. Study on the possible presence of mycoplasma in smallpox vaccine. Bull. Acad. Nat. Med. (Paris) 152:486-90.

Neufahrt, A., H, Rolly, E. Schutze. 1969. Effect of Mycoplasma on the antiviral action of 5-iodouracil-desoxyriboside (IUdR). Zentralbl. Bakteriol (Orig.) 209(4):470-7.

Nonomura, I. and S. Sato. 1971. Effect of the Newcastle disease virus TCND strain on Mycoplasma gallisepticum infection in chickens. Natl. Inst. Anim. Health Quart. (Tokyo) 11(4):184-90.

Nonomura, I. 1973. Interference of Mycoplasma gallisepticum with multiplication of Newcastle disease virus in chicken tracheal organ cultrues. Natl. Inst. Anim. Health Quart. (Tokyo) 13(3): 105-11.

Nonomura, I. and S. Sato. 1975. Interference of Mycoplasma gallisepticum with multiplication of Newcastle disease virus in chickens. Avian Dis. 19(3):603-7.

Novikova, I.S. and L.M. Kurnosova. 1970. Characteristics of mycoplasma isolated in some diseases of the urogenital tract in man. Zh. Mikrobiol. Epidemiol. Immunobiol. 47(10):137-8.

O'Reilly, K.J. and A.M. Whitaker. 1969. The development of feline cell lines for the gorwoth of feline infectious enteritis (panleucopaenia) virus. J. Hyg. 67(1):115-24.

Poten, J. 1966. Suppression of Rous virus induced transformation by an antibiotic sensitive mycoplasma-like factor. Wenner-Gren. Center Int. Symp. Ser. 6:67-71.

Reed, S.E. 1971. The interaction of mycoplasmas and influenza viruses in tracheal organ cultures. J. Infect. Dis. 124(1):18-25.

Reed, S.E. 1972. Viral enhancement of mycoplasma growth in tracheal organ cultures. J. Comp. Path. 82(3):267-78.

Romano, N., P. Brancato. 1970. Inhibition of growth of measles
   virus by mycoplasma in cell cultures and the restoring effect
   of arginine. Arch. Gesamte Virusforsch 29(1):39-43.

Rouse, H.C. and V. Bonifas. 1962. Depletion of pleuropneumonia-
   like organisms of arginine required for adenovirus plaque
   formation. In: Ann. Meeting Amer. Soc. for Microbiol.,
   Kansas City, Missouri, May 1962. Bact. Proc. 42:147.

Rouse, H.C., V.H. Bonifas and R.W. Schlesinger. 1963. Depen-
   dence of adenovirus replication on arginine and inhibition
   of plaque formation by pleuropneumonia-like organism. Virology 20(2):357-65.

Ruckdeschel, J.C., B. Kramarsky, M.R. Mardiney, Jr. 1975.
   Mycoplasma contamination of membrane associated measles antigens. Inability to demonstrate in vitro lymphocyte responsiveness to measles. Cell Immunol. 201(1):110-6.

Sato, S. 1970. Mixed infection with M. gallisepticum and the
   B1 or TCND strain of New Castle disease virus in chickens.
   Jap. Ag. Res. Quart. 5(4):48-53.

Schmidt, U., H. Hantschel, P. Schulze, H. Linsert. 1970. Mixed
   infections of avian adenovirus and the virus of infectious bronchitis. Arch. Exp. Veterinaermed. 24(2):587-607.

Scott, F.W. 1971. Comments on feline panleukopenia biologics.
   J. Am. Vet. Med. Assoc. 158(6):Suppl. 2:910-15.

Schwanz-Pfitzner, I., M. Ozel. 1973. Electron microscopy studies
   of cell cultures: demonstration of a mixed infection by Egtved
   virus of the rainbow trout and mycoplasma (Acholeplasma laidlawii) (author's transl.) Zentralbl. Bakteriol. (Orig. A)
   225(2):431-7.

Sethi, K.K. and H.F. Muller. 1972. Neuraminidase activity in
   M. gallisepticum. Infect. Immun. 5(2):260-2.

Singer, S.H. et al. 1969. Increased yields of stomatitis virus
   from hamster cells infected with mycoplasma. Nature 222:1087-8.

Singer, S.H. et al. 1970. Effect of mycoplasmas on vaccinia virus growth: requirement for arginine. Proc. Soc. Exp. Biol. Med. 133:1439-42.

Singer, S.H., M. Ford, M. Barile, R.L. Kirschstein. 1972. Effect of mycoplasmas on virus replication and plaque formation in mouse cells. Proc. Soc. Exp. Biol. Med. 139(1):56-8.

Singer, S.H., M. Ford., S. Baron. 1972. The influence of mycoplasma infection on the induction of the antiviral state by polyincsinic:polycytidilic acid. Proc. Soc. Exp. Biol. Med. 139(4):1413-6.

Singer. S.H., M. Ford and R.L. Kirschstein. 1972. Respiratory diseases in cyclophosphamide-treated mice. I. increased virulence of Mycoplasma pulmonis. Inf. Immun. 5(6):953-6.

Singer, S.H., M.F. Barile and R.L. Kirschstein. 1973. Mixed mycoplasma-virus infections in cell cultures. Ann. N.Y. Acad. Sci. 225:304-10.

Slack, P.M., D. Taylor-Robinson. 1973. The influence of mycoplasmas on the cytopathic effect of varicella virus. Arch. Gesamte Virusforsch 42(1):88-95.

Smirnova, T.D., G.Y. Kagan. 1971. Effect of mycoplasma-viral infection of a primary culture of chick embryo cells on interferon production induced by Langat virus. Zh. Mikrobiol. Epiemiol. Immunobiol. 48(12):54-8.

Smirnova., T.D. G.Y. Kagan. 1972. Stimulating effect of Langat virus on reproduction of Mycoplasma laidlawii in combined infection of a primary culture of chick embryo cells. Zh. Mikrobiol. Epidemiol. Immunobiol. 49(6):81-3.

Sorodoc, G., I. Aderca, N. Stoian, C. Surdan and P. Peiulescu. 1972. Influence of mycoplasma infection on the cultivation of some viruses in cell cultures. Rev. Roum. Virol. 9(1):77-8.

Sorodoc, Y., M. Stoian, G. Sorodoc, M. Cepleanu, C. Cernescu, N. Cajal. 1974. The influence of experimental mycoplasma infection on the cultivation of measles virus in cell cultures. Rev. Roum. Virol. 25(1):65-73.

Stock, D.A., G.A. Gentry. 1969. Mycoplasmal deoxyribonuclease activity in virus-infected L-cell cultures. J. Virol. 3(3): 313-17.

Tint, H., E.I. Rosanoff. 1969. Production and testing of rubella
    virus vaccine. Prepared on WI-38 cell cultures. Am. J. Dis.
    Child. 118(2):367-71.

Todorov, J. 1968. Interference between mycoplasmata and viruses
    (preliminary communication). Sci. Works Res. Inst. Epidemiol.
    Microbiol. (Sofia) 12:143-6.

Wahren, B. and M. Ecsenyi. 1971. Cell growth regulating factors
    in viral infections and other diseases. Exp Cell Res. 66(2):
    396-401.

Westerberg, S.C. 1971. Mycoplasma-virus interactions in mouse
    tracheal organ culture. Diss. Abstr. 32(6):3536-7-B.

Westerberg, S.C., C.B. Smith, B.B. Wiley and C. Jensen. 1972.
    Mycoplasma-virus interrelationships in mouse tracheal organ
    cultures. Infect. Immun. 5(6):840-6.

Witzleb, W. 1970. On contamination of tissue cultures with
    mycoplasmas. I. alterations of cell physiology and effects
    on virological diagnostics. (survey of literature) Arch.
    Ges. Virusforsch. 50:113-20.

Yamamoto, H., N. Ogawa and Y. Nishimura. 1969. Isolation of
    mycoplasma from fowl pox vaccine. A Rep. Natl. Vet. Assay
    Lab. Tokyo 6:169-74.

Zgorniak-Nowosielska, I.W.D. Sedwick, K. Hummeler and H. Ko-
    prowski. 1967. New assay procedure for separation of myco-
    plasmas from virus pools and tissue culture systems. J. Virol.
    1(6):1227-37.

2) Interferon

Archer, D.L. and B.G. Young. 1974. Control of interferon migrat-
    ion inhibition factor, and expression of virus capsid antigens
    in Burkitt's lymphoma-derived cell lines. Role of L-arginine.
    Infec. Immun. 9(4):684-9.

Armstrong, D. and K. Paucker, 1966. Effect of mycoplasma on
    interferon production and interferon assay in cell cultures.
    J. Bact. 92(1):97-101.

Beladi, I., R. Pusztai. 1967. Interferon-like substance produced
    in chick fibroblast cells inoculated with human adenoviruses.
    Z. Naturforsch.(B) 22(2):165-9.

Cole, B.C., J.C. Overall, Jr., P.S. Lombardi, and L.A. Glasgow. 1976. Induction of interferon in ovine and human lymphocyte cultures by mycoplasmas. Infect. Immun. 14:88-94.

Fauconnier, B. and H. Wroblewski. 1974. Interferon and antiviral activity induced in vivo by a plant mycoplasma. Acholeplasma species. Ann. Microbiol. (Paris) 125A(4):469-76.

Rinaldo, C.R., Jr., J.C. Overall, Jr., B.C. Cole, L.A. Glasgow. 1973. Mycoplasma-associated induction of interferon in ovine leukocytes. Infect. Immun. 8(5):796-803.

Rinaldo, C.R., Jr., B.C. Cole and J.C. Overall, Jr. 1974. Induction of interferon in ovine leukocytes by mycoplasma and acholeplasma. Abstracts of the Annual Meeting of the Amer. Soc. for Microbiol. 74:93.

Rinaldo. C.R., Jr., B.C. Cole, J.C. Overall, Jr., J. R. Ward, L.A. Glasgow. 1974. Induction of interferon in ovine leukocytes by species of mycoplasma and acholeplasma. Proc. Soc. Biol. Med. 146(2):613-8.

Rinaldo, C.R., Jr., B.C. Cole, J.C. Overall, Jr., L.A. Glasgow. 1974. Induction of interferon in mice by mycoplasmas. Infect. Immun. 10(6):1296-301.

Rinaldo, C.R., Jr. 1976. Mycoplasma in biological systems: induction of interferon. Health Lab. Sci. 13(2):137-43.

Singer, S.H., R.L. Kirschstein and M. Barile. 1969. Increased viral yields and decreased interferon production in mycoplasma-infected hamster cells. Bact. Proc. 1969-187.

Singer. S.H., M.F. Barile and R. L. Kirschstein. 1969. Enhanced virus yields and decreased interferon production in mycoplasma infected hamster cells. Proc. Soc. Exp. Biol. Med. 131(4): 1129-34.

Smirnova, T.C. and G.Y. Kagan. 1971. Effect of mycoplasma-viral infection of a primary culture of chick embryo cells on interferon production induced by Langat virus. Zh. Mikrobiol. Epidemiol. Immunobiol. 48(12):54-8.

Strander, H., K. Cantell. 1974. Studies on antiviral and anti-tumor effects of human leukocyte interferon in vitro and in vivo. In Vitro. (Monogr.) 0(3):49-56.

Yershov, F.I., V.M. Zhdanov. 1965. Influence of PPLO on production of interferon in virus-infected cells. Virology 27 (3):451-3.

3) Tumor Viruses and Tumor Cells

Abenova, U.A., B.V. Guschchin, K. V. Lil'in and V.M. Zhdanov. 1974. Isolation of oncornavirus type B from a continuous line of human amnion cells. Vop. Virusol. 2:216-23.

Anderson, D.R. 1965. Subcellular particles associated with human leukemia as seen with the electron microscope. Wistar Inst. Symp. Monogr. 4:113-46.

Beltran, G., J.W. Northington, E. Leiderman, W.J. Mogabgab, W.J. Stuckey. 1971. Antibody to human cell lines with and without ultrastructural evidence for Epstein-Barr virus (EBV) infection in sera from patients with diverse viral illnesses. Int. J. Cancer. 7(3):375-9.

Butler, M., R.H. Leach. 1966. Mycoplasma associated with tissue cultures, leukaemia and human tumours. Proc. R. Soc. Med. 59 (11):1116-7.

Chapman, A.L. W.J. Bopp, A.S. Brightwell, H. Cohen, A.H. Neilsen, C.R. Gravelle and A.A. Werder. 1967. Preliminary report on virus-like particles in canine leukemia and derived cell cultures. Cancer Res. 27:18-25.

Dmochowski, L., H.G. Taylor, C.E. Grey, D.A. Dreyer, J.A. Sykes, P.L. Langford, T. Rogers, C.C. Shullenberger and C.D. Howe. 1965. Viruses and mycoplasma (PPLO) in human leukemia. Cancer 18(10):1345-68.

Dvorak, R., M. Jaenner and U. Eckhardt. 1973. Ultrastructural changes of human tumors after transfer into laboratory animals. I. malignant melanoma (4 cases). Arch. Dermatol. Forsch. 246 (4):383-400.

Dvorak, R., M. Jaenner, U. Eckhardt. 1973. Changes of the ultrastructure of human tumours by transfer into laboratory animals. 3. squamous cell carcinoma (2 cases) with extracellular and intracellular mycoplasma-like bodies (author's transl.). Arch. Dermatol. Forsch. 248(1):59-77.

Dzhikidze, E.K., G.Ya. Kagan and E. Ya. Balaeva. 1973. Isolation of mycoplasma during leukemia in sacred baboons. Vestn. Akad. Med. Nauk. SSSR 28(4):48-50.

Eckner, R.J., E.S. Priori, E.A. Mirand and L. Dmochowski. 1974. Studies on the biological and antigenic properties of ESP-1 type C virus particles. Cancer Res. 34(10:2521-29.

Eckner, R.J., V. Kumar, M. Bennett. 1975. Immunogenetic analysis
  of the mechanism of induction of Friend virus leukemia. Trans-
  plant Proc. 7(2):173-84.

Fogh, J., H. Fogh and A.M. Dowling. 1970. Chromosomes of SV40
  transformed human amnion cells after mycoplasma infection. Proc.
  Soc. Exp. Biol. Med. 135(2):206-11.

Fogh, J. 1970. Mycoplasma effects on SV40 transformation of human
  amnion cells. Proc. Soc. Exp. Biol. Med. 134(1):217-24.

Fogh, J. 1971. Increased susceptibility to mycoplasma infection of
  SV40 transformed human amnion cells. Proc. Soc. Exp. Biol. Med.
  137(2):498-505.

Fogh, J. 1973. Increased mycoplasma-cell association in transformed
  human amnion cells. J. Infect. Dis. 127:Suppl.:S77-81.

Gabridge, M.D., D.D. Gamble. 1974. Independence of leukemoid potential and toxigenicity of Mycoplasma fermentans. J. Infect.
  Dis. 130(6):664-8.

Gaffney, E.V., J. Fogh, L. Ramos, J.D. Loveless, H. Fogh, A.M.
  Dowling. 1970. Established lines of SV40-transformed human amnion
  cells. Cancer Res. 30(6):1668-76.

Geldberblom, H., H. Ogura and H. Bauer. 1974. On the occurrence of
  oncornavirus-like particles in HeLa cells. Cryobiologie 8(2):
  339-44.

Gericke, D., W. Kovac and H. Flamm. 1971. Experimental studies on
  mycoplasma-induced leukemogenesis. Zentralbl. Bakt. 218(3):
  343-55.

Gerlach, F. 1971. The pathogenicity of mycoplasmas from malignant
  tumors. Wien. Tierarztl. Monatsschr. 58:1-3.

Gerlach, F. 1972. Tumors as consequences of prenatal infection
  with mycoplasma. Wien. Tierarztl. Monatsschr. 59:137-53.

Gerlach, F. 1975. Participation of mycoplasmas in oncogenesis.
  Wien. Med. Wochenschr. Suppl. 26:1-12.

Gilbey, J.G. and M. Pollard. 1967. Search for mycoplasma in germ-
  free leukemic mice. J. Nat. Cancer Inst. 38(2):113-16.

Girardi, A.J., L. Hayflick, A.M. Lewis and N.L. Somerson. 1965.
Recovery of mycoplasmas in the study of human leukaemia and other
malignancies. Nature 205(4867):188-9.

Girardi. A.J., V.M. Larson and M.R. Hilleman. 1965. Further tests
in hamsters for oncogenic quality of ordinary viruses and
mycoplasma, with correlative review. Proc. Soc. Exp. Biol. Med.
118(1):173-9.

Gogichadze, G.K., A.S. Shubin and N.P. Mazurenko. 1971. Differen-
iation of murine leukemia viruses from elementary bodies of mycoplasma by electron microscopy. Vop. Virusol. 16(5):522-6.

Grace, J.T., Jr. 1964. Relationship of viruses to leukemia and
lymphomas. Proc. Natl. Cancer Conf. 5:637-43.

Grace, J.T., Jr., J. Horoszewicz, T.B. Stim, E.A. Mirand and C.
James. 1965. Mycoplasma (PPLO) and human leukemia and lymphoma.
Cancer 18(10):1369-76.

Howell, E.V. and R.S. Jones. 1960. Role of mycoplasma (pleuropneumonia-like organism) in the regression of Murphy-Sturm
lymphosarcoma in the rat. Fed. Proc. 19(1 pt. 1):216.

Hummeler, K. 1965. Morphology of a mycoplasma isolated from
human leukemia (Negroni's agent). Wistar Inst. Symp. Monogr.
4:167-9.

Hummeler, K., D. Armstrong and N. Tomassini. 1965. Cytopathogenic
mycoplasmas associated with two human tumors. II. morphological
aspects. J. Bact. 90(2):511-16.

Hummeler, K., N. Tomassini and L. Hayflick. 1965. Ultrastructure
of a mycoplasma (negroni) isolated from human leukemia. J.
Bact. 90(2):517-23

Huppert, J., E. Delain, N. Fossar, E. May. 1974. Endonucleolytic
DNase in oncorna viruses: role of mycoplasma. Virology 57(1):
217-26.

Jasmin, G. and C.L. Richer. 1959. On the contamination of the
Murphy-Sturm lymphosarcoma with a pleuropneumonia-like organism.
Experientia 15(9):329-31.

Jasmin, C., et al. 1967. Study of mycoplasmas in patients with
leukemia or hematosarcoma. Rev. Franc. Etud. Clin. Biol.
12:599-603.

an, G.Y., et al. 1967. The effect of mycoplasma infection
on the reproduction of various RNA-containing viruses. Vop.
Virusoll 12:478-85.

Kagan, G.Y., et al. 1973. Reaction of mice on infection with
mycoplasma and leukosis viruses. J. Hyg. Epidemiol. Microbiol.
Immunol. (Praha) 17:226-36.

Klodnitskaya, L.N and N.V. Likhachev. 1970. Morphology of mycoplasma strains isolated from the spleen of cows with lymphosarcoma. Dokl. Vses. Akad. Sel.-Khoz. Nauk. 1970(9):24-6.

Klodnitskaya, S.N., N.V. Likhachev and V.A. Odinokova. 1975.
Pathogenicity of mycoplasmas isolated from cows with leucosis.
Dokl. Vses. Akad. Sel'sk. Nauk. 7:38-9, 47.

Kohler, W. 1962. Behaviour of avian and human PPLO in mice infected with ectromelia virus and in mice bearing an ascites
tumor. Zentrlbl. Bakt. I(Orig.) 185:243-51.

Koshimizu, K., K. Yamamoto and M. Ogata. 1973. Mycoplasmas isolated from dogs with malignant lymphoma. Jap. J. Vet. Sci.
35(2):123-32.

Kraemer, P.M., V. Defendi, L. Hayflick and L.A. Manson. 1963.
Mycoplasma (PPLO) strains with lytic activity for murine
lymphoma cells in vitro. Proc. Soc. Exp. Biol. Med. 112
(2):381-7.

Kraemer, P.M. 1964. Mycoplasma (PPLO) from covertly contaminated
tissue cultures: differences in arginine degradation between
strains of mouse lymphoma cells. Proc. Soc. Exp. Biol. Med.
117(3):910-18.

Lazarus, H., K.M.K. Beckett, D. Cuppels and G.F. Foley. 1967.
Relationship of mycoplasma to acute leukemia in children
(cause incidental). J. Bact. 94(5):1797.

Leach, R.H., M. Butler. 1966. Comparison of mycoplasmas associated
with human tumors, leukemia, and tissue cultures. J. Bacteriol.
91(3):934-41.

Lozinskii, T.F., M. Ya. Volkova, U.A. Abenova, N.N. Mazurenko,
G.G. Miller, I.A. Irlin, K.V. Il'in, A.F. Bukovskii, B.V.
Gushchin, et al. 1974. Production of oncornaviruses from human
cell cultures. Vop. Onkol. 20(1):56-62.

Lozzio, C B. and B.B. Lozzio. 1975. Human chronic myelogenous
leukemia cell-line with positive Philadelphia chromosome.
Blood 45(3):321-34.

Macpherson, I., W. Russell. 1966. Transformations in hamster
cells mediated by mycoplasmas. Nature 210(43):1343-5.

Magrassi, F.G. 1968. Critical evaluation and current prospects
of research on the relations between mycoplasma and neoplasms.
G. Mal. Infett. 20:591-4.

Markarian, D.S., E.K. Dzhikidze, E.Ia. Balaeva, A.I. Trots. 1975.
Changes in transplantable cultures infected with mycoplasmas
isolated from leukemic monkeys. Tsitologiia 17(7):822-8.

Maruyama, K., L. Dmochowski, J.M. Bowen, R.L. Hales. 1968.
Studies of human leukemia and lymphoma cells by membrane im-
munofluorescence and mixed hemadsorption tests. Tex. Rep.
Biol. Med. 26(4):545-65.

McClain, K., W.H. Kirsten. 1974. Mouse leukemia virus growth in
mouse cells contaminated with Mycoplasma. Cancer Res. 34(2):
281-5.

Millian, S.J. and I. Spigland. 1966. Antibodies for mycoplasmas
in normal individuals and patients with neoplasias. Cancer
19(12):1820-24.

Miller, G., J. Emmons, D. Stitt. 1971. Susceptibility of human
lymphoblastoid cell lines to a cytopathic effect induced by
an arginine-utilizing mycoplasma strain. J. Infect. Dis. 124(3):
322-6.

Miller, G., H. Lisco, H.I. Kohn, D. Stitt, J.F. Enders. 1971.
Establishment of cell lines from normal adult human blood leukocytes by exposure to Epstein-Barr virus and neutralization by
human sera with Epstein-Barr virus antibody. Proc. Soc. Exp.
Biol. Med. 137(4):1459-65.

Morgunova, T.D., Z.A. Postnikova, I.V. Rakovskaya and G. Y.
Kagan. 1974. Mixed infection with Rauscher virus and Mycoplasma
laidlawii in BALB/cDe mice. Vop. Virusol. 2:144-8.

Morton, D.L., F.R. Eilber, R.A. Malmgren, K.O. Cooke. 1970. Evidence for a virus in human sarcomas. Bibl. Haematol. (36):754-60.

Murphy, W.H., I.J. Ertel, C.J. Zarafonetis. 1965. Virus studies
  of human leukemia. Cancer 18(10):1329-44.

Murphy, W.H., C. Bullis, E.J. Ertel and C.J. Zarafonetis. 1967.
  Mycoplasma studies of human leukemia. Ann. N.Y. Acad. Sci.
  143(1):544-56.

Murphy, W.H., C. Bullis, E.J. Ertel and C.J. Zarafonetis.
  1967. Antibodies to mycoplasma in sera of leukemic patients.
  Proc. Soc. Exp. Biol. Med. 124(2):366-72.

Murphy, W.H., C. Bullis, L. Dabich, R. Heyn, C.J. Zarafonetis.
  1970. Isolation of mycoplasma from leukemic and non-leukemic
  patients. J. Natl. Cancer Inst. 45(2):243-51.

Negroni, G. 1966. The causes of human leukemia - viruses or
  mycoplasmas? p.91-101 20th Ann. Symp. of Fundamental Cancer
  Research, 1966, Williams and Wilkins Co., Baltimore, Md.

Negroni, G. 1966. The role of mycoplasmas and viruses in human
  leukemia. Proc. Roy. Soc. Med. 59:662-3.

Nigro, N., et al. 1966. Mycoplasmas and acute infantile leukemia.
  Minerva Pediat. 18:1238-44.

Niwayama, G. and J.T. Grace, Jr. 1971. Mycoplasmas (PPLO) and human
  neoplasms. Tohoku J. Exp. Med. 105(3):257-80

Ogata, M. and K. Koshimizu. 1967. Isolation of mycoplasmas
  from tissue cell lines and transplantable tumor cells. Jap.
  J. Microbiol. 11(4):289-303.

Panem, S., W.H. Kirsten. 1975. Secondary scanning electron
  microscopy of cells infected with murine oncornaviruses.
  Virology 63(2):447-58.

Pirtle, E.C., W.L. Mengeling, N.F. Cheville. 1970. Initiation and
  characterization of two porcine embryonal nephroma cell lines.
  Am. J. Vet. Res. 31(9):1601-8.

Plata, E.J. 1968. Induction of leukemoid disease in mice by mycoplasma isolated from leukemic patients. Diss. Abstr. 29(1-3):
  1106B.

Plata, E.J., M.R. Abell and W.H. Murphy. 1973. Induction of leukemoid disease in mice by Mycoplasma fermentans. J. Infect. Dis.
  128(5):588-97.

Ponten, J., I. Macpherson. 1966. Interference with Rous sarcoma
    virus focus formation by a mycoplasma-like factor present in
    human cell cultures. Ann. Med. Exp. Biol. Fenn. 44(2):260-4.

Pope, J.H., B.G. Achong, M.A. Epstein, J. Biddulph. 1967. Burkitt
    lymphoma in New Guinea: establishment of a line of lymphoblasts
    in vitro and description of their fine structure. J. Nat.
    Cancer Inst. 39(5):933-45.

Postnikova, Z.A., T.D. Morgunova, I.V. Rakovskaya and G.Y. Kagan.
    1973. Reproduction of the Rauscher virus in virus-resistant
    mice in mono infection and mixed mycoplasma and virus infection.
    Vestn. Akad. Med. Nauk. SSSR 28(2):75-9.

Poten, J. 1966. Suppression of Rous virus induced transformation
    by an antibiotic sensitive mycoplasma-like factor. Wenner-Gren
    Center Int. Symp. Ser. 6:67-71.

Priori, E.S., L. Dmochowski, B. Myers, T. Shigematsu, J.R. Wilbur.
    1973. Studies on a human cell line (ESP-1) producing type C virus
    particles. Bib. Haematol. 39:720-31.

Rosanova, A.R., et al. 1966. Preliminary report on finding of myco-
    plasma in malignancy. Med. Sci. Hist. 9:141-7.

Rose, N.R., V. Milisauskas, G. Zeff. 1975. Antigenic and enzymatic
    changes in infected and transformed human diploid cells. Immunol.
    Commun. 4(1):1-16.

Sabin, A.B. 1967. Search for viral etiology of human leukemia and
    lymphomas: past efforts and future perspectives. Ann. 1st Super.
    Sanita 3(1):86-100.

Schendler, S., R.J. Harris. 1967. The effect of Rous sarcoma virus
    (Schmidt-Ruppin strain) on the chromosomes of human leucocytes
    in vitro. Int. J. Cancer 2(2):109-15.

Scolnick, E.M., W.P. Parks, G.J. Todaro, S.A. Aaronson. 1972.
    Immunological characterization of primate C-type virus reverse
    transcriptases. Nature (New Biol.) 235(54):35-40.

Schramm, T. 1968. Mycoplasmas (PPLO) and oncogenesis. Arch.
    Geschwulstforsch. 32(1):168-78.

Sethi, K.K. and H. Brandis. 1970. Oncolytic effect of a M. galli-
    septicum strain on solid Ehrlich carcinoma. Path. Microbiol. 37
    (2):105-12.

Shepard, M.C. 1958. Growth and development of T-strain pleuro-
    pneumonia-like organisms in human epidermoid carcinoma cells
    (HeLa). J. Bact. 75(5):351-5.

Simmons, D.G., P.D. Lukert. 1972. Isolation of an anaerobic mycoplasma from avian cell cultures and some of its effects on
Marek's disease virus. Avian Dis. 16(3):521-8.

Sinkovics, J.G., G.F. Groves, B.A. Bertin, C.C. Shullenberger.
1969. A system of tissue cultures for the study of a mouse leukemia
virus. J. Infect. Dis. 119(1):19-38.

Somerson, N.L. and M.K. Cook. 1965. Suppression of Rous sarcoma
virus growth in tissue cultures by Mycoplasma orale. J. Bact. 90
(2):534-40.

Spence, I.M. 1972. Studies on Burkitt's lymphoma. I. A preliminary report on the presence of mycoplasma-like organisms in
specimens examined by electron microscopy. S. Afr. J. Med. Sci.
37:27-32.

Stevens, D.A., T.W. Pry, E.A. Blackham. 1970. Prevalence of precipitating antibody to antigens derived from Burkitt lymphoma
cultures infected with herpes-type virus (EB virus). Blood 35
(2):263-75.

Sutton, R.N.P. 1966. Mycoplasma and leukemia in childhood: a
brief report. Brit. Med. J. 5528:1496-8.

Tallgren, L.G., R. Wegelius, L.C. Andersson and E. Jansson. 1974.
Eosinophilic leukaemia: recovery of Mycoplasma orale from the
bone marrow. Acta Med. Scand. 195(1/2):87-92.

Tully, J.G. and R. Rask-Nielsen. 1967. Mycoplasma in leukemic
and nonleukemic mice. Ann. N.Y. Acad. Sci. 143(1):345-52.

VanDiggelen, O.P., S. Shin and D.M. Phillips. 1977. Reduction
and elimination of mycoplasma from infected cultures by
passage in nude mice. Cancer Res. 37:2680-7.

Vasileva, V.A., B.A. Lapin, L.A. Iakovleva, M.T. Ivanov, D.S.
Markarian. 1971. Obtaining a transplantable line from a culture
of leukocytes from a pavian hamadrils with leukosis-reticulosis.
Vopr. Virusol. 16(3):312-6.

Weissenbacher, E.R. 1973. Demonstration of mycoplasma in uterine
neoplasms. Med. Klin. 68:1006-9.

Wu, A.M., R.C. Ting, S.S. Yang, R.C. Gallo, M. Paran. 1973.
RNA tumor virus and reverse transcriptase. I. Biochemical studies on the ESP-1 particles. II. Role of the reverse transcriptase in murine RNA tumor virus. Bibl. Haematol. 39:506-17.

Young, R.K., R.M. Cailleau, B. Mackay and W.J. Reeves, Jr. 1974.
Establishment of epithelial cell line MDA-MB-157 from metastatic
pleural effusion of human breast carcinoma. In Vitro (Rockville)
9(4):239-45.

Zhdanov, V.M., V.D. Soloviev, T.A. Bektemirov, K.V. Ilyin, A.F.
Bykovsky, N.P. Mazurenko, I.S. Irlin, F.I. Yershov. 1973.
Isolation of oncornaviruses from continuous human cell cultures.
Intervirology 1(1):19-26.

Zhdanov, V.M., A.F. Bykovski, T.A. Bektemirov, K.V. Ilyin, M.P.
Mazurenko. 1974. Biochemical methods of demonstrating latent
oncornaviruses and mycoplasma. Vopr. Med. Khim. 20(4):396-400.

4) Mycoplasma Viruses

Cole, R.M., J.G. Tully, T.J. Popkin et al. 1973. Morphology,
ultrastructure and bacteriophage infection of the helical
mycoplasma-like organism (Spiroplasma citri gen. nov. sp. nov.)
cultured from "Stubborn disease" of citrus. J. Bacteriol. 15:
367-84.

Das, J. and J. Maniloff. 1975. Replication of mycoplasmavirus
MVL51. I. replicative intermediates. Biochem. Biophys. Res.
Commun. 66(2):599-605.

Fraser, D. and J. Crum. 1975. Enhancement of mycoplasma virus
plaque visibility by tetrazolium. Appl. Microbiol. 29(2):
305-6.

Gourlay, R.N. 1971. Mycoplasmatales virus-laidlawii 2, a new
virus isolated from Acholeplasma laidlawii. J. Gen. Virol.
12:65-7.

Gourlay, R.N., J. Bruce and D.J. Garwes. 1971. Characterization
of mycoplasmatales virus laidlawii I. Nature New Biol. 229:
118-19.

Gourlay, R.N. and S.G. Wyld. 1971. Some biological characteristics of Mycoplasmatales virus-laidlawii 1. J. Gen.
Virol. 14(1):15-23.

Gourlay, R.N. and S.G. Wyld. 1973. Isolation of Mycoplasmatales virus-laidlawii 3, a new virus infecting Acholeplasma laidlawii. J. Gen. Virol. 19(2):279-83.

Liska, B. 1972. Isolation of a new mycoplasmatales virus. Studia Biophysica 34:151.

Liska, B. and L. Tkadlecek. 1975. Electron-microscopic study of a Mycoplasmatales virus, strain MVLgpS2-L 172. Folia Microbiol. 20(1):1-7.

Liss, A. and J. Maniloff. 1972. Transfection mediated by Mycoplasmatales viral DNA. Proc. Natl. Acad. Sci. USA 69(11): 3423-7.

Liss, A. and J. Maniloff. 1973. Characterization of Mycoplasmatales virus DNA. Biochem. Biophys. Res. Commun. 51(1): 214-18.

Liss, A. and J. Maniloff. 1973. Infection of Acholeplasma laidlawii by MVL51 virus. Virology 55(1):118-26.

Liss, A. and J. Maniloff. 1974. Intracellular replication of mycoplasma-virus MVL51. J. Virol. 13(4):769-74.

Liss, A. and J. Maniloff. 1974. Effect of EDTA and competitive DNA on mycoplasmavirus trasnsfection of Acholeplasma laidlawii. Microbiol. 11A(46):107-14.

Liss, A. 1975. Mycoplasmatales virus, group L1: isolation, characterization, growth and transfection studies. Diss. Abstr. 35(8):4055-B.

Maniloff, J. and A. Liss. 1973. The molecular biology of mycoplasma viruses. Ann. N.Y. Acad. Sci. 225:149-58.

Robertson, J., et al. 1972. Virus-like particles in Mycoplasma hominis. Can. J. Microbiol. 18:1971-2.

Swartzendruber, D.C., J. Clark and W.H. Murphy. 1967. Detection of phage-like particles by electron microscopy in a human strain of mycoplasma. Bact. Proc. 1967-151.

Tkadlecek, L. and B. Liska. 1973. Electron microscopy of the Mycoplasmatales virus, strain MV-Lg-pS2-L172. Folia Microbiol. 18:188.

H. Amniocentesis and Amnionitis

Altucci, P., G.L. Varone, G. Catalano and L. Manguso. 1971.
Mycoplasmas in human genito-urinary pathology. Pathol. Microbiol. 37(2):89-98.

Bredt, W., P.S. Lam, P. Fiegel and D. Hoffler. 1974. Demonstration of mycoplasma in suprapubic vesical puncture urine.
Deut. Med. Wochenschr. 99:1553-6.

Caspi, E., E. Herczeg, F. Soloman and D. Sompolinsky. 1971
Amnionitis and T strain mycoplasmemia. Am. J. Obstet. Gynecol.
111(8):1102-6.

Caspi, E., F. Solomon and D. Sompolinsky. 1972. Early abortion
and mycoplasma infection. Isr. J. Med. Sci. 8(2):122-7.

Decker, K., et al. 1974. Amnionitis due to Mycoplasma hominis
with intact membranes. Geburtshilfe Frauenheilkd. 34:269-71.

Romano, N., F. Romano and F. Carollo. 1971. T-strains of mycoplasma in broncho-pneumonic lungs of an aborted fetus. New
Eng. J. Med. 285(17):950-2.

Schneider, E.L., E.J. Stanbridge, C.J. Epstein, M. Golbus,
G. Abbo-Halbasch, G. Rodgers. 1974. Mycoplasma contamination
of cultured amniotic fluid cells: potential hazard to prenatal chromosomal diagnosis. Science. 194(135):477-80.

Shurin, P.A., S. Alpert, D. Rosner, S.G. Driscoll, Y.-H. Lee,
W.M. McCormack, B.A.G. Santamarina and E.H. Kass. 1975.
Chorioamnionitis and colonization of the newborn infant with
genital mycoplasmas. New Engl. J. Med. 293(1):5-8.

Weissenbacher, E.R. 1973. Demonstration of mycoplasma in uterine
neoplasms. Med. Klin. 68:1006-9.

5. ORGAN CULTURES

Butler, M. 1969. Isolation and growth of mycoplasma in human embryo trachea cultures. Nature 224(219):605-6.

Butler, M. 1969. Pathogenesis of respiratory mycoplasma studied
in human embryo trachea cultures. J. Gen. Microbiol. 59:vii.

Butler, M., W.J. Ellaway. 1971. Growth and cytopathogenicity
of mycoplasma in human and chicken trachea explants. J. Comp.
Pathol. 81(3):359-64.

Cherry, J.D., D. Taylor-Robinson. 1970. Large quantity production
of chicken embryo tracheal organ cultures and use in virus and
mycoplasma studies. Appl. Microbiol. 19(4):658-62.

Cherry, J.D., D. Taylor-Robinson. 1970. Peroxide production by
mycoplasmas in chicken tracheal organ cultures. Nature 228
(276):1099-100.

Cherry, J.D. and D. Taylor-Robinson. 1971. Mycoplasma pathogenicity studies in chicken tracheal organ cultures. J. Pediat.
78(6):1064-5.

Cherry, J.D. and D. Taylor-Robinson. 1972. A non-pathogenic
mycoplasma inhibiting the effect of a pathogenic mycoplasma
in organ culture. In: Abstr. 72nd Ann. Meet. Am. Soc. Microbiol.
Washington, D.C.

Cherry, J.D. and D. Taylor-Robinson. 1973. Mycoplasma pathogenicity studies in organ cultures. Ann. N.Y. Acad. Sci. 225:
290-303.

Collier, A.M., W.A. Clyde, Jr. and F.W. Denny. 1969. Biologic
effects of Mycoplasma pneumoniae and other mycoplasmas from
man on hamster tracheal organ culture. Proc. Soc. Exp. Biol.
Med. 1 2(3):1153-8.

Collier, A.M. and J.B. Baseman. 1973. Organ culture techniques
with mycoplasmas. Ann. N.Y. Acad. Sci. 225:277-89.

Gabridge, M.G. 1975. Oxygen consumption by trachea organ cultures
infected with Mycoplasma pneumoniae. Infect. Immun. 12(3):
544-9.

Gabridge, M.G. 1976. Microrespirometer chamber for determinations of viability in and organ cultures. J. Clin. Microbiol. 3
(6):560-65.

Gabridge, M.G. Polisky, R.B. 1976. Quantitative reduction of 2,3,
4-triphenyl tetrazolium chloride by hamster trachea organ cultures: effects of Mycoplasma pneumoniae cells and membranes.
Infect. Immun. 13(1):84-91.

Howard, C.J. and L.H. Thomas. 1974. Inhibition by Mycoplasma
    dispar of ciliary activity in tracheal organ cultures. Infect.
    Immun. 10(2):405-8.

Hu, P.C., A.M. Collier, and J.B. Baseman. 1975. Alterations
    in the metabolism of hamster tracheas in organ culture after
    infection by virulent Mycoplasma penumoniae. Infect. Immun.
    11(4):704-10.

Hu, P.C., A.M. Collier, J.B. Baseman. 1976. Interaction of
    virulent Mycoplasma pneumoniae with hamster tracheal organ
    cultures. Infect. Immun. 14(1):217-24.

Nonomura, I. 1973. Interference of Mycoplasma gallisepticum
    with multiplication of Newcastle disease virus in chicken
    tracheal organ culturs. Natl. Inst. Anim. Health Quart.
    (Tokyo). 13(3):105-11.

Pijoan, C.D., H. Roberts and J.D.J. Harding. 1972. The effect
    of porcine mycoplasmas on pig tracheal organ cultures.
    J. App. Bact. 35(3):361-5.

Pijoan, C. 1974. The effect of Mycoplasma hyorhinis strain S$_7$
    on pig tracheal organ cultures. Brit. Vet. J 130(1):xxii-
    xxiii.

Reed, S.E. 1971. The interaction of mycoplasmas and influenza
    viruses in tracheal organ cultures. J. Infect. Dis. 124
    (1):18-25.

Reed, S.E. 1972. Viral enhancement of mycoplasma growth in
    tracheal organ cultures. J. Comp. Path. 82(3):267-78

Stalheim, O.H.V. and J.E. Gallagher. 1975. Effects of Myco-
    plasma spp., Trichomonas fetus, and Campylobacter fetus
    on ciliary activity of bovine uterine tube organ cultures.
    Am. J. Vet. Res. 36(8):1077-80.

Taylor-Robinson, D., et al. 1974. Growth and effect f myco-
    plasmas in Fallopian tube organ cultures. Brit. J. Vener.
    Dis. 50:212-16.

Taylor-Robinson, D. 1976. The use of organ cultures and animal
    models in the study of Mycoplasma pneumoniae infections.
    Infection 4(1 suppl.):4-8.

Westerberg, S.C. 1971. Mycoplasma-virus interactions in mouse
    tracheal organ culture. Diss. Abstr. 32(6):3536-7-B.

6. ANTIBIOTIC SENSITIVITIES AND METHODS OF ELIMINATION

Arai, S., Y. Yuri, A. Kudo, M. Kikuchi, K. Kumagai. 1967. Effect of antibiotics on the growth of various strains of mycoplasma. J. Antibiot.(A) (Tokyo) 20(5):246-53.

Arisoy, F., J.R. Etheridge and A. Foggie. 1969. The effect of oxytetracycline, erythromycin and tylosin on the growth in vitro of 15 mycoplasma strains isolated from sheep and goats in Turkey. Pendik Vet. Kontrol Ara. Enst. Derg. 2(1):137-49.

Balduzzi, P. and R.J. Charbonneau. 1964. Decontamination of PPLO infected tissue cultures. Experientia 20(11):651-652.

Bothig, B., G. Schliepe. 1970. Influence of mycoplasma infections in permanent cell cultures on the propagation of enteroviruses and the elimination of mycoplasma infections using antibiotic therapy. Dtsch. Gesundheitsw. 25(27):1278-82.

Buogo, A., G. Zanuso. 1975. Anti-mycoplasmatic activity of 2 antracyclinic antibiotics. Boll. 1st Sieroter Milan 54(5):378-81.

Brunnemann, H.Z. 1967. Effect of disinfectants on mycoplasma. Ges. Hyg. 13:529-33.

Buskirk, H.H. 1967. Control of pleuropneumonia-like organisms in cell culture. Appl. Microbiol. 15(6):1442.

Crook, L.E., K.R. Rees and A. Cohen. 1972. The action of dauno-mycin on mycoplasma infected HeLa cells in culture. Chem. Biol. Interact. 4:343-50.

Cross, G.F., M.R. Goodman and F.J. Shaw. 1967. Detection and treatment of contaminating mycoplasmas in human cell culture. Aust. J. Exp. Biol. Med. Sci. 45(2):201-12.

Dinter, Z., D. Taylor-Robinson. 1969. Susceptibility and resistance of various strains of Mycoplasma hyorhinis to antisera, polymyxins and low pH values. J. Gen. Microbiol. 57(2):263:72.

Dolan, M.M., D.S. Ziv., J.F. Pagano and K.J. Ferlanto. 1963. In vitro and in vivo effect of various antibiotics on pleuro-pneumonia-like organisms. In: J.C. Sylvester, ed. Antimicrobial Agents and Chemotherapy -191163. Proceedings of a Conference. Am. Soc. for Microbiol. pp. 434-8.

Domermuth, C.H. 1960. Antibiotic resistance and mutation rates of mycoplasma. Avian Dis. 4:456-66.

Donker-Vost, J. and S.C. Goelst. 1972. Mycoplasma in stallion
    semen and their sensitivity to some antibiotics and chemo-
    therapeutic drugs. Tijdschr. Diergeneesk. 97(7):412-17.

Drew, W.L., R. Love. 1968. Production of herpes simplex virus by
    HeLa Cells treated with 5-fluoro-2'-deoxyuridine. Am. J. Pathol.
    53(1):169-82.

Fallon, R.J. 1970. The effect of cephaloridine and a cephalospor-
    in derivative on mycoplasmas. J. Appl. Bacteriol. 33(4):744-9.

Fogh, J. and C. Hacker. 1960. Elimination of pleuropneumonia-like
    organisms from cell cultures. Exp Cell Res. 21:242-4.

Friend, C., M.C. Patuleia and J.B. Nelson. 1966. Antibiotic ef-
    fect of tylosin on a mycoplasma contaminant in a tissue culture
    leukemia cell line. Proc. Soc. Exp. Biol. Med. 121(4):1009-10.

Gori, G.B. and D.Y. Lee. 1964. A method for eradication of myco-
    plasma infections in cell cultures. Proc. Soc. Exp. Biol. Med.
    117(3):918-21.

Hlinak, P. and D. Schimmel. 1968. Contamination of cell cultures
    by mycoplasma. 3. controlling mycoplasma in cell cultures.
    Munchen, Vet. Med. 23:259-64.

Holland, J.F., R. Korn, J. O'Malley, H.J. Minnemeyer, H. Tieckel-
    mann. 1967. 5-allyl-2'-deoxyuridine inhibition of nucleoside
    phosphorylase in HeLa cells containing mycoplasma. Cancer Res.
    27(10):1867-73.

Hoshino, Y., T. Maekawa, I. Umezawa, T. Hata. 1970. Effect of
    antibiotics on mycoplasma. J. Antibiot. (Tokyo) 23(11):
    531-6.

Howard, C.J., J. Brownlie, R.N. Gourlay and J. Collins. 1975.
    Presence of a dialysable fraction in normal bovine whey
    capable of killing several species of bovine mycoplasmas.
    J. Hyg. 74(2):261-70.

Inglis, J.M. and J.K.A .Cook. 1964. Comparison of in vitro and
    in vivo activity of spiramycin and erythromycin against My-
    coplasma gallisepticum. J. Comp. Path. Therap. 74(2):101-7.

Johnson, R.W., M.D. Orlando. 1967. Elimination of pleuropneumonia-
    like organisms from tissue culture. Appl. Microbiol. 15(1):
    209-10.

Keller, R., P.F. Smith and H.E. Morton. 1952. Susceptibility of pleuropneumonia-like organisms from human genital tract to the action of soaps. J. Gen Microbiol. 7(3/4):313-19.

Kenny, G.E. 1962. The effect of pleuropneumonia-like organisms (mycoplasma) on growth of mammalian cells in vitro. Diss. Abstr. 22(11):3815-16.

Kihara, K., et al. 1971. Effect of antiseptics and detergents on mycoplasma. Med. Biol. (Tokyo) 83:5-8.

Kikava, E.M. 1970. Study of virus cultures with regard to mycoplasma contamination and development of purification methods. Vopr. Virusol. 15:241-4.

Klen, R., H. Skalska, V. Srb and J. Heger. 1973. The influence of rifamycin on the chromosomes of HeLa cells. Folia. Biol. (Prague) 19(5):354-8.

Kondo, F., N. Kitano, H. Domon, M. Arai, T. Haneishi. 1974. Aspiculamaycin, a new cytosine nucleoside antibiotic. IV. antimycoplasma activity of aspiculamycin in vitro and in vivo. J. Antibiot. (Tokyo) 27(7):529-34.

Koostra, W.L., J.N. Adams and P.F. Smith. 1966. In vitro selection and identification of antibiotic-resistant mycoplasma mutants. J. Bact. 91(6):2386.

Koski, T.A., G.G. Christianson, F.L. Cole. 1976. Inactivation of mycoplasmas by use of phenol, formalin and beta-propiolactone. J. Biol. Stand. 4(2):151-4.

Kuzmina, S.V. 1972. The ratio of the phases of mitosis in decontaminated cell lines and in cell lines contaminated with mycoplasma. Biull. Eksp. Biol. Med. 72:101-3.

Larin, N.M., N.V. Saxby, G.M. Williamson, D. Buggey, N.S. Kenwright. 1967. In vitro susceptibility of Mycoplasma pneumoniae to tetracyclines. Antimicrob. Agents Chemother. 7: 680-6.

Leberman, P.R., P.F. Smith and H.E. Morton. 1950. The susceptibility of pleuropneumonia-like organisms to the in vitro action of antibiotics: Aureomycin, chloramphenicol, dihydiostrepomycin, streptomycin, and sodium penicillin. G. J. Urol. 64(1):167-73.

Leberman, P.R., P.F. Smith and H.E. Morton. 1952. Susceptibility of pleuropneumonia-like organisms to action of antibiotics.
II. Terramycin and neomycin. J. Urol. 68(1):399-402.

Levashov, V.S. and Y.Y. Tsilinskii. 1964. The degree of contamination of tissue cultures by pleuropneumonia-like organism and
a technique for purifying these cultures. TR Inst. Poliomelita
Virusn. Ente falitov. 5:150-3.

Lyon, T.C., Jr., et al. 1971. Antibiotic sensitivities of oral
mycoplasma. J. Dent. Res. 50 (6 Part 2):1678-81.

Mardh, P.H. 1975. Elimination of mycoplasmas from cell cultures
with sodium polyanethol sulphonate. Nature 254(5500):515-6.

Nasemann, T. and H. Rockl. 1960. Pleuropneumonia-like organisms:
their effect on chicken chorioallantoic membrane and the resistance to antibiotics. Ann. N.Y. Acad. Sci. 79(10):588-92.

Neustroeva, V.V. and I.V. Rakovskaya. 1968. Use of lincomycin
for decontamination of tissue cultures infected with mycoplasma. Zh. Microbiol. Epidemiol. Immunobiol. 45(3):67-9.

Norman, A.W., R.A. Demiel, B. DeKruyff and L.L.M. Van Deenen.
1972. Studies on the biological properties of polyene antibiotics: evidence for the direct interaction of Filipin
with cholesterol. J. Biol. Chem. 247(6):1918-29.

Ogata, M., et al. 1971. In vitro sensitivity of mycoplasmas
isolated from various animals and sewage to antibiotics and
nitrofurans. J. Antibiot. (Tokyo) 24:443-51.

Omura, S., et al. 1972. Antimycoplasma activities of macrolide
antibiotics J. Antibiot. (Tokyo) 25:105-8.

Oswald, E.J., et al. 1968. Survival of mycoplasma in dry state,
semisynthetic antibiotics. Antimicrob. Agents Chemother.
8:471-3.

Pallanza, R. 1967. Sensitivity of L-forms and mycoplasma to
various antibiotics. Boll. Chim. Farm 106(12):855-60.

Perlman, D. and S.A. Brindle. 1965. Antibiotic control of mycoplasma in tissue culture. Bact. Proc. V136, p. 120.

Perlman, D., S.B. Rahman and J.B. Semar. 1967. Antibiotic control
of mycoplasma in tissue culture. Appl. Microbiol. 15(1):82-5.

Perlman, D., et al. 1968. An agar diffusion method for evalu-
    ation of antimycoplasma substances. J. Antibiot. (Tokyo)
    21:300-401.

Perlman, D., C.C. Fraterrigo and J.L. Schwartz. 1972. Antibiotics
    from mycoplasma I. Acholeplasma laidlawii B. J. Antibiotics 25
    (9):535-6.

Pollock, M.F., and J.T. Syverton. 1960. Time and concentration
    of kanamycin for elimination of pleuropenumonia-like organism
    from mammalian cell cultures. Bact. Proc. 60:121.

Pollock, M.E., G.E. Kenny and J.T. Syverton. 1960. Isolation and
    elimination of pleuropneumonia-like organism from mammalian cell
    cultures. Proc. Soc. Exp. Biol. Med. 105(1):10-15.

Pollock, M.E. and G.E. Kenny. 1963. Mammalian cell cultures con-
    taminated with pleuropneumonia-like organisms. III. elimination
    of pleuropneumonia-like organism with specific antiserumm.
    Proc. Soc. Exp. Biol. Med. 112(1):176-81.

Provost, A., 1969. Cytotoxic effect of anti-mycoplasma mycoides
    serum on bovine lung cells in vitro. Rev. Immunol. (Paris) 33
    (1):1-6.

Provost, A., and R. Queval. 1972. Note on the mycoplasmocidal
    activity of trypanocidal drugs. Bull. Epizoot. Dis. Afr. Special
    Issue 77-8.

Rahman, S.B., J.B. Semar and D. Perlman. 1967. Antibiotic resis-
    tance in mycoplasma isolates from (contaminated) tissue cultures.
    Appl. Microbiol. 15(4):970.

Rakovskaya, I.V. and V.V. Neustroeva. 1967. Some aspects of de-
    contamination of tissue cultures from mycoplasma. Zh. Micro-
    biol. Epidemiol. Immunobiol. 44(9):51-4.

Reynolds, R.K. and F.M. Hetrick. 1969. Potential use of surface-
    active agents for controlling mycoplasma contamination in
    animal cell cultures. Appl. Microbiol. 17(3):405-11.

Roberts, D.H. 1964. The inactivation of mycoplasma by B-propiolac-
    tone. Brit. Vet. J. 120(10):479-80.

Robinson, L.B., T. McP. Brown and R.H. Wichelhausen. 1959.
    Studies on the effect of erythromycin and antimalarial compounds
    on pleuropneumonia-like organsims. Antibiot. Chemother. 9(2):
    111-14.

Roger, F. and A.Roger. 1960. Importance of hamsters for the elimination of a contaminant of the pleuropneumonia group in Ricket-
tsiales cultures. Ann. Inst. Pasteur (Paris) 98:151-3.

Rooney, W.F. 1970. Effects of antibiotics on turkey fertility,
hatchability, sperm metabolism, and microbial content of semen.
Diss. Abstr. 31:3095-6-B.

Sakai, T. and D. Perlman. 1975. Antibiotics from mycoplasma.
III. characteristics of two broad spectrum antibiotics produced
by mycoplasma species RP III. J. Antiobiot. 28(10):749-56.

Schutze, E. 1968. Modification of mycoplasmas with antibiotics
in vitro and in vivo. Zentralbl. Bakt. 208:320-29.

Schutze, E., D. Gericke. 1969. Experiments on elimination of mycoplasmas from transplantation tumours. Zentralbl. Bakteriol.
(Orig.) 209(4):536-44.

Schwartz, J.L. and D. Perlman. 1972. Antibiotic resistance
mechanism in mycoplasma species. J. Antibiotics 24(9):575-82.

Schweizer, H., et al. 1970. On contamination of tissue cultures
with mycoplasmas. 3. elimination of mycoplasmas from contaminated tissue cultures. Arch. Ges. Virusforch. 30:130-6.

Scrina, M. 1968. Studies towards the elimination of mycoplasma contaminations in cell cultures with the aid of antibiotics. Z. Med.
Mikrobiol. Immunol. 154(3):267-76.

Shepard, M.C., C.D. Lunceford and R.L. Baker. 1966. T-strain
mycoplasma: selective inhibition by erythromycin in vitro.
Brit. J. Vener. Dis. 42(1):21-4.

Shedden, W.I.H. and B.C. Cole. 1966. The use of sodium aurothiomalate in the eradication of pleuropneumonia-like organisms
(PPLO) from a chronically infected strain of hamster kidney
cells (BHK21C13). J. Path. Bact. 92:574-76.

Smith, P.F., H.E. Morton and P.R. Leberman. 1950. Susceptibilities
of pleuropneumonia-like organisms to some selective bacterio-
static agents. Proc. Soc. Exp. Biol. Med. 74:552.

Sprossig, M., P. Wutzler, H. Schweizer and H. Mickel. 1976. Cold
sterilization of serums with peracetic acid. J. Hyg. Epidemiol.
Microbiol. Immunol. (Praha) 20:157-63.

Sylvestre, M.A. and D. Perlman. 1975. Antibiotics from mycoplasma: ii. Characterization of antibiotics produced by Mycoplasma
sp. RPIII. J. Antibiot. 28(1):73-4.

Taylor-Robinson, D. 1967. Mycoplasmas of various hosts and their
    antibiotic sensitivities. Postgrad. Med. J. 43:Suppl. 43:100-4.

Trapeznikova, T.M. and D.F. Osidze. 1971. Sensitivity of mycoplas-
    mas to antibiotics and the decontamination of cell cultures.
    Veterinariya, Moscow 3:43-4.

VanDiggelen, O.P., S. Shin and D.M. Phillips. 1977. Reduction in
    cellular tumorigenicity after mycoplasma infection and elimin-
    ation of mycoplasma from infected cultures by passage in nude
    mice. Cancer Res. 37:2680-7.

Vogelzang, A.A. and G. Compeer-Dekker. 1969. Elimination of myco-
    plasma from various cell cultures. AvLJ. Microbiol. Serol. 35
    (4):393-408.

Ward, J.R., S. Madoff and L. Dienes. 1955. In vitro sensitivity
    of some bacteria, thier L-forms and pleuropneumonia-like organisms
    to antbiotics. Proc. Soc. Exp. Biol. Med. 97(1):132-5.

Weedon, D.d., W.J. Martin, A.G. Karlson, R.G. Shorter. 1973.
    In vitro effect of human lymphotoxin on microorganisms. Mayo
    Clin. Proc. 48(8):560-4.

Westrom, L., et al. 1971. The effect of antibiotic therapy on
    mycoplasma in the female genital tract. In vitro and in vivo
    studies on the sensitivity of Mycoplasma hominis and T-myco-
    plasmas to tetracyclines and other antibiotics. Acta Obstet.
    Gynecol. Scand. 50-25-31.

Wolford, R.G. and F.M. Hetrick. 1972. Elimination of mycoplasma
    contaminants from virus stocks by treatment with nonionic deter-
    gents. Appl. Microbiol. 24(1):18-21.

Yamanaka, T., H. Yoshizawa, S. Hashizume. 1974. Isolation of myco-
    plasma from mammalian cell lines and its elimination by treat-
    ment with antibiotics (author's transl.) virus (Tokyo) 24(1):
    42-50.

Yeber, P., K. Jurmanova, J. Leska and L. Hana. 1975. Drying and
    irradiation of calf and horse serum. I. influence on the growth
    of cell cultures and mycoplasma. Zentralbl. Bacteriol. 231:
    508-13.

Zgorniak-Nowosielska, I. 1970. Detection of mycoplasma in cell
    cultures and the antibiotic resistance of the isolated strains.
    Med. Dosw. Mikrobiol. 22:195-203.

7. PREVENTIVE MEASURES

Boone, C.W., N. Mantel, T.D. Caruso, Jr., E. Kazam, R.E. Stevenson. 1971. Quality control studies on fetal bovine serum used
in tissue culture. In Vitro 7(3):174-89.

Buskirk, H.H. 1967. Control of pleuropneumonia-like organisms in
cell culture. Appl. Microbiol. 15(6):1442.

Dolan, M.M., D.S. Ziv, J.F. Pagano and R.J. Ferlanto. 1963. In
vitro and in vivo effect of various antibiotics on pleuropneumonia-like organisms. In: J.C. Sylvester, ed. Antimicrobial
Agents and Chemotherapy - 1963. Proceedings of a Conference.
Am. Soc. for Microbiol. pp. 434-8.

Fogh, J., H. Fogh. 1969. Procedures for control of mycoplasma contamination of tissue cultures. Ann. N.Y. Acad. Sci. 172(2): 15-30.

Fogh, J., N.B. Holmgren and P.O. Ludovici. 1971. A review of cell
culture contaminations. In Vitro 7(1):26-41.

Hearn, H.J., Jr., J.E. Officer, V. Elsner and A. Brown. 1959. Detection, elimination and prevention of contamination of cell cultures with pleuropneumonia-like organisms. J. Bact 78(4): 575-82.

Hlinak, P. and D. Schimmel. 1968. Contamination of cell cultures
by mycoplasma. 3. controlling mycoplasmas in cell cultures.
Munchen. Vet. Med. 23:259-64.

McGarrity, G.J. and L.L. Coriell. 1971. Procedures to reduce
contamination of cell cultures. In Vitro 6(4):257-65.

McGarrity, G.J. 1975. Control of microbiological contamination.
Tissue Culture Manual1:181-4.

McGarrity, G.J. 1975. Serum quality control. Tissue Culture
Manual 1:167-9.

McGarrity, G.J. 1976. Spread and control of mycoplasmal infection of cell cultures. In Vitro 12(9):643-8.

McGarrity, G.J. 1977. Cell culture facilities. Tissue Culture
Manual. in press.

Rothblatt, G.H. and H.E. Morton. 1959. Detection of possible source
of contaminating pleuropneumonia-like organisms in cultures of
tissue cells. Proc. Soc. Exp. Biol. Med. 100(1): 87-90.

Spendlove, R.S., R.B. Crosbie, S.F. Hayes, R.F. Keeler. 1971.
Tricine-buffered tissue culture media for control of mycoplasma contaminants. Proc. Soc. Exp. Biol. Med. 137(1):258-63.

SUBJECT INDEX

Abortion, 184
Acetate, as energy source, 6
Aceto-orcein staining, 184
Acholeplasmas, 2, 14-16, 19, 21-22
Acholeplasma species, 6, 14-15, 37, 62-63, 67, 127
A. axanthum, 23-24, 37, 39, 62, 137
A. equifoetale, 24
A. granularum, 24, 62
A. laidlawii, 6, 11, 15-16, 22, 23, 24, 37, 39, 43, 53, 62, 63, 67, 95, 106, 109, 110, 117, 128, 137, 143, 144, 163, 170, 188, 201, 207-208 209, 216, 224, 229
A. modicum, 23, 24
A. oculi, 24
Acholeplasmataceae, 5
Achromatic gap, 127
Acid soluble oligonucleotides, 124
Acridine orange, 47, 76
Actin-like protein, 14
Acute respiratory disease, 21
Aerosolization, 18, 44, 224
Agar, 48, 49, 50, 57, 58, 60, 68, 71
Agglutination, 52, 135, 138
Airborne route of transmission, 18, 232
Air filtration, 232, 234
Amino acid metabolism, 16, 17, 123, 124, 125, 129-130, 138
Ammonia, 16, 51, 125
Amniocentesis, 159, 164, 184

Amniotic fluid, 152, 159-160, 161, 162, 183-184, 187
Anaerobic atmospheres, 48, 61
An. abactoclasticum, 23
Anaeroplasmas, 5, 7, 15-16
Aneuploidy, 187
Anionic detergents, 18
Antibiotics, 2, 4, 19
    in cell cultures, 40, 50, 66, 100, 151-152, 189, 222, 229, 231, 235
    amphoteracin B, 19
    ampicillin, 19
    aureomycin, 151
    bacitracin, 19
    chloramphenicol, 129, 130
    chlorotetracycline, 189
    erythromycin, 129, 130
    gentamycin, 229
    kanomycin, 93
    oxacillin, 229
    penicillin, 2, 19, 40, 229
    polymyxin, 19
    streptomycin, 40, 229
    tetracycline, 20-21, 93
    tylocine, 93
Antibodies, 51, 138, 221-222
Arginine, 2, 16, 25, 47, 48, 58, 76, 121, 139, 143-145, 152, 173
Arginine effect, 119, 120, 121 122, 123, 125, 127, 135, 138, 143, 144, 152, 171, 173
Aseptic technique, 232
Autoantibodies, 135, 137-138, 143
Autoradiography, 73-74, 88-89, 139-140, 153, 197-199

335

QR
352
I57
1977

Institute for Medical Research
    Workshop on Mycoplasma Infection
    of Cell Cultures, Camden, N.J.,
    1977.
    Mycoplasma infection of cell
cultures : [proceedings] / edited by
Gerard J. McGarrity, Donald G. Murphy,
and Warren W. Nichols. -- New York :
Plenum Press, c1978.
    x, 342 p. : ill. ; 26 cm. --
(Cellular senescence and somatic cell
genetics ; v. 3)

    Includes index.
    Bibliography: p. 243-334.
    ISBN 0-306-32603-5

MUNION ME
C000998

830614
KW /EW

(Cont'd on next card)
830608 CStoC
A*   83-B4623
77-25003